PRIMARY INTRAOCULAR LYMPHOMA

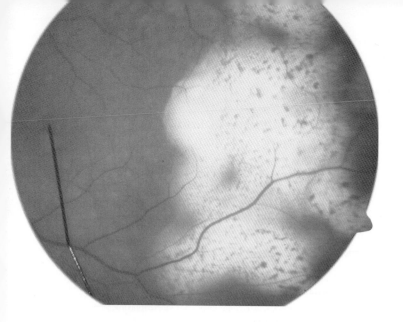

PRIMARY
INTRAOCULAR
LYMPHOMA

Chi-Chao Chan
National Eye Institute, USA

John A. Gonzales
University of Southern California, Los Angeles, USA

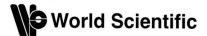 **World Scientific**

NEW JERSEY • LONDON • SINGAPORE • BEIJING • SHANGHAI • HONG KONG • TAIPEI • CHENNAI

Published by

World Scientific Publishing Co. Pte. Ltd.

5 Toh Tuck Link, Singapore 596224

USA office: 27 Warren Street, Suite 401-402, Hackensack, NJ 07601

UK office: 57 Shelton Street, Covent Garden, London WC2H 9HE

Library of Congress Cataloging-in-Publication Data
Chan, Chi-Chao
  Primary intraocular lymphoma / by Chi-Chao Chan & John A Gonzales.
    p. ; cm.
  Includes bibliographical references and index.
   ISBN-13 978-981-270-407-8 -- ISBN-10 981-270-407-8
   1. Reticulo-endothelial system--Tumors. 2. Lymphomas. 3. Eye Neoplasms.
  4. Lymphoma. I. Gonzales, John A. II. Title.

  RC280.R4 C43 2007
  616.99'446--dc22

                                                    2007011847

British Library Cataloguing-in-Publication Data
A catalogue record for this book is available from the British Library.

Typeset by Stallion Press
Email: enquiries@stallionpress.com

Printed by FuIsland Offset Printing (S) Pte Ltd, Singapore

— This book is dedicated to our families —

Winifred Mao and Eugene Chan

Chung and Henry Eng

John, Manuela, and Joseph Gonzales

Foreword

by Professor W. R. Green

Drs. Chan and Gonzales have provided an excellent and comprehensive review of primary intraocular lymphoma, including clinical, histopathologic and immunologic features and the history of nosologic changes and evidence of possible etiology. In addition, the authors have presented molecular characteristics of the lymphoma, many of which are based on their own research using up-to-date molecular pathological techniques, including microdissection, *immunoglobulin gene* rearrangements, *bcl-2* translocations, molecular signals, and certain infectious DNA involvements.

There are many remaining unanswered problems in primary intraocular lymphoma; this book is a major step forward in summarizing the ophthalmic, immunological, pathological and oncological information that exists today. *Primary Intraocular Lymphoma* is an indispensable and invaluable reference and guide for any professional faced with the challenge of caring for patients with this disease. Ophthalmologists, neurologists, pathologists, oncologists, and medical students will benefit from reading the book to better understand and manage this malignancy.

W. Richard Green, M.D.
Professor of Ophthalmology and Pathology
Wilmer Ophthalmological Institute
The Johns Hopkins School of Medicine
Baltimore, MD
USA

December 2006

Foreword

by Professor R. B. Nussenblatt

Ocular inflammatory diseases such as uveitis include many different disorders. One disorder that is usually not considered as part of these diseases is lymphoma. Indeed, primary intraocular lymphoma (PIOL), probably a subgroup of primary central nervous system lymphoma (PCNSL), is one such disease. Usually characterized as a masquerade syndrome, PIOL will present clinically as an intraocular inflammation or uveitis. To distinguish between PIOL and a non-infectious uveitis can have life and death consequences for the patient, since treatments for each are clearly very different. PIOL often presents as a chronic, smoldering inflammation. The clinician's ability to recognize the sometimes subtle differences between PIOL and uveitis is critical. To identify this disorder and to adequately treat it are major challenges.

Dr. Chan is one of the world's leaders in the pursuit of our understanding of intraocular lymphoma. She has published very extensively in this field and has made important diagnostic observations as well as those leading to a better understanding of the basic mechanistic characteristics of this disease. This book represents a unique compendium of Dr Chan's extensive and profound expertise in this field. She and her co-author, Dr Gonzales, provide the clinician and the researcher with a wealth of up-to-date information covering all aspects of this disorder.

The chapters offer a comprehensive review of the subject. The information provided here reflects the most up-to-date information about PIOL, including practical clinical information. It also reflects the comments and thoughts that were expressed at the National Institutes of

Health meeting on PIOL, held in September 2004*. This volume will be indispensable to any clinician dealing with posterior segment diseases and the researcher who is interested in the challenge of curing what many of us believe is a curable cancer that for now still has a high mortality and very significant morbidity.

Robert B. Nussenblatt, M.D.
Chief, Laboratory of Immunology
National Eye Institute
National Institutes of Health
Bethesda, MD
USA

September 2006

---

*R.B. Nussenblatt, C.C. Chan, W.H. Wilson, J. Hochman, M. Gottesman for the Ocular Lymphoma Workshop Group: International central nervous system and ocular lymphoma workshop: Recommendations for the future. *Ocul Immunol Inflam* 14:139–144, 2006.

Preface

In medicine and science, two inseparable sisters, a modern renaissance has occurred in which the pursuit of knowledge has provided the world with fascinating discoveries and answers to age-old questions. Perhaps one of the most shining and striking moments in this modern renaissance was the elucidation of the human genome. From this momentous project were produced tools and knowledge that could be put to use to solve other problems and answer other questions. We find, however, that in seeking out an answer, we instead discover that we have more questions than when we started out. Moreover, answers that are found in chemistry, physics, insect genetics, and so forth frequently provide researchers in seemingly unrelated fields with clues that may prove to be important in their own hunts. It is important, then, that as true renaissance scientists, we open ourselves to the knowledge that is transmitted (literally on a daily basis now) in the world of science and medicine.

The world of ophthalmology is certainly partaking in this renaissance with ever new advancements in the field. Ocular immunopathology is at the forefront of these new advancements. The immune system, involved in diverse processes from inflammation to cancer, has proven to play a central role in many diseases. Even when an organ system is seemingly tucked away from the immune system, as are the brain and intraocular structures, dysfunctions involving components of the immune system can nonetheless manifest themselves. Yet again we are left with more questions than answers in attempting to understand disease.

It is with a sense of excitement and hunger for new knowledge that we present this book, the first to be published on the subject, on primary intraocular lymphoma (PIOL). This is exciting because it is within recent memory when the first histopathological presentations of PIOL were presented in the literature. Moreover, as we acquired knowledge of the inner workings of the immune system, we were able to modify our thoughts on the precise cell involved in this cancer. As genetics burgeoned into a powerful science, we were able to uncover ever more information on this rare tumor. Our appetite, however, is not abated. We are perhaps more hungry now for answers than in our first descriptions of this tumor in the literature of the 1940s and 1950s.

One might think of this book, then, as a menu. In the first four chapters we seek to stimulate the appetite with discussion of the definition of primary intraocular lymphoma, historical reviews and cases of PIOL, the classification systems that once existed and those in use today, and the epidemiology in PIOL. The next two chapters deal with the clinical presentation of the disease and ways that we image PIOL. As the disease often masquerades as a uveitis, it is important to recognize the salient features of this lymphoid malignancy, especially when it occurs in patients who fit the disease profile. We then turn our attention to the pathology and immunology involved in PIOL, in two respective chapters. It is perhaps here that we ought to pause during our feast of knowledge and reflect on just how much information we have acquired on PIOL in the past six decades. No longer are we dealing with the abstract reticulum cell sarcoma, but rather an immunologically and genetically distinct entity.

From the important main courses of clinical, pathological, and immunological presentations, we then turn to the important subject of diagnostic techniques and then to the unsettled business, but absolutely essential concepts, of therapy in PIOL. It has been noted by some gastronomic connoisseurs that a dinner ending without cheese is like a beautiful woman with only one eye. Something integral is missing. Similarly, our knowledge of the best therapeutic approaches to this tumor is not complete. Yet, while perfect treatment regimens for PIOL are missing, we have made important advancements in treating this tumor and we strive to make even further developments in this arena. The more effect we have on treating this tumor, the more we can affect the prognostics associated with the disease. Prognosis is dealt with in its own chapter and it is important to recognize here that PIOL is a malignant disease where we as ophthalmologists have the opportunity to extend or save our patients' lives. With manifestations limited to the eye (unless the brain is involved) patients will seek out, or be referred to, ophthalmologists. Therefore, it is of the utmost importance that ophthalmologists be able to identify possible presentations of PIOL and in appropriate cases seek out diagnostic procedures. Furthermore, it is important to consider what testing should be performed when attempting to diagnose PIOL with limited tissue specimens. Ocular pathologists and cytologists will certainly play an important role in drawing out the diagnostic plan for a patient. Finally, the ophthalmologist must guide his or her patient into appropriate care and management that is coordinated with neurooncologists. Thus, a great responsibility is shouldered by the ophthalmologist for the very quality of life of patients with PIOL.

There are hypotheses for the origin of PIOL, which are discussed in another chapter and it is here that we are struck with the fact that we still have much to learn about the fundamental problems that allow for a lymphoma to occur in the eye. This chapter is followed by another describing animal models of the disease developed at the National Eye Institute, in order to begin to understand some of the fundamental mechanisms involved in PIOL.

We end our book with illustrative cases that presented at the National Eye Institute. Some of these cases are classical presentations of PIOL, while others proved to be more challenging, both diagnostically and therapeutically. These cases are useful in that they allow the reader to follow some of the typical diagnostic and therapeutic techniques that are commonly employed.

The topic of PIOL is certainly a full plate and not always easy to digest. We feel that we have presented the important concepts and future directions in this disease in a manner that will allow the reader to better understand this most interesting cancer. We also wish to inform the reader that this story is far from complete. We and others around the world continue to work on elucidating the factors and mediators involved in this cancer and ways that important components of the disease might be modulated for therapeutic benefit. We hope that this book will whet the appetite of our readers and produces in them a hunger similar to ours for understanding PIOL.

We wish to thank the National Eye Institute and the Howard Hughes Medical Institute Research Scholars Program for their support. We also thank our colleagues, the physicians who refer patients to the NEI and the staff who work on the PIOL cases at the NEI. We are deeply indebted to the more than 100 patients who have contributed to our understanding of the disease, and to their families for their support during such a challenging time. Finally, we save our most profound thanks to our families and friends, whose love and encouragement helped us through the writing process of this book.

Chi-Chao Chan, M.D.
John Alexander Gonzales, M.D.

Contents

Chapter 1

Definition of Primary Intraocular Lymphoma

Primary intraocular lymphoma (PIOL) is a neoplasm, most frequently of B-cell, and rarely, T-cell, origin arising from or initially presenting in the sub-retinal pigment epithelium (RPE), retina and vitreous.[1–6] PIOL of the B-cell type is a non-Hodgkin's lymphomatous process of the diffuse large B-cell histologic type and its distinction lies in the fact that it is a subtype of primary central nervous system lymphoma (PCNSL). The neurosensory retina is, in fact, an extension of the CNS. Indeed, the neurosensory retina and retinal pigment epithelium are derived from the same neuroectoderm that forms the CNS during embryogenesis. And, like the retina, the CNS is an immunologically privileged organ as well.

PIOL is distinct from the other lymphomatous processes inside the eye much more commonly including metastatic systemic lymphoma to the eye, which typically affects the uveal tract and ocular adnexa via hematogenous routes; and the extremely rare extranodal marginal zone B-cell lymphoma (mucosa-associated lymphoid tissue lymphoma) that affects the choroid.[7–9] In addition, although a subtype of PCNSL, PIOL may arise *de novo* in the neurosensory retina rather than metastasizing from a primary non-ocular CNS structure.

As an immunologically privileged organ, the internal tissues of the eye are normally protected from inflammatory processes mediated by the immune system's B- and T-cells. Thus, the induction of inflammatory conditions within the eye is intriguing, as inflammatory B- and T-cells are not typically found there. Equally intriguing is the development of lymphomatous processes involving these same cells from which the eye is normally protected.

What is most curious about PCNSL and PIOL is the recent increase in prevalence in these malignancies. Certainly the rising prevalence of immunodeficiency states can explain part of this phenomenon,[10] but concurrent rises in the prevalence rate in immunocompetent patients warrant an in-depth look into this fascinating disease process. To that end, this book serves to be a guide into the history, diagnosis, management and treatment of PIOL, as well as providing insights into the future progress yet to be made in this most interesting and fatal malignancy.

References

1. Levy-Clarke GA, Chan CC, Nussenblatt RB. (2005) Diagnosis and management of primary intraocular lymphoma. *Hematol Oncol Clin North Am* **19**(4): 739–749.
2. Chan CC. (2003) Primary intraocular lymphoma: clinical features, diagnosis, and treatment. *Clin Lymphoma* **4**(1): 30–31.
3. Chan CC. (2003) Molecular pathology of primary intraocular lymphoma. *Trans Am Ophthalmol Soc* **101**: 275–292.
4. Chan CC, Buggage RR, Nussenblatt RB. (2002) Intraocular lymphoma. *Curr Opin Ophthalmol* **13**(6): 411–418.
5. Chan CC, Wallace DJ. (2004) Intraocular lymphoma: update on diagnosis and management. *Cancer Control* **11**(5): 285–295.
6. Merle-Beral H, Davi F, Cassoux N, *et al.* (2004) Biological diagnosis of primary intraocular lymphoma. *Br J Haematol* **124**(4): 469–473.
7. Coupland SE, Joussen A, Anastassiou G, Stein H. (2005) Diagnosis of a primary uveal extranodal marginal zone B-cell lymphoma by chorioretinal biopsy: case report. *Graefes Arch Clin Exp Ophthalmol* **243**(5): 482–486.
8. Coupland SE, Foss HD, Hidayat AA, *et al.* (2002) Extranodal marginal zone B cell lymphomas of the uvea: an analysis of 13 cases. *J Pathol* **197**(3): 333–340.
9. Colovic MD, Jankovic GM, Cemerikic-Martinovic V, *et al.* (1998) Primary intraocular marginal zone B-cell (MALT) lymphoma. *Eur J Haematol* **60**(1): 61–62.
10. Eby NL, Grufferman S, Flannelly CM, *et al.* (1988) Increasing incidence of primary brain lymphoma in the US. *Cancer* **62**(11): 2461–2465.

Chapter 2

History of Primary Intraocular Lymphoma (1950s–1970s)

Though rare, lymphomatous processes affecting the intraocular structures have been reported since the 1940s and early 1950s.[1-3]

To understand the historical significance of primary intraocular lymphoma, we need to consider one of the first widely accepted classification systems of lymphomas in general. In 1966, Henry Rappaport classified tumors
of the hematopoietic system according to their characteristic morphology
and their resemblance to normal, non-neoplastic cellular components (see
Chapter 3, "Classification of Lymphomas"). At that time, lymphomas were
divided into three groups based on cytology: reticulum cell sarcoma, lymphosarcoma, and Hodgkin's disease.[4] In addition, a follicular form of
lymphoma was also noted that recapitulated normal follicles in the lymph
nodes. Rappaport's description of the salient features of reticulum cell sarcoma, was based upon the malignant cells' resemblance to the reticular cell (a
pluripotent stem cell, according to Rappaport) or its histiocytic or lymphocytic derivatives. In Rappaport's definition, a reticulum cell sarcoma was a
"tumor of reticular tissue composed predominantly of neoplastic histiocytes
in various stages of maturation and differentiation." In its more differentiated
form, the reticulum cell sarcoma was composed of cells with distinct cell borders harboring a pale cytoplasm and nuclei resembling those of epithelioid
histiocytes (oval), fibroblasts (ovoid or elongated), or monocytes (indented
and lobulated). Less differentiated reticulum cell sarcomas were noted to
have round or oval nuclei, occasionally with indentations or irregular borders, and containing prominent nucleoli. The vacuolated cytoplasm in either
form of differentiation could be variable, sometimes being scant and at other
times abundant. As for the origin of reticulin fibers, Rappaport speculated

3

that the neoplastic histiocytes may have played a role in the production of this type of immature collagen. Indeed, in describing the more differentiated form, each histiocyte appeared to have surrounded itself with reticulin fibers and the degree of reticulin fiber formation was obvious with silver impregnation of histology slides. Other reticulum cell sarcomatous nodules were practically devoid of reticulin fibers, but occasionally exhibited compression of such fibers at the periphery of their growth. Rappaport noted that, in addition to reticulin stains and cytology, this feature in a lymph node aided one in distinguishing subtle cases of malignant growth from mere reactive follicular centers. Despite the fact that such neoplastic histiocytes (also known as reticulum cells) were associated with reticulin fibers, it was pointed out later by others that the only similarity between reticulin fibers and reticulum cells was in similar names.[5] Pathologists at the Armed Forces Institute of Pathology (AFIP) in Washington, D.C. noted that reticulin was a form of pre-collagen that had been shown by others to be produced by fibroblasts,[6] while reticulum cells belonged to the lymphoreticular system. Thus, histologic diagnoses made from hematoxylin and eosin (H&E) stains were of primary importance for the AFIP pathologists while staining for reticulin fibers was a secondary issue.[5]

Rappaport related that the malignant lymphomas occurred within lymph nodes or extranodally, but rarely in the central nervous system. No mention is made of intraocular lymphoma in Rappaport's descriptions.

The first case of the so-called intraocular reticulum cell sarcoma involved a Caucasian male 27 years of age.[3] Slit lamp examination revealed mutton fat keratic precipitates, with cells noted in the anterior chamber, and the iris was thickened with engorged blood vessels. Examination of the fundus revealed an edematous optic nerve head with surrounding retinal edema. There was engorgement of the retinal blood vessels and numerous retinal hemorrhages. The patient was diagnosed with neuroretinitis, retinal hemorrhage and periphlebitis, iridocyclitis, and glaucoma. The patient was treated with standard therapy for uveitis at that time (corticosteroids), yet his condition progressed with the anterior chamber becoming shallower and an increase in iris thickness with development of nodules and posterior synechiae. Eventually, his eye became blind and painful and because of this, in addition to difficulty in establishing a satisfactory diagnosis, the eye was enucleated. Pathologic inspection revealed conjunctival, episcleral, uveal, retinal pigment epithelial, retinal, and optic nerve infiltration with closely packed cells. The diagnosis of intraocular reticulum cell sarcoma was made. Shortly thereafter, and interestingly so, a new and rapid increase in the right testicular size (equivalent to a "peach") warranted excision of that organ. Pathologic inspection here showed replacement of normal testicular tissue with closely packed cells resulting in the diagnosis of lymphosarcoma of the testicle. Despite receiving radiotherapy to the orbit, testicle, and abdomen, the patient succumbed to his malignancies 11 months after first presenting to Cooper and Ricker. Aside from being the first reported case of intraocular reticulum cell sarcoma, what makes this case so fascinating is the concurrent involvement of the testicle in a neoplastic process. The testicle, like the eye, is an immunoligically privileged organ. Unlike the eye's close relationship to the tissues of the CNS, the reason for the testicle's immunoprivilege can be related to the antigenicity that is produced by its inherent function of generating gametocytes with half the chromosomal content compared with the rest of the cells of the body. This patient was never noted to suffer from CNS manifestations such as ataxia, altered mental status, or neuropathy. As computerized tomography (CT) and magnetic resonance imaging (MRI) were not available at that time, it is difficult to ascertain whether this patient truly had primary intraocular lymphoma versus a metastasis from either his testicular cancer or elsewhere. Histopathology of the eye revealed tumor cells in the uvea and retina. Immunophenotyping was not available at this time so Cooper and Ricker were unable to deduce the probable B-cell origin of this tumor. However, they well knew that despite the lack of intraocular lymphoid tissue, lymphomatous processes somehow were able to occur intraocularly[3] and they went on to note that the lymphomatous processes occurred in other tissues devoid of lymph nodes, including the skin. Today, this type of lymphoma is known as cutaneous T-cell lymphoma (mycosis fungoides).

Several factors make the so-called reticulum cell sarcoma in this patient an unlikely primary process, though Cooper and Ricker put forth this possibility. One factor is the patient's young age, although it is not impossible for very young people to be afflicted with primary intraocular lymphoma.[7,8] Another factor is the infiltration of non-intraocular structures, including the conjunctiva and episclera, which seldom occurs in the natural process of the disease. The pathology of the uveal involvement suggests a metastatic malignancy and Cooper and Ricker conceded that this was likely the most probable event. Subsequent literature brought forth other cases of intraocular reticulum cell sarcoma and Currey and Deutsch are credited with describing the first true case of primary intraocular disease.[9]

It was not until the late 1970s and early 1980s that the term "reticulum cell sarcoma" became a misnomer as researchers demonstrated the lymphocytic origin of these tumors.[10–13] In fact, even during the late 1980s, some were noting, almost foretellingly, that "When the ocular/CNS form of the disease [reticulum cell sarcoma] is more clearly defined immunocytologically, a change in the name of the disease will likely be in order".[14] Table 2.1

Table 2.1 First Historical Accounts of Ocular Reticulum Cell Sarcoma in the English Literature

Author	Year	Age	Sex	Race	Diagnosis
Cooper & Ricker[3]	1951	27	M[a]	C[c]	RCS[f] of the choroid, retina, conjunctiva, iris, ciliary body OD[g]
Cook[15]	1953	59	F[b]	NR[d]	Primary choroidal lymphosarcoma with involvement of the ciliary body, subarachnoid space invasion, and optic nerve infiltration
Reese[16]	1956	47	M	NR	RCS with intraocular involvement
Reese[16]	1956	62	F	NR	RCS with intraocular involvement; involvement of the abdomen
Reese[16]	1956	58	M	NR	RCS with intraocular involvement; previous visceral malignant lymphoma
Beasley[17]	1961	51	M	C	Lymphosarcoma, lymphocytic type of choroid with extension through retina OD
Currey & Deutsch[9]	1965	50	M	AA[e]	RCS of the uveal tract and optic nerve OS[h]
Vogel, et al.[18]	1968	67	M	C	Intraocular RCS OU[i]
Vogel, et al.[18]	1968	71	F	C	RCS of the retina OD
Vogel, et al.[18]	1968	40	F	C	RCS of the retina OD
Vogel, et al.[18]	1968	46	M	C	RCS of the retina and uvea OS
Vogel et al.[18] / Nevins et al.[19]	1968	64	F	C	Primary, solitary RCS OD
Vogel, et al.[18]	1968	58	F	C	RCS of the retina, vitreous and subretinal space OS

[a]M = male; [b]F = female; [c]C = Caucasian; [d]NR = not reported; [e]AA = African-American; [f]RCS = reticulum cell sarcoma; [g]OD = right eye; [h]OS = left eye; [i]OU = both eyes.

summarizes the reports of PIOL in the 1950s and 1960s in the English literature.

References

1. McGavic JS. (1943) Lymphomatoid diseases involving the eye and its adnexa. *Arch Ophthalmol* **30**: 179–193.
2. Heath P. (1948) Ocular lymphomas. *Trans Am Ophthalmol Soc* **46**: 385–398.
3. Cooper EL, Ricker JL. (1951) Malignant lymphoma of the uveal tract. *Am J Ophthalmol* **34**: 1153–1158.
4. Rappaport H. (1966) *Atlas of Tumor Pathology, Section III-Fascicle 8, Tumors of the Hematopoietic System.* Armed Forces Institute of Pathology, Washington, D.C.
5. Henry JM, Heffner RR, Jr, Dillard SH, *et al.* (1974) Primary malignant lymphomas of the central nervous system. *Cancer* **34**(4): 1293–1302.
6. Puchtler H. (1964) On the original definition of the term "reticulin". *J Histochem Cytochem* **12**: 552.
7. Wender A, Adar A, Maor E, Yassur Y. (1994) Primary B-cell lymphoma of the eyes and brain in a 3-year-old boy. *Arch Ophthalmol* **112**(4): 450–451.
8. Young TL, Himelstein BP, Rebsamen SL, *et al.* (1996) Intraocular Ki-1 lymphoma in a 2-year-old boy. *J Pediatr Ophthalmol Strabismus* **33**(5): 268–270.
9. Currey TA, Deutsch AR. (1965) Reticulum cell sarcoma of the uvea. *Southern Med J* **58**: 919.
10. Horning SJ, Doggett RS, Warnke RA, *et al.* (1984) Clinical relevance of immunologic phenotype in diffuse large cell lymphoma. *Blood* **63**(5): 1209–1215.
11. Taylor CR, Russell R, Lukes RJ, Davis RL. (1978) An immunohistological study of immunoglobulin content of primary central nervous system lymphomas. *Cancer* **41**(6): 2197–2205.
12. Warnke R, Miller R, Grogan T, *et al.* (1980) Immunologic phenotype in 30 patients with diffuse large-cell lymphoma. *N Engl J Med* **303**(6): 293–300.
13. Warnke R, Miller R, Levy R. (1980) Immunologic phenotype in large-cell lymphoma. *N Engl J Med* **303**(22): 1303.
14. Freeman LN, Schachat AP, Knox DL, *et al.* (1987) Clinical features, laboratory investigations, and survival in ocular reticulum cell sarcoma. *Ophthalmology* **94**: 1631–1639.
15. Cook C. (1954) Uveal lymphosarcoma. *Br J Ophthalmol* **38**(3): 182–185.
16. Reese AB. (1963) *Tumors of the Eye.* Hoeber, New York.
17. Beasley H. (1961) Lymphosarcoma of the choroid. *Am J Ophthalmol* **51**: 1294–1296.

18. Vogel MH, Font RL, Zimmerman LE, Levine RA. (1968) Reticulum cell sarcoma of the retina and uvea. Report of six cases and review of the literature. *Am J Ophthalmol* **66**(2): 205–215.
19. Nevins RC, Jr, Frey WW, Elliott JH. (1968) Primary, solitary, intraocular reticulum cell sarcoma (microgliomatosis). (A clinicopathologic case report). *Trans Am Acad Ophthalmol Otolaryngol* **72**(6): 867–876.

Chapter 3

Classification of Lymphomas

Until 1997, classifying lymphomas proved to be frustrating for pathologists and clinicians. Much of the early problems with categorizing lymphomas lay in the fact that it was simply not clear for certain from what normal tissues or cells the particular tumor had arisen, making it difficult for pathologists to define a unifying nomenclature. Clinicians sought out systems of classification that held prognostic and treatment utility. Various classification systems were developed resulting in different centers using different schemata, and making diagnoses that were inconsistent or had no similar counterpart in another institution's classification pattern. Differing classification systems set the stage for differing methods of diagnosing and treating what could very well be the same disease process. In addition, it was difficult to compare prognoses or uniform treatment modalities between the lymphomas classified by the various systems. Interestingly, all lymphomatous processes, even Hodgkin's disease, were considered manifestations of the same disease[1] at one time.

Attempts at creating a uniform classification system for non-Hodgkin's lymphomas had their beginnings with Gallo and Malory,[2] who developed a clinicopathologic classification criterion. Later, Rappaport produced a lymphoma classification system with subtypes that were based on cellular features such as size and amount of cytoplasm, as well as the overall morphology of the tumor, such as nodularity.[3] Though his system was a purely morphologic approach to the categorization of lymphomas, the great progress that was provided by the Rappaport system was recognizing the prognostic significance of nodular lymphomas.[3] However, as time passed and as information about lymphomatous cells themselves accumulated, modifications were made to the Rappaport classification system,

9

producing a complicated, unwieldly, and often non-intuitive nomenclature. The major piece of information that had been discovered during the 1960s and 1970s was that of immunologic markers on the surfaces of lymphoid cells. The identification of lymphocyte surface markers harkens back to the work of Bach,[4] Coombs,[5] Brain,[6–8] and Lay[9] in the early 1970s. They each showed that human lymphocytes would bind to sheep red blood cells, spontaneously producing erythrocyte (E) rosettes. Jondal and colleagues showed that T lymphocytes were involved in mediating the rosette formation.[10,11] Taylor applied immunoperoxidase methods, which had been used previously to uncover the immunoglobulin surface markers expressed on the lymphoma cells, to stain CNS lymphomas for immunoglobulin components.[12]

Lukes and Collins, echoing the voices of others, noted that the advancements made in immunology made it apparent that lymphomas could and should be classified according to their immunologic markers in addition to their morphologic appearance[13–15] and proposed their own system to reflect this new knowledge. The Lukes-Collins system made use of the developing advancements in immunologic differentiation in B and T lymphocytes. Thus, the Lukes-Collins system was an immunologic *and* morphologic classification. An important development from the Lukes-Collins classification system was the realization that many tumors previously described as histiocytic lymphomas, reticulum cell sarcomas (PIOL had previously been known as ocular reticulum cell sarcoma), and other types of historical sarcomas were actually lymphomas derived from malignantly transformed B- and T-cells.[15] Lukes and Collins vented their frustration with the previous nomenclature by noting that "(t)he terms 'reticulum cell sarcoma' and 'lymphosarcoma' in addition have been applied in an extraordinarily variable fashion and achieved a meaningless status, by preventing effective comparison of results from different centers."[13]

At around the same time, a histopathological classification system, the Kiel System, was introduced.[16] Then, in the early 1980s, the National Cancer Institute at the National Institutes of Health sponsored a study of the lymphomas which led to the production of the Working Formulation, reminiscent of the Rappaport system, that was especially useful to clinicians as it held power in its ability to typify treatment and prognostic features.[17] However, even further progress in the fields of immunology and genetics were being accomplished that would make it necessary yet again for a more relevant classification system.

The advancements made in immunology and genetics allow pathologists to discriminate between reactive and malignant lymphocytic processes. The malignant nature of a lymphoid neoplasm is discovered by noting the clonality of the antigen receptor gene rearrangement. This seemingly common and simple task today harkens back to the early 1980s when researchers were beginning to elucidate the monoclonality of diffuse large B cell lymphomas.[18] In B lymphocytes, rearrangements in the variable (V), diversity (D), and joining (J) gene segments of the immunoglobulin heavy chain gene precede transformation in both malignant and reactive processes. Malignant processes churn out the same type (or clone) of tumor cell, identical to the progenitor that initially went awry. Thus, all the progeny produced from a malignant progenitor B lymphocyte will share the identical immunoglobulin gene configuration and will be monoclonal. In reactive processes where B lymphocytes respond normally to the different peptides that compose an antigen by proliferation and production of various immunoglobulins with different rearrangements in VDJ gene segments (telltale signs that affinity maturation is occurring in order to effectively and specifically eradicate a pathogen that contains many different antigens), the daughter cells will have *different* immunoglobulin gene configurations from each other and from their progenitor. These daughter cells will belong to different clone subsets (are of multiple clonalities) and are thus, polyclonal. Stages of B- and T-cell differentiation in lymphomas are determined by noting the configuration of their respective antigen receptor genes (or lack thereof as in precursor B-/T-cell acute lymphoblastic leukemias/lymphomas) and correlating that with the corresponding normal B- and T-cell counterpart. In addition, leukocyte surface antigens (such as the cluster of differentiation (CD)), genotypic abnormalities (such as chromosomal translocations), and karyotypic anomalies (such as chromosomal duplications) further enable pathologists to molecularly and/or immunohistochemically characterize a lymphoma quite specifically by its stage of differentiation and state of activation. For example, progenitor and early lymphocytes express an array of CD molecules that denote where along the timeline of maturation they exist. In addition, the expression of these CD molecules is independent of antigen exposure, a hallmark of lymphocyte immaturity. However, lymphocytes that have been exposed to an antigen exist on a different timeline of maturity and activation and will therefore express different CD molecules on their cell surfaces. In the laboratory, pathologists are able to visualize the characteristic membrane-bound CD molecules and receptors (immunoglobulins in the case of B-cells and T-cell receptors in the case of T-cells), as well as co-receptors that neoplastic lymphoid cells express using immunohistochemistry with specific monoclonal and/or polyclonal antibodies.[19]

These advancements in characterization led to an algorithm in classifying lymphomas adopted by the World Health Organization (WHO). The WHO classification system was arrived at after acceptance and amendment of the Revised European-American Classification of Lymphoid Neoplasms (REAL), which itself was originally introduced in 1994. In November 1997, a summit was held at Arlie House, Virginia to devise an approach for classifying neoplastic processes of the hematopoietic system.[20] An advisory committee that was composed of American and European co-chairs (comprising pathologists, hematologists, and oncologists) met to evaluate the REAL classification and consider its adoption, producing the WHO/REAL classification system of lymphomas we use today. The WHO/REAL classification immunophenotypically identifies three types of lymphomas: B-cell neoplasms, T-cell and natural killer (NK) cell neoplasms, and Hodgkin's disease. B- and T-cell neoplasms are further subclassified according to diseases of precursor (lymphoblastic) neoplasms or diseases of mature (peripheral) neoplasms. Moreover, cytogenetic features (such as chromosomal translocations) were used to further characterize lymphomas. Unlike non-Hodgkin's lymphoma, in which 10–30% of the disease may present initially at an extranodal site,[21] Hodgkin's disease has a very characteristic and predictable occurrence. Hodgkin's disease usually starts at a single site within the lymphatic system, most often a cervical or supraclavicular lymph node or a mediastinal lymph node. Hodgkin's disease represents a distinct clinical entity with its own histologic subtypes, staging system,[22,23] and treatments. Hodgkin's disease, unlike diffuse large B-cell lymphoma, has a very good cure rate.[24,25]

Considering where PIOL fits into the scheme of things, we turn to the WHO/REAL classification system. PIOL is, in fact, a sub-type of primary central nervous system lymphoma (PCNSL) and non-Hodgkin's lymphoma

(NHL). Recall that the neuraxis consists of not only the brain and spinal cord, but the neurosensory retina as well (see Chapter 1). PCNSL is most commonly a B-cell tumor, though T-cell PCNSL has been described.[26,27] As an NHL B-cell disease, PCNSL is most frequently a subtype of diffuse large B-cell lymphoma (DLBCL). DLBCLs are the most common non-Hodgkin's malignancy and represent 31% to 40% of all NHLs.[28]

With the sequence of the human genome,[29,30] the potential for a new era in lymphoma taxonomy has emerged. From gene expression profiling using genome scan microarray techniques, it has been shown that there is significant and characteristic genetic heterogeneity within DLBCLs,[31,32] which in turn appears to account for the clinical heterogeneity seen within this histological subtype[33,34]; 40% of DLBCL patients respond to current treatment modalities, while the remainder die from the disease. Thus, the ability to determine genetic signatures expressed by subtypes of DLBCL is important for developing and using specific therapies aimed at target genes, their transcription factors, and their products. The therapeutic prowess that oncologists acquire against the subtypes of DLBCL, then, dictates prognosis.

There are three major subtypes of DLBCL: activated B-cell DLBCL (ABC DLBCL), germinal center B-cell (GCB DLBCL), and primary mediastinal (thymic large) B-cell DLBCL (PMB DLBCL) also known as type 3 based on the gene signature profiling. Some signatures include genes expressed in a particular type of cell or stage of differentiation, whereas other signatures include genes expressed during a particular biologic response, such as cellular proliferation or the activation of a cellular signaling pathway.[35] GCB DLBCL responds to a foreign antigen within the germinal center microenvironment of secondary lymphoid organs. In general, this group has a high rate of overall survival after chemotherapy.[34,36] ABC DLBCL (comprising 30% of DLBCL) is induced by mitogenic stimulation of blood B cells and has a poor rate of overall survival.[34,36] The type 3 DLBCL does not express genes characteristic of the other two groups and may yet be found to be heterogeneous.[37,38]

From gene expression profiling, it has been found that some subtypes of DLBCLs express certain types of genes more than other subtypes. For example, some GCB DLBCLs overexpress the BCL2 protein (a mitochondrial outer membrane protein that protects cells, such as B cells, from apoptosis) and this can be due to the translocation t(14;18)(q32;q21)[39] or amplification of the *bcl2* gene. In addition, some GCB DLBCLs exhibit amplification of the c-REL locus.[40,41] The c-REL protein is a member of the NF-kB/REL family of transcription factors and is involved in transcribing NF-kB-responsive genes,[42] a potential mechanism leading to cell survival and tumorogenesis. ABC DLBCLs seem to demonstrate constitutive activation of the IkB kinase, which can lead to the translocation of the transcription regulator NF-kB into the nucleus and the transcription of genes that promote cellular proliferation and survival.[43] The constitutive activity of IkB kinase is not seen in GCB DLBCL. Type 3 DLBCLs, like ABC DLBCLs, seem to also show constitutive activation of the NF-kB pathway.[44] Thus, this pathway seems to be an important target in treating ABC and PMB DLBCLs. This new found knowledge regarding genetic signatures has already resulted in therapy aimed at interfering with the activation of this pathway, namely an IkB kinase inhibitor, PS-1145, which has been shown to be effective against ABC DLBCLs and PMBLs, but not GCB DLBCLs.[45]

Gene expression profiling may allow us to classify lymphomatous diseases more specifically than our current taxonomy and offers prognostic utility.[31] Indeed, there is currently no perfect prognostic indicator and the development of such a tool is tantalizing. However, there is substantial heterogeneity of gene expression even within each of the three subgroups of DLBCL[31,32,46] and there is no single gene that can distinguish one subgroup from another. In addition, currently there is no standardization for the nomenclature offered by gene expression profiling. While there is no doubt that PCNSL is an NHL DLBCL, gene expression profiling is now underway to elucidate the different signatures that potentially exist within this subtype. For example, recent gene expression profiling work seems to indicate that some PCNSLs belong to GCB DLBCLs.[47] Due to the paucity of PIOL cases and materials, it is almost impossible to evaluate the pattern of gene expression using gene expression profiling to classify PIOL in this fashion currently. However, as our ability to classify lymphomas based upon their gene expression profiles improves and molecular technology to analyze small samples advances, we will likely see PIOL being more specifically defined by this system in the future as well.

In its DLBCL form, PCNSL is an aggressive tumor that is usually fatal (see Treatment, Chapter 11). Less frequently, primary lymphomas of the CNS can be derived from other B-cell lymphomas, such as marginal zone B-cell lymphomas (MZBCL).[48] However, in these cases, the disease is not intraparenchymal (being most often associated with the leptomeninges) and is clinically low-grade in nature. PIOL, like PCNSL, seems to be most often a DLBCL.

References

1. Custer RP, Bernhard WG. (1948) The interrelationship of Hodgkin's disease and other lymphatic tumors. *Am J M Sc* **216**: 625–642.
2. Gallo EA, Mallory TB. (1942) Malignant lymphoma: a clinicopathological survey of 618 cases. *American J Pathol* **18**: 381–429.
3. Rappaport H. (1966) *Atlas of Tumor Pathology, Section III-Fascicle 8, Tumors of the Hematopoietic System.* Armed Forces Institute of Pathology, Washington, D.C.
4. Bach MK, Brashler JR. (1970) Isolation of subpopulations of lymphocytic cells by the use of isotonically balanced solutions of Ficoll. I. Development of methods and demonstration of the existence of a large but finite number of subpopulations. *Exp Cell Res* **61**(2): 387–396.
5. Coombs RR, Gurner BW, Wilson AB, *et al.* (1970) Rosette-formation between human lymphocytes and sheep red cells not involving immunoglobulin receptors. *Int Arch Allergy Appl Immunol* **39**(5–6): 658–663.
6. Brain P, Gordon J, Willetts WA. (1970) Rosette formation by peripheral lymphocytes. *Clin Exp Immunol* **6**(5): 681–688.
7. Brain P, Gordon J. (1971) Rosette formation by peripheral lymphocytes. II. Inhibition of the phenomenon. *Clin Exp Immunol* **8**(3): 441–449.
8. Brain P, Marston RH. (1973) Rosette formation by human T and B lymphocytes. *Eur J Immunol* **3**(1): 6–9.
9. Lay WH, Mendes NF, Bianco C, Nussenzweig V. (1971) Binding of sheep red blood cells to a large population of human lymphocytes. *Nature* **230**(5295): 531–532.
10. Jondal M, Klein E, Yefenof E. (1975) Surface markers on human B and T lymphocytes. VII. Rosette formation between peripheral T lymphocytes and lymphoblastoid B-cell lines. *Scand J Immunol* **4**(3): 259–266.
11. Jondal M. (1976) SRBC rosette formation as a human T lymphocyte marker. *Scand J Immunol* **Suppl 5**: 69–76.
12. Taylor CR, Russell R, Lukes RJ, Davis RL. (1978) An immunohistological study of immunoglobulin content of primary central nervous system lymphomas. *Cancer* **41**(6): 2197–2205.
13. Lukes RJ, Collins RD. (1974) Immunologic characterization of human malignant lymphomas. *Cancer* **34**(4 Suppl): suppl:1488–1503.

14. Lukes RJ, Collins RD. (1974) A functional approach to the classification of malignant lymphoma. *Recent Results in Cancer Research* **46**: 18–30.
15. Lukes RJ, Collins RD. (1975) New approaches to the classification of the lymphomata. *Br J Cancer* **31 SUPPL 2**: 1–28.
16. Lennert K, Mohri NS, H, Kaiserling E. (1975) The histopathology of malignant lymphoma. *Br J Haematol* **31**(Suppl): 193–203.
17. National Cancer Institute sponsored study of classifications of non-Hodgkin's lymphomas: summary and description of a working formulation for clinical usage. (1982) The Non-Hodgkin's Lymphoma Pathologic Classification Project. *Cancer* **49**(10): 2112–2135.
18. Warnke R, Miller R, Levy R. (1980) Immunologic phenotype in large-cell lymphoma. *N Engl J Med* **303**(22): 1303.
19. Diamond BA, Yelton DE, Scharff MD. (1981) Monoclonal antibodies. A new technique for producing serologic reagents. *N Engl J Med* **304**(22): 1344–1349.
20. Harris NL, Jaffe ES, Diebold J, *et al.* (1999) The World Health Organization classification of neoplastic diseases of the hematopoietic and lymphoid tissues. Report of the Clinical Advisory Committee meeting, Airlie House, Virginia, November, 1997. *Ann Oncol* **10**(12): 1419–1432.
21. Anderson T, Chabner BA, Young RC, *et al.* (1982) Malignant lymphoma. 1. The histology and staging of 473 patients at the National Cancer Institute. *Cancer* **50**(12): 2699–2707.
22. Carbone PP, Kaplan HS, Musshoff K, *et al.* (1971) Report of the Committee on Hodgkin's Disease Staging Classification. *Cancer Res* **31**(11): 1860–1861.
23. Lister TA, Crowther D, Sutcliffe SB, *et al.* (1989) Report of a committee convened to discuss the evaluation and staging of patients with Hodgkin's disease: Cotswolds meeting. *J Clin Oncol* **7**(11): 1630–1636.
24. DeVita VT, Jr (2003) A selective history of the therapy of Hodgkin's disease. *Br J Haematol* **122**(5): 718–727.
25. Donaldson SS, Hancock SL, Hoppe RT. (1999) The Janeway lecture. Hodgkin's disease — finding the balance between cure and late effects. *Cancer J Sci Am* **5**(6): 325–333.
26. Choi JS, Nam DH, Ko YH, *et al.* (2003) Primary central nervous system lymphoma in Korea: comparison of B- and T-cell lymphomas. *Am J Surg Pathol* **27**(7): 919–928.
27. Gijtenbeek JM, Rosenblum MK, DeAngelis LM. (2001) Primary central nervous system T-cell lymphoma. *Neurology* **57**(4): 716–718.
28. A clinical evaluation of the International Lymphoma Study Group classification of non-Hodgkin's lymphoma. (1997) The Non-Hodgkin's Lymphoma Classification Project. *Blood* **89**(11): 3909–3918.

29. Lander ES, Linton LM, Birren B, *et al.* (2001) Initial sequencing and analysis of the human genome. *Nature* **409**(6822): 860–921.
30. Venter JC, Adams MD, Myers EW, *et al.* (2001) The sequence of the human genome. *Science* **291**(5507): 1304–1351.
31. Alizadeh AA, Eisen MB, Davis RE, *et al.* (2000) Distinct types of diffuse large B-cell lymphoma identified by gene expression profiling. *Nature* **403**(6769): 503–511.
32. Chan WC, Huang JZ. (2001) Gene expression analysis in aggressive NHL. *Ann Hematol* **80 Suppl 3**: B38–41.
33. Lossos IS, Czerwinski DK, Alizadeh AA, *et al.* (2004) Prediction of survival in diffuse large-B-cell lymphoma based on the expression of six genes. *N Engl J Med* **350**(18): 1828–1837.
34. Wright G, Tan B, Rosenwald A, Hurt EH, *et al.* (2003) A gene expression-based method to diagnose clinically distinct subgroups of diffuse large B cell lymphoma. *Proc Natl Acad Sci USA* **100**(17): 9991–9996.
35. Staudt LM. (2003) Molecular diagnosis of the hematologic cancers. *N Engl J Med* **348**(18): 1777–1785.
36. Rosenwald A, Wright G, Chan WC, *et al.* (2002) The use of molecular profiling to predict survival after chemotherapy for diffuse large-B-cell lymphoma. *N Engl J Med* **346**(25): 1937–1947.
37. Rosenwald A, Wright G, Leroy K, *et al.* (2003) Molecular diagnosis of primary mediastinal B cell lymphoma identifies a clinically favorable subgroup of diffuse large B cell lymphoma related to Hodgkin lymphoma. *J Exp Med* **198**(6): 851–862.
38. Savage KJ, Monti S, Kutok JL, *et al.* (2003) The molecular signature of mediastinal large B-cell lymphoma differs from that of other diffuse large B-cell lymphomas and shares features with classical Hodgkin lymphoma. *Blood* **102**(12): 3871–3879.
39. Iqbal J, Sanger WG, Horsman DE, *et al.* (2004) BCL2 translocation defines a unique tumor subset within the germinal center B-cell-like diffuse large B-cell lymphoma. *Am J Pathol* **165**(1): 159–166.
40. Bentz M, Barth TF, Bruderlein S, *et al.* (2001) Gain of chromosome arm 9p is characteristic of primary mediastinal B-cell lymphoma (MBL): comprehensive molecular cytogenetic analysis and presentation of a novel MBL cell line. *Genes Chromosomes Cancer* **30**(4): 393–401.
41. Joos S, Otano-Joos MI, Ziegler S, *et al.* (1996) Primary mediastinal (thymic) B-cell lymphoma is characterized by gains of chromosomal material including 9p and amplification of the REL gene. *Blood* **87**(4): 1571–1578.
42. Ghosh S, May MJ, Kopp EB. (1998) NF-kappa B and Rel proteins: evolutionarily conserved mediators of immune responses. *Annu Rev Immunol* **16**: 225–260.

43. Davis RE, Brown KD, Siebenlist U, Staudt LM. (2001) Constitutive nuclear factor kappaB activity is required for survival of activated B cell-like diffuse large B cell lymphoma cells. *J Exp Med* **194**(12): 1861–1874.
44. Feuerhake F, Kutok JL, Monti S, *et al.* (2005) NFkappaB activity, function, and target-gene signatures in primary mediastinal large B-cell lymphoma and diffuse large B-cell lymphoma subtypes. *Blood* **106**(4): 1392–1399.
45. Lam LT, Davis RE, Pierce J, *et al.* (2005) Small molecule inhibitors of IkappaB kinase are selectively toxic for subgroups of diffuse large B-cell lymphoma defined by gene expression profiling. *Clin Cancer Res* **11**(1): 28–40.
46. Bea S, Zettl A, Wright G, *et al.* (2005) Diffuse large B-cell lymphoma subgroups have distinct genetic profiles that influence tumor biology and improve gene expression-based survival prediction. *Blood.*
47. Braaten KM, Betensky RA, de Leval L, *et al.* (2003) BCL-6 expression predicts improved survival in patients with primary central nervous system lymphoma. *Clin Cancer Res* **9**(3): 1063–1069.
48. Tu PH, Giannini C, Judkins AR, *et al.* (2005) Clinicopathologic and genetic profile of intracranial marginal zone lymphoma: a primary low-grade CNS lymphoma that mimics meningioma. *J Clin Oncol* **23**(24): 5718–5727.

Chapter 4

Epidemiology of Primary Intraocular Lymphoma

Incidence and Prevalence Within the Immunocompetent Population

Incidence of PCNSL in Immunocompetent Patients. Of the newly diagnosed primary intracranial tumors, PCNSL makes up from 6 to 7% of those cases.[1–5] While the reported incidence of all primary brain and CNS tumors is about 11.5 to 13.8 cases per 100,000 person years,[6,7] others have reported that primary brain tumors have an annual incidence of 130.8 per 100,000 persons.[6] The incidence of PCNSL has been reported as being 0.3 to 0.43 cases per 100,000 person years.[3,7,8] Previously, Freeman,[9] Jellinger,[10] and Zimmerman[11] reported on PCNSL in the mid-1970s as representing only about 1 to 2% of all NHLs and less than 5% of all intracranial tumors. The incidence in PCNSL has been noted to be increasing since the 1980s with Eby's examination of the disease by using the National Cancer Institute's (NCI) Surveillance, Epidemiology, and End Results (SEER) program data.[12] Later, as the year 2000 approached, Corn reported that over two decades, from 1973 to 1992, the incidence of PCNSL increased more than 10-fold from 2.5 cases to 30 cases per 10 million population.[13] Moreover, Corn projected that the incidence rate would increase to approximately 51.1 cases per 10 million population in the year 2000. PCNSL is also associated with other parts of the neuraxis, notably the eye (as PIOL) and approximately 15 to 25% of patients with PCNSL will have secondary intraocular involvement.

Prevalence of PCNSL in Immunocompetent Patients. According to the National Cancer Institute's (NCI) Surveillance, Epidemiology, and End

Results (SEER) program data, the United States Estimated Complete Prevalence Counts for brain and other CNS tumors is 105,960 cases (as of 1 January 2002, http://seer.cancer.gov/about; site accessed 15 November 2005). This can be compared with reports noting that the incidence of PCNSL ranges from 0.48 to 1 per 100,000 population in developed countries, such as the United States.[14] Based on a conservative estimate, there are approximately 1,500 cases annually of PCNSL in the United States.

Elsewhere in the world, immunocompetent patients were noted to have PCNSL with increased frequency. Schabet reported in 1999 that during the period 1984–1985, the University of Tuebingen in Germany diagnosed one immunocompetent patient with PCNSL.[15] Diagnoses were made in increasing numbers over the years at the University, with 14 being diagnosed during the period 1995–1996. Better recognition of PCNSL could play a minor role in an increase of disease prevalence.

Incidence of PIOL in Immunocompetent Patients. The incidence of PIOL is estimated to range from 30 to 200 people annually in the United States.[16,17] Most patients (60 to 90%) who present initially with PIOL will eventuate to CNS disease[16,18–21] and approximately 20% of PCNSL patients will have intraocular lymphomatous involvement.[22,23] Considering that PIOL is a subset of PCNSL, as the incidence of CNS disease increases, intraocular lymphomatous processes have the potential to increase as well and it is undeniable that various centers have noted an increased rate of incidence or diagnosis at this anatomic site in the immunocompetent population. Therefore, if we consider that the United States population estimate is 295,734,134 (July 2005 estimate, http://www.indexmundi.com/united_states/population.html; site accessed 17 November 2005), and considering that the incidence of PCNSL in Americans is approximately 51 cases per 10 million, we conservatively estimate that approximately 1500 cases of PCNSL occur annually. Based on the conservative estimate that 20% of patients with PCNSL have ocular involvement, the annual prevalence of PIOL is approximately 300 cases (either alone or in association with PCNSL) in the United States.

Demographics Within the Immunocompetent Population

Age of Immunocompetent Patients in PCNSL and PIOL. PCNSL and PIOL typically affect people in their fifth to sixth decade of life. The youngest reported age has been a child of 2 years in Europe, though the clinical history and findings were not presented in any detail.[24] The rising incidence in PCNSL has been seen in all age groups, suggesting that the increased incidence is independent of age. However, the greatest increase in incidence has been noted in patients over 60 years of age. Surawicz *et al.* examined the incidence rates over 8 age groups.[7] The incidence rates for people 0 to 19 years of age were found to be 0.02 per 100,000 person-years; 0.37 for 20- to 34-year-olds; 0.63 for 35- to 44-year-olds; 0.46 for 45- to 54-year-olds; 0.97 for 55- to 64-year-olds; 1.46 for 65- to 74-year-olds; 1.57 for 75- to 84-year-olds; and for those over 85 years of age the incidence rate was 0.68 per 100,000 person-years.[7] Age appears to be important in terms of prognosis, as patients under 60 years of age with PCNSL fare better than those over 60 years of age.[24-26] In India, the mean age of PCNSL patients has been reported as 39.5 to 44.4 years,[27] with no statistically significant change in age trend for the period of time examined (1980 through 2003). It appears, then, that PCNSL patients in India are not developing the disease at a younger age now than in the past. One of the patients from this study was 3 years of age at the time of diagnosis. What could be the explanation for the lower mean age of PCNSL patients in India compared with the more developed countries such as the United States? Sarkar *et al.* brings up the point that there are important differences in the population demographics in India compared with that in Western geographic locales and the United States. The life expectancy of the population of India is 64.35 years; in the United States, it is 77.71 years; in France, 79.6 years; Germany, 78.65 years; the United Kingdom, 78.38 years; and in Japan, 81.15 years.[27] Also, only 4.9% of India's population are 65 years of age or older, while in the United States 12.4% of the population are over the age of 65. On the other hand, the mean age of immunocompetent patients in the developed countries of France and Belgium has been reported as 61 years, which is similar to that in other developed nations. In a study of 32 cases of PCNSL from Japan, the median age of the patients was 61.3 years.[28] Previously, Hayakawa and colleagues examined 170 patients with PCNSL in 1994.[29] The mean age for Hayakawa's particular patients was 56.7 years.

Gender. Brain tumors in general seem to exhibit a male predilection (although meningiomas show a female preponderance).[7] For example, one

study reported that glioblastomas, anaplastic astrocytomas, oligoden-
rogliomas, anaplastic oliogdendrogliomas, ependymomas, mixed gliomas,
astrocytomas not otherwise specified, medulloblastomas, and germ cell
tumors are more common in men than in women.[7] PCNSLs also predominate in men, with the incidence of CNS lymphomas in men being
reported as 0.60 per 100,000 person years; in women, the rate is 0.28 per
100,000 person years.[7] Other studies have yielded male to female ratios of
1.4 to 2:1. Male to female relative risk has been described as being approximately 2.25.[7] Though a male preponderance seems to be the rule, there
have been studies in which a decidedly female predominance exists. In a
study of ocular and cerebral lymphomas from France, Cassoux and colleagues retrospectively reviewed 44 cases of PIOL with and without CNS
involvement, 36 being female and eight being male (male to female ratio
of 1 to 4.5).[30] However, another study looking at an immunocompetent
PCNSL population from France and Belgium, had a male to female ratio
of practically 1:1 (127 female patients and 121 male patients over a 15-year
period, from 1980 to 1995).[24]

Ethnics. Examination of the incidence rates of CNS lymphoma in
American whites and African-Americans has shown that there seems to be
no ethnical preference with respect to these two major ethnicities in the
United States.[7] Whites were shown to have a brain lymphoma incidence
rate of 0.42 per 100,000 person-years, while African-Americans had an
incidence rate of 0.49, a difference that was not statistically significant.[7]

Using the Lymphoma Study Group classification system,[31] Shibamoto
from Hayabuchi's group[32] looked at trends in PCNSL in Japan (between
1995 and 1999) as a follow-up to their previous examination during the
period from 1985 to 1994. The four-years study revealed 101 patients with
PCNSL, while the study from 1985 to 1994 yielded 157 immunocompetent
patients. Kuratsu[33] reported an annual overall age-adjusted incidence rate
for all intracranial tumors of nearly 11/100,000, with 4.6% of the 2129
patients with primary CNS tumors having malignant lymphoma.
Meanwhile, Hayakawa and colleagues examined 170 patients with PCNSL
in 1994.[29] The mean age for Japanese patients was 56.7 years and 93
patients were male (54.7%) while 77 were female (45.3%). Hayabuchi and
colleagues reported on findings obtained from the CNS Lymphoma Study
Group Members, a PCNSL consortium of medical centers throughout

Japan.[34] This group analyzed 466 cases of PCNSL in patients testing HIV-negative, obtained during the period from of 1985 to 1994. The researchers found that the male to female ratio was 1.45:1 and that the median age was 60 years, the parameters being similar to those in the United States. Interestingly, 20 tumors (8.5%) were of the T cell immunophenotype, while from other studies such tumors made up less than 2% of all PCNSLs.[35] Another 214 tumors (45.9%) and 232 (49.8%) were unclassifiable or unknown.

In Korea, an analysis of 3221 CNS tumors yielded 76 cases of PCNSL, with a median age of 54 years and a male to female ratio of 1.3:1.[36] These cases made up 2.4% of the total number of cases from the study carried out from 1997 to 1998. A prior study, from 1983 to 1987, had yielded 23 cases out of 894 (or 0.9%). Thus, Korea showed a trend of increasing incidence of PCNSL.

In India, it has been reported that diagnoses of PCNSL have exhibited an increasing trend.[27] Sarkar retrospectively analyzed 116 cases of PCNSL from two clinical centers, one in Northern India and the other in Southern India over a 24-year period. PCNSL cases increased in incidence 3.5-fold from two cases per year in the early 1980s to 7 in the early 2000s. The disease affected males more than females, with a male to female ratio up to 2.3:1.

Although amongst some geographic locations, e.g. the United States and some Western European countries, the incidence rates of PCNSL have increased, in other areas this has not been the case. In Alberta, Canada, PCNSL incidence rates were reported not to have increased.[37] PCNSL patients were retrospectively reviewed over a two-decade period covering the years from 1975 to 1996. PCNSLs were found to represent 0.96% of all the cases of NHL during the period of time studied. The late 1970s showed an incidence rate of 0.178 immunocompetent cases per million population, compared with 1.642 cases in 1996, though there was no statistically significant change in this incidence rate. The median age of patients studied in this population was 64 years and a male to female ratio of 3:2 was found. Similar findings have been reported in Scotland.[38]

Table 4.1 summarizes the epidemiology of several large PIOL case series in the literature. PIOL is a malignancy for which the average age of the patients is the late 50s and with no gender preference reported in predominately white population studies.[30,39-44] However, reports from some centers have noted a female preponderance in their cases.[30,40]

Table 4.1 Epidemiology from PIOL Case Series

| Author | Year | Number of Patients | M:F Ratio[1] | Demographics | |
				Mean Age (years)	Ethnicity
Freeman	1987	32	1:2.2	60	91% white 9% black
Whitcup	1993	12	1:5	57	NS[2]
Peterson	1993	24	1:2	58	NS
Akpek	1995	10	1.5:1	59	90% white 10% black
Cassoux	2000	42	1:4.5	54	97.6% white 2.4% Asian
Hoffman	2003	10	1.5:1	61.1	NS
Hormigo	2004	31	1:1.4	59 (median)	NS

[1]M:F Ratio = male-to-female ratio; [2]NS = not stated.

Prevalence and Incidence Within the AIDS Population

Prevalence of PCNSL in AIDS Patients. Approximately 2 to 10% of AIDS patients have PCNSL.[45] The prevalence of AIDS in the adult populations in various geographic locations is as follows: 0.61% in the United States; 0.2% in the United Kingdom; 0.4% in France; 0.1% in Germany; 0.1% in Japan; 0.9% in India; and 37.3% in Botswana (2003 estimate). In some locales, PCNSL is diagnosed only postmortem, such as in East Africa.[46] Poor access to healthcare and limited diagnostic resources are key factors that give rise to such postmortem diagnoses. In addition, the assumption that behavior or mental status changes may be due to cerebral edema, can prompt the usage of corticosteroids leading to a partial regress of PCNSL or PIOL, thereby masking the lymphomatous process.[47,48] Prior to the AIDS epidemic, transplant patients were the group most likely to develop PCNSL.

Incidence of PCNSL in AIDS Patients. HIV patients are at increased risk for developing both HD and NHL. Indeed, the development of an NHL in an HIV-infected patient is an AIDS-defining illness[49] and is associated with CD4 lymphocyte counts of less than 50/μL. While the cause PCNSL in immunocompetent patients has failed to reveal any clear etiological factor, latent Epstein Barr Virus (EBV) infection is identified as the causative agent in most AIDS patients.[26] Like AIDS-associated systemic NHL (accounting for 3–4% of primary AIDS-defining illnesses in developed countries[50,51]) the development of CNS lymphoma in AIDS patients occurs late in the disease, although it occurs as an AIDS-defining illness less often than systemic NHL.[52–55] AIDS patients have been reported to have an incidence rate of 0.32 per 1000 person years[56] as well as having a 2 to 6% risk of developing clinically significant PCNSL.[57–62] However, pathologically diagnosed AIDS (based upon autopsy examinations) has revealed that the risk for PCNSL in AIDS patients is 12%, with the risk increasing corresponding to the duration of the disease (the risk being as high as 57% in patients suffering from AIDS for more than three years).[55,63] The acquisition of a systemic or CNS AIDS-associated NHL late in the course of the disease indicates that a decimated immune system sets the stage for lymphomatous development.

Though the incidence of PCNSL is higher in AIDS patients than in immunocompetent patients, the incidence rates for this group have declined. One of the factors that seems to have had the greatest impact on the improvement of incidence rates in AIDS patients, is the use of highly active antiretroviral therapy (HAART).[64,65] Wolf examined a retrospective cohort of HIV-positive patients in Germany.[56] A total of 214 patients were studied and 61% of them had NHL as their first AIDS-defining disease. Five time periods (from 1982 to 2002) were involved. Three time periods (1982–1986, 1987–1990, and 1991–1994) occurred prior to the introduction and widespread use of HAART (pre-HAART era), while two time periods (1995–1998 and 1999–2002) came after that. The incidence of NHL in the AIDS patients studied by Wolf increased during the pre-HAART era from 8.24 per 1000 person years during the 1983–1986 period to 14.83 per 1000 person years during the 1991–1994 time period. The post-HAART era saw incidence rates for NHLs decline, first to 8 per 1000 person years during the 1995–1998 time period and then to 3.7 per 1000 person years during 1999–2002. Although the incidence rates for CNS lymphoma in these patients have always been less than that of systemic NHL, rises and falls in the incidence rates of CNS disease during the time periods examined mirrored that of the systemic disease. The incidence of CNS lymphoma in Wolf's examined patients was 2.75 per 1000 person years during the 1983–1986 pre-HAART period and rising to a high of 5.33 per 1000 person years during 1991–1994. However, during the post-HAART era, the incidence rates declined to 1.53 per 1000 person years during 1995–1998. A further decline in incidence to 0.32 per 1000 person years was seen during the 1999–2002 period. Thus, while some initially speculated that because AIDS patients live longer with lower CD4 counts and higher concentrations of virons due to improvements in treatment, allowing for an accumulation of "hits" to build up and produce lymphoma, recent data seem to suggest that HAART cannot only improve survival with AIDS, but also reduce the incidence of major complications, namely, the development of extranodal NHL, like PCNSL.[66]

While HAART has improved survival and PCNSL incidence rates in AIDS patients, an interesting possibility has arisen. Prior to HAART, opportunistic infections were able to get a better footing at establishing disease in AIDS patients. In addition, pre-HAART AIDS patients suffered especially from decimated CD4 lymphocyte levels, leaving mainly B cells as the major immunologic guardians of the body. However, opportunistic infections could easily have set the stage for the activation of such B cells which we postulate could then have allowed for the expansion of certain malignant clones of B cells. This scenario is very much like that involved in the activated B cell (ABC) type of diffuse large B cell lymphoma (DLBCL) described in Chapter 3. However, the current use of HAART has certainly decreased the incidence of opportunistic infections in AIDS patients. For example, hospital admissions in 12 states in the United States for opportunistic infections in patients infected with HIV decreased from 47% to 20% over a four-year period between 1996 and 2000.[67] In addition, HAART is able to maintain higher CD4 lymphocyte counts than would be possible without HAART.[68] We expect that it would not be unreasonable for a possible shift from the ABC DLBCLs that could possibly have characterized AIDS-associated PCNSLs in the pre-HAART era to a genotype like that in germinal center B cell (GCB) DLBCLs today in the HAART/post-HAART era. Developments in gene microarray technology will undoubtedly provide us with insights into the genotypic DLBCL that produces most PCNSLs in AIDS patients.

Demographics Within the AIDS Population

Age of AIDS patients with PCNSL. Patients with AIDS develop PCNSL at a younger age than their immunocompetent counterparts. AIDS patients are typically diagnosed with PCNSL in their third or fourth decade of life, whereas patients with intact immune systems are diagnosed with the brain malignancy during their fifth or sixth decade.[22,26,59,62] In the pre-HAART era, the median age at baseline was 36.7 years, while the median age of patients in the post-HAART era is 39.4 years.[56] In developing countries with limited diagnostic and therapeutic resources (such as HAART) and limitations in the access to healthcare, such as India, opportunistic infections may shorten the lives of patients prior to the development of PCNSL or PIOL.[27]

Gender in AIDS-associated PCNSL. The development of PCNSL in AIDS patients shows an overwhelmingly male predilection of 7.38:1[26] in Western countries, where homosexual intercourse is a major mode of transmission. However, in developing continents, such as Africa and Asia, heterosexual intercourse is the major route of transmission of HIV. This is reflected in the country of Botswana, Africa where the prevalence rate of AIDS in 2003 was 37.3% and where 37% of pregnant females are infected with HIV.[69]

PCNSL and PIOL in Other Immunocompromised Populations

PCNSL in Organ Transplant Recipients. The transplantation of solid organs has been reported to be associated with increased risk of developing lymphomas. This syndrome is known as post-transplant lymphoproliferative disorder (PTLD) and two factors are associated with the occurrence of PTLD — iatrogenic immunosuppresion and EBV.[70] Thus, PCNSL that arises in PTLD patients is quite similar to that in AIDS patients. Unlike these two immunocompromised conditions, EBV seems not to play a major role at all in the occurrence of PCNSLs in the immunocompetent population.[71,72] Interestingly, the second most common type of malignancy in transplant patients after non-melanoma skin cancer is PCNSL.[73] The risk of developing PCNSL is approximately 2.5% in such patients, but increases with the use of certain immunosuppressive agents, especially the use of multiple agents together like cycolosporin A, azathioprine, and prednisone.[74] Certain organ transplants may require more rigorous use of immunosuppresants. For example, renal transplant patients typically are treated with cyclosporine or azathioprine (more recently, however, with tacrolimus and mycophenolate mofetil)[75] and biologics, and have a 1–2% risk of developing PCNSL. On the other hand, cardiac, pulmonary, or hepatic transplantation can require more intensive immunosuppression and these patients have a 2 to 7% risk of developing PCNSL.[74,76–78] Indeed, a patient who had undergone heart transplant surgery received cyclosporine, azathioprine, and prednisone immunosuppression later developed symptoms of dementia as well as vitreous cells and retinal infiltrates in the left eye.[78] Magnetic resonance imaging (MRI) scan showed an orbital apical mass in the left eye with extension to the brain. Craniotomy with biopsy showed a probable lymphoma. At autopsy, she was found to have B-cell PCNSL in the left orbitofrontal cortex, hypothalamus, corpus striatum, mammillary body, and posterior lobe of the pituitary and PIOL involving the vitreous, retina, RPE, optic nerve, iris and ciliary body. Most of the NHLs and PCNSLs that develop in transplant patients are DLBCLs, but T cell PCNSLs have been described before. For example, the first case of T cell PCNSL in a renal transplant patient was described by Hacker and colleagues.[79] In this case, a 33-year-old female received a kidney transplant for end-stage renal failure due to renal dysplasia. She received azathioprine and prednisone and was found to have developed a T cell PCNSL at 51 years of age.

PCNSL in Congenital Immunodeficiency States. Those born with immunodeficiency states carry a 4% risk of developing PCNSL at a median age of 10 years.[80,81] Cerebral lymphomas can occur in diseases such as severe combined immunodeficiency[82] and Wiskott-Aldrich syndrome.[12,15,83]

PCNSL in Patients with Iatrogenic Immunosuppression. Conditions requiring immunosuppressant therapy for treatment have been reported to be associated with increased risk for developing PCNSL. Recently, a patient receiving mycophenolate mofetil for myasthenia gravis was reported to develop PCNSL after three years of treatment. After withdrawal of the immunosuppressant, the lymphoma regressed.[84]

Understanding the Rise in Incidence of PCNSL

The Changing Incidence in PCNSL and PIOL. Two factors that can account for part of the increasing incidence of PCNSL and PIOL are increasing awareness and recognition of these malignant processes. As ophthalmologists became increasingly aware of the existence of these malignancies (PCNSL not having been reported in the literature before 1929[85] and PIOL being reported during the 1950s and 1960s),[86,87] mounting reports evidenced the fact that cases that would have previously been diagnosed as simply uveitis were being properly diagnosed as PIOL.

An example of the increasing awareness and recognition of cancers in general is evidenced by the actions taken by the United States Congress in the 1970s.

United States Congress and Cancer. The prevention, diagnosis, and treatment of cancer has been an important goal of the United States government for over three decades. To this end, the National Cancer Act of 1971 (Public Law 92–218; 92nd Congress, S. 1828; December 23, 1971) was signed into law by United States President Richard Nixon. The Act was an amendment to the Public Health Service Act and was created specifically to enable the NCI to combat cancer. In Findings and Declaration of Purpose, Section 2 of the Act, the United States Congress recognizes not only the increasing incidence in cancer, but the far reaching effects the disease has on the citizens of the United States. The fact that cancer is a leading cause of death in the United States is also recognized by Congress with a desire for advancements in the arenas of prevention and therapy through scientific research and discovery. The Act mandates in Section 407 (a) that, "The Director of the National Cancer Institute shall coordinate all of the activities of the National Institutes of Health relating to cancer with the National Cancer Program." In addition, there are explicit mandates that efforts be expanded, intensified, and coordinated through a cancer program such that data and discoveries and advancements are disseminated in an expeditious manner for the purpose of improving cancer detection, treatment, and survival. In addition, collaborations between foreign researchers are encouraged, fostering benefits for people with cancer worldwide. The President of the United States is given power to select the three members that make up the President's Cancer Panel, two of whom must be scientists. The Cancer Act also calls for the establishment of a National Cancer Advisory Board within the National Cancer Institute (NCI). The President of the United States is charged with reviewing the administrative procedures of the National Cancer Program and reporting to Congress, "the findings of such review and the actions taken to facilitate the conduct of the Program, together with recommendations for any needed legislative changes." The mandates set forth by the Cancer Act of 1971 have helped seed the growing advancements in the realm of cancer research not only in the Unites States, but throughout the world.

The SEER Program. One of the myriad accomplishments brought forth by the NCI's new responsibilities and powers is the Surveillance, Epidemiology and End Results (SEER) report. This report is a compilation and profile of data concerning cancer, including the incidence, mortality, and survival data of the various cancers. Furthermore, the SEER program tracks the changes that occur in the incidence, mortality, and survival for each type of cancer. Non-profit medical-related organizations are contracted with the NCI's SEER program and these organization keep a "cancer information reporting system" that includes data such as cancer patients that are seen, diagnostic services that are performed, histologic reports of cancers, cancer sites, therapy, and patient demographics. Mortality data is recorded and population estimates are obtained from the United States Bureau of the Census. The result of collecting this data is that long-term trends in the incidence and mortality of various types of cancer can be identified. The SEER program initially tracked the incidence in cancer of eight United States geographic locations and later expanded to include 13 geographic locations within the United States.

Findings and Data Supporting the Increasing Incidence in PCNSL and PIOL. PCNSL was and still is a relatively rare malignancy. However, the rising incidence in some areas and outside the context of AIDS is cause for concern. The rising incidence in PCNSL and PIOL can be traced by the paths taken by others since the 1970s. For example, Freeman and colleagues examined 1467 cases of extranodal NHL obtained from the End Results Group of United States cancer registries at over 100 hospitals between the years 1950–1964[9] (recall the first account of intraocular lymphoma was in 1951,[86] which is described in Chapter 2). Twenty-three cases (1.57%) and 32 cases (2.18%) were lymphomas of the CNS (brain and spinal cord) and eye (eye and orbit), respectively. There were 23 cases (1.57%) of lymphomas occurring in another immunologically privileged organ, the testis. Whether the ocular lymphomas were primary intraocular or adnexal is not examined. In 1975, Jellinger and colleagues examined 80 cases of CNS lymphoma from a series of approximately 8000 intracranial tumors and found the incidence of CNS lymphoma to be 0.85%.[10] Zimmerman examined 7000 cases of intracranial tumors and found that 208 (3%) had a lymphoma. Evidence gathered over the past half century indicates the incidence of the malignancy is increasing.

Data Supporting the Increasing Incidence in PCNSL and PIOL. Eby and colleagues were the first to report on the increasing incidence of PCNSL.[12] Eby *et al.* turned to the National Cancer Institute's (NCI) Surveillance, Epidemiology, and End Results (SEER) Program's report covering the years 1973 through 1984[88] and the Third National Cancer Survey covering the years 1969 through 1971.[89] Though the SEER program data did not provide information on the immune status of PCNSL patients, Eby attempted to minimize the influence AIDS patients (an immunocompromised group at high risk for developing PCNSL) have on data concerning PCNSL rates by excluding never-married men. Previously, Daling and colleagues had described that, compared with men currently married or who have wed in the past, never-married men are a high risk group for harboring AIDS.[90] Eby *et al.* found that the age-adjusted rate per 10 million people in the United States was 2.7 for the years 1973 through 1975. The years 1976 through 1978 and years 1979 through 1981 saw an increase in incidence rates to 4.8 and 5.8 in 10 million population, respectively. The last time period studied by Eby and colleagues, 1982 through 1984, saw the incidence rate increased to 7.5 in 10 million, an almost three-fold rise over a decade. The Chi-square trend was 15.25 and this increase was statistically significant (P value < 0.001). The incidence rates for both men and women increased over the same time periods. The time period 1973 to 1975 saw an incidence rate of 1.8 in 10 million and 3.5 in 10 million for men and women, respectively. The last time period studied, years 1982 through 1984, saw an incidence rate of 6.5 in 10 million for men and 8.9 in 10 million for women.

Certainly improvements and advancements in diagnostic techniques can account for increases in the incidence of certain diseases, and Eby's group conceded that this could be the case with PCNSL. Also, one must remember that PCNSL was not always known to be a lymphomatous process. Indeed, in Chapter 3 on "Classification of Lymphoma," the change in the nomenclature of PCNSL was explored. Aside from being known as a reticulum cell sarcoma, lymphoma of the brain was also known as microglioma.[91] Eby *et al.* attempted to follow the trends for microgliomas in addition to the PCNSL finding for both synonymous diseases that the incidence rate per million population increased over the first three time periods examined (1973 through 1975, 1976 through 1978, and 1979 through 1981). Microgliomas showed a statistically significant increase in incidence from 3.8 in 10 million population during the 1973 through 1975 time period, to 8.5 in 10 million during the 1982 through 1984 time period. The period of 1982 through 1984 saw a decrease in incidence rate of microglioma to zero in 10 million population, reflecting the change in nomenclature resultant from the developing cognizance of the lymphomatous nature of the malignancy. When Eby combined the incidence of brain lymphoma with microglioma (including earlier data covering the period 1969 through 1971 from the Third National Cancer Survey) there was an increased incidence. Eby was curious to see if other immunologically privileged organs also showed similar increases in incidence rates. Interestingly, neither eye nor testis showed an increased incidence over the time periods examined.[12]

Fine and Mayer performed a retrospective analysis of the literature describing cases of PCNSL reported between January 1980 and September 1992, finding 40 series of PCNSL occurring in patients without AIDS and 32 series of PCNSL that had developed in AIDS patients.[26] The two researchers found that the immunodeficient state brought about by AIDS was the major contributor to the rise in incidence rates of PCNSL in immunocompromised patients. Both Fine and Mayer also found that the incidence rate for those with immunocompetency increased as well, but for an unknown reason. The male to female ratio in immunocompetent patients was found to be 1.35:1, while in AIDS patients this ratio showed an overwhelmingly male predilection, 7.38:1.

Fine and Mayer pointed out that the work of Eby and colleagues[12] had excluded never-married men as a means of excluding AIDS patients.[26] However, as Fine notes, men who have been married, in addition to women and children, can have the disease and that it is not exclusive to any lifestyle. Thus, one must assume that there are indeed some AIDS patients still left in Eby's data even after exclusion of never-married men. Oleson and colleagues also brought up the point that AIDS patients can be attempted to be controlled for in the numerator of calculations made in the determination of the incidence rates, but it is impossible to exclude these patients from the denominator, which represent the total population.[14] Thus, the incidence rates might actually be higher than determined in the supposedly immuno-competent populations. Of course, Eby and colleagues desire to exclude AIDS patients makes sense when one considers differences in the pathobiology of the disease between AIDS and immunocompetent patients. This difference is the Epstein Barr virus (EBV), which will be discussed in detail in Chapters 7 and 8. Instead of using the SEER data, Fine and Mayer performed a MEDLINE database search of articles on PCNSL printed in English between January 1980 and September 1992 and then searched the same database for the literature with the terms, "AIDS," "human immunodeficiency virus (HIV)," "lymphoma," and "central nervous system." By performing these searches, Fine was able to identify 792 non-AIDS patients with PCNSL and 315 AIDS patients with the malignancy. Both Eby *et al.* and Fine and Mayer recognized that improved diagnostics (e.g. the introduction of MRI) and increased screening, recognition, and awareness could account for the increased incidence. However, Eby *et al.* followed the incidence of microgliomas, another primary brain tumor that is diagnosed in much the same was as PCNSL.[12] Interestingly, Eby *et al.* found that the incidence of microgliomas had not increased even after the introduction of the MRI. In addition, the increased incidence of PCNSL had already started to occur prior to the common utilization of MRI scanning for brain lesions. Fine and Mayer supported the reasoning that improved diagnostics could be the explanation for the increased incidence by noting that over the mid-1980s to mid-1990s there was a higher percentage of PCNSLs identified in resected or biopsied CNS malignancy specimens.[26] Perhaps the increased incidence of PCNSL was due to a similar increase in NHLs in general. Eby *et al.* found that although the incidence of NHLs had increased since the SEER program had started, it had actually leveled off during the early to mid-1980s. However, this was not the case for PCNSLs.

Corn *et al.* and colleagues also turned to the SEER program's data to analyze the attributes of the increased incidence of PCNSL.[13] Their analysis was performed in much the same way as Eby and colleagues.[12] Corn reported the incidence rates for NHLs, all gliomas, glioblastoma, and PCNSL from the SEER data during the time period 1973 through 1992. Like Eby and colleagues, Corn *et al.* analyzed the incidence rates for patients with never-married men excluded and for all patients (with never-married men included). The trends in the age-adjusted crude incidence rates for PCNL in the two groups; the group with exclusion of never-married males; and the group with inclusion of never-married males, showed that the incidence rate was still increasing since the report by Eby *et al.* in 1988. For the group with inclusion of never-married males, the incidence rate in patients below 60 years of age was 1.7 per 10 million population, and in those over 60 years of age it was 7.3 per 10 million in population for the period 1973–1975. The period 1991–1993 saw the incidence rate increased to 16.9 in 10 million and 100.9 in 10 million for those under 60 years and those over 60 years, respectively. With the inclusion of never-married men, the incidence rates started at 1.9 and 8.5 in 10 million for those less than 60 years and those greater than 60 years, respectively. By 1993, the incidence rates had increased to 59.6 (for patients less than 60 years of age) and 103.6 (for those over the age of 60 years) in 10 million population. Corn and colleagues showed their findings graphically for PCNSL with non-PCNSL NHLs, gliomas, and glioblastoma. PCNSL certainly showed a lesser incidence rate for all periods of time than the other three tumors analyzed, but the rate of increase in incidence was greater than that for non-PCNSL NHLs. While Fine and Mayer and Eby *et al.* recognized that advancements in imaging of intracranial lesions and screening had been made that might explain in part the rise in incidence, Corn and colleagues also mentioned that perhaps the incidence of the disease would have been underestimated, at least in AIDS patients. The reason for this is due to a disinclination of surgeons to biopsy AIDS patients with brain masses.[92] Since the diagnosis of PCNSL is based on histopathology (i.e. tissue must show evidence of a lymphomatous process), the lack of biopsies in AIDS patients could certainly leave many cases of PCNSL in this population underdiagnosed. In addition, after extrapolation to the year 2000, PCNSL showed no decline or leveling off. The trends for other tumors, including non-PCNSL NHLs, gliomas, and glioblastomas showed a modest increase in incidence. The rate of diagnosis for PCNSL had also increased over the interval of time analyzed.

The Role of Infectious Agents in PCNSL and PIOL. Investigators have suggested a role involving oncogenic viral infections. Though infectious agents could potentially play a role in causing PCNSL in immunocompetent patients, no definitive association has been made. EBV has been associated with Burkitt's lymphoma and PCNSL.[22,93,94] Intriguingly, Corboy *et al.* found that DNA of the human herpes virus 8 (HHV-8), an infectious agent associated with Kaposi's sarcoma, primary effusion lymphomas, Castleman's disease, and multiple myeloma, was detected in the 56% of PCNSLs from 36 patients with and without AIDS.[95] Unlike the lymphomatous cells, the surrounding normal brain tissue was negative for the viral DNA. Others have described findings of infectious agents in PCNSLs, including PIOLs, occurring in non-AIDS patients. Chan and colleagues from the National Eye Institute (NEI) discovered that in four ocular samples of PIOL cells of 13 examined, there was DNA from HHV-8; among these specimens only one from a patient with AIDS contained EBV DNA.[96] Later, Shen and colleagues reported that two ocular specimens of 10 PIOL immunocompetent patients contained *Toxoplasma gondii* DNA.[97] Though these findings in immunocompetent patients are captivating, there has been no definitive link of infectious agents causing PCNSLs or PIOLs in this population.

Other infectious agents may be associated with other ocular lymphomatous processes. For example, some extranodal marginal zone lymphomas of mucosa-associated lymphoid tissue (MALT), specifically gastric MALTs (arising from the major causative agent in gastric ulcers) have been found to arise due to infection by the bacterium *Helicobacter pylori*.[98,99] Indeed, *Helicobacter pylori* DNA is found in conjuncitval MALT lymphoma.[100] Currently, 15% of NHLs in patients infected with HIV are PCNSLs, while this malignancy makes up 1% of NHLs in immunocompetent patients. Certainly in AIDS patients, latent EBV infection is associated with the development of PCNSL and PIOL.[26] However, as noted previously, the use of HAART may have the potential to affect what genotypic subtype of PCNSL and PIOL develops within the AIDS patients. As HAART decreases the ability of opportunistic infections to cause disease in AIDS patients and as this important therapy is able to maintain a B and T cell milieu that is more similar to an immunocompetent patient, we may find that a shift from ABC DLBCL toward GCB DLBCL type PCNSLs occurs. This is important because as we direct therapy towards PCNSLs and PIOLs, targeting the genes or gene products that are expressed in genotypic subtypes of CNS lymphomas will more specifically eradicate the disease.

References

1. Shah GD, DeAngelis LM. (2005) Treatment of primary central nervous system lymphoma. *Hematol Oncol Clin North Am* **19**(4): 611–627.
2. Cote TR, Biggar RJ, Rosenberg PS, *et al.* (1997) Non-Hodgkin's lymphoma among people with AIDS: incidence, presentation and public health burden. AIDS/Cancer Study Group. *Int J Cancer* **73**(5): 645–650.

3. Cote TR, Manns A, Hardy CR, *et al.* (1996) Epidemiology of brain lymphoma among people with or without acquired immunodeficiency syndrome. AIDS/Cancer Study Group. *J Natl Cancer Inst* **88**(10): 675–679.
4. Miller DC, Hochberg FH, Harris NL, *et al.* (1994) Pathology with clinical correlations of primary central nervous system non-Hodgkin's lymphoma. The Massachusetts General Hospital experience 1958–1989. *Cancer* **74**(4): 1383–1397.
5. DeAngelis LM. (1991) Primary central nervous system lymphoma: a new clinical challenge. *Neurology* **41**(5): 619–621.
6. Davis FG, Kupelian V, Freels S, *et al.* (2001) Prevalence estimates for primary brain tumors in the United States by behavior and major histology groups. *Neuro-oncol* **3**(3): 152–158.
7. Surawicz TS, McCarthy BJ, Kupelian V, *et al.* (1999) Descriptive epidemiology of primary brain and CNS tumors: results from the Central Brain Tumor Registry of the United States, 1990–1994. *Neuro-oncol* **1**(1): 14–25.
8. Behin A, Hoang-Xuan K, Carpentier AF, Delattre JY. (2003) Primary brain tumours in adults. *Lancet* **361**(9354): 323–331.
9. Freeman C, Berg JW, Cutler SJ. (1972) Occurrence and prognosis of extranodal lymphomas. *Cancer* **29**(1): 252–260.
10. Jellinger K, Radaskiewicz TH, Slowik F. (1975) Primary malignant lymphomas of the central nervous system in man. *Acta Neuropathol Suppl (Berl)* **Suppl 6**: 95–102.
11. Zimmerman HM. (1975) Malignant lymphomas of the nervous system. *Acta Neuropathol Suppl (Berl)* **Suppl 6**: 69–74.
12. Eby NL, Grufferman S, Flannelly CM, *et al.* (1988) Increasing incidence of primary brain lymphoma in the US. *Cancer* **62**(11): 2461–2465.
13. Corn BW, Marcus SM, Topham A, *et al.* (1997) Will primary central nervous system lymphoma be the most frequent brain tumor diagnosed in the year 2000? *Cancer* **79**(12): 2409–2413.
14. Oleson JE, Janney CA, Rao RD, *et al.* (2002) The continuing increase in the incidence of primary central nervous system non-Hodgkin lymphoma: a surveillance, epidemiology, and end results analysis. *Cancer* **95**(7): 1504–1510.
15. Schabet M. (1999) Epidemiology of primary CNS lymphoma. *J Neurooncol* **43**(3): 199–201.
16. Baehring JM, Androudi S, Longtine JJ, *et al.* (2005) Analysis of clonal immunoglobulin heavy chain rearrangements in ocular lymphoma. *Cancer* **104**(3): 591–597.
17. Chan CC. (2003) Molecular pathology of primary intraocular lymphoma. *Trans Am Ophthalmol Soc* **101**: 275–292.

18. Char DH, Ljung BM, Miller T, Phillips T. (1988) Primary intraocular lymphoma (ocular reticulum cell sarcoma) diagnosis and management. *Ophthalmology* **95**: 625–630.
19. Char DH, Margolis L, Newman AB. (1981) Ocular reticulum cell sarcoma. *Am J Ophthalmol* **91**(4): 480–483.
20. Rockwood EJ, Zakov ZN, Bay JW. (1984) Combined malignant lymphoma of the eye and CNS (reticulum-cell sarcoma). *J Neurosurg* **61**: 369–374.
21. Chan CC, Buggage RR, Nussenblatt RB. (2002) Intraocular lymphoma. *Curr Opin Ophthalmol* **13**(6): 411–418.
22. Hochberg FH, Miller DC. (1988) Primary central nervous system lymphoma. *J Neurosurg* **68**(6): 835–853.
23. Buggage RR, Chan CC, Nussenblatt RB. (2001) Ocular manifestations of central nervous system lymphoma. *Curr Opin Oncol* **13**(3): 137–142.
24. Bataille B, Delwail V, Menet E, *et al.* (2000) Primary intracerebral malignant lymphoma: report of 248 cases. *J Neurosurg* **92**(2): 261–266.
25. Abrey LE, DeAngelis LM, Yahalom J. (1998) Long-term survival in primary CNS lymphoma. *J Clin Oncol* **16**(3): 859–863.
26. Fine HA, Mayer RJ. (1993) Primary central nervous system lymphoma. *Ann Intern Med* **119**(11): 1093–1104.
27. Sarkar C, Sharma MC, Deb P, *et al.* (2005) Primary central nervous system lymphoma — a hospital based study of incidence and clinicopathological features from India (1980–2003). *J Neurooncol* **71**(2): 199–204.
28. Yamanaka R, Morii K, Shinbo Y, *et al.* (2005) Modified ProMACE-MOPP hybrid regimen with moderate-dose methotrexate for patients with primary CNS lymphoma. *Ann Hematol* **84**(7): 447–455.
29. Hayakawa T, Takakura K, Abe H, *et al.* (1994) Primary central nervous system lymphoma in Japan — a retrospective, co-operative study by CNS-Lymphoma Study Group in Japan. *J Neurooncol* **19**(3): 197–215.
30. Cassoux N, Merle-Beral H, Leblond V, *et al.* (2000) Ocular and central nervous system lymphoma: clinical features and diagnosis. *Ocul Immunol Inflamm* **8**(4): 243–250.
31. Mikata A. (1981) A new histological classification of malignant lymphomas (LSG classification) and its significance. *Nippon Ketsueki Gakkai Zasshi* **44**(7): 1401–1410.
32. Shibamoto Y, Tsuchida E, Seki K, *et al.* (2004) Primary central nervous system lymphoma in Japan 1995–1999: changes from the preceding 10 years. *J Cancer Res Clin Oncol* **130**(6): 351–356.
33. Kuratsu J, Takeshima H, Ushio Y. (2001) Trends in the incidence of primary intracranial tumors in Kumamoto, Japan. *Int J Clin Oncol* **6**(4): 183–191.

34. Hayabuchi N, Shibamoto Y, Onizuka Y. (1999) Primary central nervous system lymphoma in Japan: a nationwide survey. *Int J Radiat Oncol Biol Phys* **44**(2): 265–272.

35. Ferreri AJ, Reni M, Villa E. (1995) Primary central nervous system lymphoma in immunocompetent patients. *Cancer Treat Rev* **21**(5): 415–446.

36. Suh YL, Koo H, Kim TS, *et al.* (2002) Tumors of the central nervous system in Korea: a multicenter study of 3221 cases. *J Neurooncol* **56**(3): 251–259.

37. Hao D, DiFrancesco LM, Brasher PM, *et al.* (1999) Is primary CNS lymphoma really becoming more common? A population-based study of incidence, clinicopathological features and outcomes in Alberta from 1975 to 1996. *Ann Oncol* **10**(1): 65–70.

38. Yau YH, O'Sullivan MG, Signorini D, *et al.* (1996) Primary lymphoma of central nervous system in immunocompetent patients in south-east Scotland. *Lancet* **348**(9031): 890.

39. Freeman LN, Schachat AP, Knox DL, *et al.* (1987) Clinical features, laboratory investigations, and survival in ocular reticulum cell sarcoma. *Ophthalmology* **94**: 1631–1639.

40. Whitcup SM, de Smet MD, Rubin BI, *et al.* (1993) Intraocular lymphoma. Clinical and histopathologic diagnosis. *Ophthalmology* **100**: 1399–1406.

41. Peterson K, Gordon KB, Heinemann MH, DeAngelis LM. (1993) The clinical spectrum of ocular lymphoma. *Cancer* **72**(3): 843–849.

42. Akpek EK, Ahmed I, Hochberg FH, *et al.* (1999) Intraocular-central nervous system lymphoma: clinical features, diagnosis, and outcomes. *Ophthalmology* **106**(9): 1805–1810.

43. Zaldivar RA, Martin DF, Holden JT, Grossniklaus HE. (2004) Primary intraocular lymphoma: clinical, cytologic, and flow cytometric analysis. *Ophthalmology* **111**(9): 1762–1767.

44. Hormigo A, Abrey L, Heinemann MH, DeAngelis LM. (2004) Ocular presentation of primary central nervous system lymphoma: diagnosis and treatment. *Br J Haematol* **126**(2): 202–208.

45. Forsyth PA, DeAngelis LM. (1996) Biology and management of AIDS-associated primary CNS lymphomas. *Hematol Oncol Clin North Am* **10**(5): 1125–1134.

46. Otieno MW, Banura C, Katongole-Mbidde E, *et al.* (2002) Therapeutic challenges of AIDS-related non-Hodgkin's lymphoma in the United States and East Africa. *J Natl Cancer Inst* **94**(10): 718–732.

47. Basso U, Brandes AA. (2002) Diagnostic advances and new trends for the treatment of primary central nervous system lymphoma. *Eur J Cancer* **38**(10): 1298–1312.

48. Herrlinger U. (1999) Primary CNS lymphoma: findings outside the brain. *J Neurooncol* **43**(3): 227–230.
49. (1986) Classification system for human T-lymphotropic virus type III/lymphadenopathy-associated virus infections. *MMWR Morb Mortal Wkly Rep* **35**(20): 334–339.
50. Biggar RJ, Rabkin CS. (1992) The epidemiology of acquired immunodeficiency syndrome-related lymphomas. *Curr Opin Oncol* **4**(5): 883–893.
51. Serraino D, Franceschi S, Tirelli U, Monfardini S. (1992) The epidemiology of acquired immunodeficiency syndrome and associated tumours in Europe. *Ann Oncol* **3**(8): 595–603.
52. Anders KH, Guerra WF, Tomiyasu U, *et al.* (1986) The neuropathology of AIDS. UCLA experience and review. *Am J Pathol* **124**(3): 537–558.
53. Levy RM, Bredesen DE, Rosenblum ML. (1985) Neurological manifestations of the acquired immunodeficiency syndrome (AIDS): experience at UCSF and review of the literature. *J Neurosurg* **62**(4): 475–495.
54. Morgello S, Petito CK, Mouradian JA. (1990) Central nervous system lymphoma in the acquired immunodeficiency syndrome. *Clin Neuropathol* **9**(4): 205–215.
55. Welch K, Finkbeiner W, Alpers CE, *et al.* (1984) Autopsy findings in the acquired immune deficiency syndrome. *Jama* **252**(9): 1152–1159.
56. Wolf T, Brodt HR, Fichtlscherer S, *et al.* (2005) Changing incidence and prognostic factors of survival in AIDS-related non-Hodgkin's lymphoma in the era of highly active antiretroviral therapy (HAART). *Leuk Lymphoma* **46**(2): 207–215.
57. Formenti SC, Gill PS, Lean E, *et al.* (1989) Primary central nervous system lymphoma in AIDS. Results of radiation therapy. *Cancer* **63**(6): 1101–1107.
58. Levy RM, Janssen RS, Bush TJ, Rosenblum ML. (1988) Neuroepidemiology of acquired immunodeficiency syndrome. *J Acquir Immune Defic Syndr* **1**(1): 31–40.
59. Ling SM, Roach M, 3rd, Larson DA, Wara WM. (1994) Radiotherapy of primary central nervous system lymphoma in patients with and without human immunodeficiency virus. Ten years of treatment experience at the University of California San Francisco. *Cancer* **73**(10): 2570–2582.
60. MacMahon EM, Glass JD, Hayward SD, *et al.* (1991) Epstein-Barr virus in AIDS-related primary central nervous system lymphoma. *Lancet* **338**(8773): 969–973.
61. Rosenblum ML, Levy RM, Bredesen DE, *et al.* (1988) Primary central nervous system lymphomas in patients with AIDS. *Ann Neurol* **23 Suppl:** S13–16.

62. Baumgartner JE, Rachlin JR, Beckstead JH, *et al.* (1990) Primary central nervous system lymphomas: natural history and response to radiation therapy in 55 patients with acquired immunodeficiency syndrome. *J Neurosurg* 73(2): 206–211.
63. Goplen AK, Dunlop O, Liestol K, *et al.* (1997) The impact of primary central nervous system lymphoma in AIDS patients: a population-based autopsy study from Oslo. *J Acquir Immune Defic Syndr Hum Retrovirol* 14(4): 351–354.
64. Goedert JJ. (2000) The epidemiology of acquired immunodeficiency syndrome malignancies. *Semin Oncol* 27(4): 390–401.
65. (2000) Highly active antiretroviral therapy and incidence of cancer in human immunodeficiency virus-infected adults. *J Natl Cancer Inst* 92(22): 1823–1830.
66. Sacktor N. (2002) The epidemiology of human immunodeficiency virus-associated neurological disease in the era of highly active antiretroviral therapy. *J Neurovirol* 8 Suppl 2: 115–121.
67. Gebo KA, Fleishman JA, Moore RD. (2005) Hospitalizations for metabolic conditions, opportunistic infections, and injection drug use among HIV patients: trends between 1996 and 2000 in 12 states. *J Acquir Immune Defic Syndr* 40(5): 609–616.
68. Autran B. (1999) Effects of antiretroviral therapy on immune reconstitution. *Antivir Ther* 4 Suppl 3: 3–6.
69. (2004) Introduction of routine HIV testing in prenatal care — Botswana, 2004. *MMWR Morb Mortal Wkly Rep* 53(46): 1083–1086.
70. Levine AM. (1994) Lymphoma complicating immunodeficiency disorders. *Ann Oncol* 5 Suppl 2: 29–35.
71. Paulus W, Jellinger K, Hallas C, *et al.* (1993) Human herpesvirus-6 and Epstein-Barr virus genome in primary cerebral lymphomas. *Neurology* 43(8): 1591–1593.
72. Schiff D, Suman VJ, Yang P, *et al.* (1998) Risk factors for primary central nervous system lymphoma: a case-control study. *Cancer* 82(5): 975–982.
73. Penn I. (1983) Lymphomas complicating organ transplantation. *Transplant Proc* 15(4, Suppl. 1): 2790–2797.
74. Boubenider S, Hiesse C, Goupy C, *et al.* (1997) Incidence and consequences of post-transplantation lymphoproliferative disorders. *J Nephrol* 10(3): 136–145.
75. Gentil MA, Gonzalez-Roncero F, Cantarell C, *et al.* (2005) Effect of new immunosuppressive regimens on cost of renal transplant maintenance immunosuppression. *Transplant Proc* 37(3): 1441–1442.
76. Penn I. (1993) Incidence and treatment of neoplasia after transplantation. *J Heart Lung Transplant* 12(6 Pt 2): S328–336.

77. Penn I. (1996) Posttransplantation de novo tumors in liver allograft recipients. *Liver Transpl Surg* 2(1): 52–59.
78. Johnson BL. (1992) Intraocular and central nervous system lymphoma in a cardiac transplant recipient. *Ophthalmology* 99(6): 987–992.
79. Hacker SM, Knight BP, Lunde NM, *et al.* (1992) A primary central nervous system T cell lymphoma in a renal transplant patient. *Transplantation* 53(3): 691–692.
80. Filipovich AH, Heinitz KJ, Robison LL, Frizzera G. (1987) The Immunodeficiency Cancer Registry. A research resource. *Am J Pediatr Hematol Oncol* 9(2): 183–184.
81. Perry GS, 3rd, Spector BD, Schuman LM, *et al.* (1980) The Wiskott-Aldrich syndrome in the United States and Canada (1892–1979). *J Pediatr* 97(1): 72–78.
82. Kaufman DA, Hershfield MS, Bocchini JA, *et al.* (2005) Cerebral lymphoma in an adenosine deaminase-deficient patient with severe combined immunodeficiency receiving polyethylene glycol-conjugated adenosine deaminase. *Pediatrics.*
83. Heidelberger KP, LeGolvan DP. (1974) Wiskott-Aldrich syndrome and cerebral neoplasia: report of a case with localized reticulum cell sarcoma. *Cancer* 33(1): 280–284.
84. Vernino S, Salomao DR, Habermann TM, O'Neill BP. (2005) Primary CNS lymphoma complicating treatment of myasthenia gravis with mycophenolate mofetil. *Neurology* 65(4): 639–641.
85. Bailey P. (1929) Intracranial sarcomatous tumors of leptomeningeal origin. *Arch Surg* 18: 1359–1402.
86. Cooper EL, Ricker JL. (1951) Malignant lymphoma of the uveal tract. *Am J Ophthalmol* 34: 1153–1158.
87. Vogel MH, Font RL, Zimmerman LE, Levine RA. (1968) Reticulum cell sarcoma of the retina and uvea. Report of six cases and review of the literature. *Am J Ophthalmol* 66(2): 205–215.
88. (1981) Surveillance, epidemiology, and end results: incidence and mortality data, 1973–77. *Natl Cancer Inst Monogr* (57): 1–1082.
89. (1975) Third national cancer survey: incidence data. *Natl Cancer Inst Monogr* (41): I–x, 1–454.
90. Daling JR, Weiss NS, Klopfenstein LL, *et al.* (1982) Correlates of homosexual behavior and the incidence of anal cancer. *Jama* 247(14): 1988–1990.
91. Russell DS, Marshall AHE, Smith FB. (1948) Microgliomatosis. *Brain* 71: 1–15.
92. Corn BW, Trock BJ, Curran WJ, Jr. (1995) Management of primary central nervous system lymphoma for the patient with acquired immunodeficiency syndrome. Confronting a clinical catch-22. *Cancer* 76(2): 163–166.

93. Burkitt DP. (1983) The discovery of Burkitt's lymphoma. *Cancer* **51**(10): 1777–1786.

94. Tao Q, Robertson KD, Manns A, *et al.* (1998) Epstein-Barr virus (EBV) in endemic Burkitt's lymphoma: molecular analysis of primary tumor tissue (published erratum appears in *Blood* 1998 Apr 15; 91(8):3091). *Blood* **91**(4): 1373–1381.

95. Corboy JR, Garl PJ, Kleinschmidt-DeMasters BK. (1998) Human herpesvirus 8 DNA in CNS lymphomas from patients with and without AIDS (see comments). *Neurology* **50**(2): 335–340.

96. Chan CC, Shen DF, Whitcup SM, Nussenblatt RB, *et al.* (1999) Detection of human herpesvirus-8 and Epstein-Barr virus DNA in primary intraocular lymphoma. *Blood* **93**(8): 2749–2751.

97. Shen DF, Herbort CP, Tuaillon N, *et al.* (2001) Detection of toxoplasma gondii DNA in primary intraocular b-cell lymphoma. *Mod Pathol* **14**(10): 995–999.

98. Sung JJ, Chung SC, Ling TK, *et al.* (1995) Antibacterial treatment of gastric ulcers associated with Helicobacter pylori. *N Engl J Med* **332**(3): 139–142.

99. Veldhuyzen van Zanten SJ, Sherman PM. (1994) Helicobacter pylori infection as a cause of gastritis, duodenal ulcer, gastric cancer and nonulcer dyspepsia: a systematic overview. *Can Med Assoc J* **150**(2): 177–185.

100. Chan CC, Smith JA, Shen DF, *et al.* (2004) *Helicobacter pylori* (*H. pylori*) molecular signature in conjunctival mucosa-associated lymphoid tissue (MALT) lymphoma. *Histol Histopathol* **19**(4): 1219–1226.

Chapter 5

Clinical Manifestations of PIOL

Historical Account

The clinical manifestations of reticulum cell sarcoma (now known as PIOL) often resemble that of uveitis and, occasionally, infectious ocular diseases. Thus, PIOL is a masquerade syndrome.

By 1988 nearly 100 cases of intraocular reticulum cell sarcoma (PIOL) had been reported in the literature. It was in the late 1980s that most of the literature recognized the lymphomatous origin of this ocular malignancy.

First Cases of Lymphoma in the Eye. The first patient with intraocular lymphoma (though most likely to be a systemic metastasis to the eye) to be reported in the literature[1] showed ocular symptoms before the systemic disease was discovered. What brought this rather young (27 years of age) gentleman to his ophthalmologist (prior to being referred to Cooper and Ricker) were complaints of ocular pain and blurred vision in the right eye (Table 5.1). Not unusual even today, the patient was diagnosed initially with iritis and was prescribed corticosteroid treatment. When he was referred to Cooper and Ricker, visual acuity in the right eye was good, being 20/25. A mild ciliary flush was noted, and slit lamp biomicroscopy revealed mutton fat keratic precipitates. In addition, the iris stroma was thickened with engorged vessels. Fundus examination revealed an edematous optic nerve head and surrounding retina. Periphlebitis and engorged retinal veins also characterized the fundus examination. The retina exhibited retinal hemorrhages. Topical and systemic corticosteroid therapy for presumed uveitis was instituted, and, as is all too commonly the case with even modern descriptions of PIOL, the inflammation exhibited by the patient's right eye was refractory to treatment.

Table 5.1 The First Cases of PIOL

Author	Year	Patient Information	Initial Complaints	Other Complaints	Oucular Examinations							
					Slit Lamp				Dilated Fundus			
					Cornea	Anterior Chamber	Iris	Lens	Vitreous	Retina	Optic Nerve	
Cooper & Ricker	1951	27-year-old male	Pain and blurred VA[6] right eye. VA measured as 20/25 Later VA right eye became hand motion	3 years earlier, swollen lymph nodes of groin; 2 years earlier jaundice, headaches, decrease in weight by 19 pounds Six months later right testicle became swollen to size of a peach, liver and spleen became palpable	Mild ciliary flush	Keratic precipitates IOP right eye, 50 mHG AC became more shallow as iris became thicker IOP eventually became subnormal	Iris OD[4] eventually became thickened and posterior synechiae developed Large nodules (3–4 mm in diameter), also developed in the iris; these nodules grew larger and then became smaller	Not stated	Free of hemorrhage	Numerous retinal hemorrhages throughout fundus Retinal veins engorged with preiphlebitic changes	Edema of optic nerve head	

(Continued)

Table 5.1 (*Continued*)

Author	Year	Patient Information	Initial Complaints	Other Complaints	Ocular Examinations								
					Slit Lamp					Dilated Fundus			
					Cornea	Anterior Chamber	Iris	Lens	Vitreous	Retina	Optic Nerve		
Currey & Deutsch	1965	50-year-old African-American male	Pain, redness, loss of vision OS[5] × 3 months	Not stated	Not stated	Not stated	Rubeosis iridis	Dense, cloudy lens	Not stated	No view of fundus due to lens	Not stated		
Vogel	1968	67-year-old Caucasian male	Not stated	Not stated	Not stated	Not stated	Ciliary body and iris infiltrated by RCS[1]	Not stated	Not stated	Retina infiltrated by RCS	Not stated		
Nevins	1968	64-year-old Caucasian female	Blurred and decreased vision	Patient suffered from nocardiosis prior to death	WNL[2]	WNL	WNL	Minimal nuclear sclerosis OU[3]	Vitreous stranding OU	Posterior chronic non-granulomatous uveitis OU RCS right eye of choroid and subretina	RCS infiltration		

[1]RCS = reticulum cell sarcoma; [2]WNL = within normal limits; [3]OU = both eyes; [4]OD = right eye; [5]OS = left eye; [6]VA = visual acuity.

Currey and Deutsch described a middle-aged patient of 50 years who presented with a painful and red left eye that had a decline in vision to the point of being noted as "blind" (Table 5.1).[2] Slit lamp examination revealed many keratic precipitates and anterior chamber flare. Rubeosis iridis was also noted, and funduscopic examination was difficult to perform due to a dense cataract. Treatment with atropine, hydrocortisone and antibiotic ointment, and a carbonic anhydrase inhibitor was initiated, but the eye was intractable to such treatment. For this reason, the left eye was enucleated and submitted for pathologic inspection. The tissues surrounding the cornea exhibited infiltration by lymphocytes, and the cornea showed some lymphocytes within the stroma. The iris, ciliary body, pars plana and choroid all showed thickening on gross examination. Microscopic examination revealed that the trabecular meshwork and canal of Schlemm, iris and ciliary body were densely infiltrated with lymphocytic cells. (Intraocular pressure prior to enucleation had been described as being 60 mm of Hg.) The retina exhibited some degeneration of the rod and cone processes as well as the outer nuclear layer, but no lymphocytic infiltrate. The choroid, however, was thickened by a cellular infiltrate. These cells also filled the lumen of the choroidal vessels. Fibrotic areas with obliterated choriocapillaris and necrosis of the RPE were revealed. The lamina cribrosa was infiltrated by the neoplastic cells as well. The diagnosis of reticulum cell sarcoma of the uveal tract and optic nerve was made. As we know, uveal infiltration by neoplastic lymphocytes is the characteristic of a systemic metastasis to the intraocular tissues,[3] whereas PIOL characteristically localizes between the sub-RPE and Bruch's membrane.[4,5]

Could this patient have harbored a systemic lymphoma that metastasized to the eye? Currey and Deutsch noted on the basis of clinical examination as well as X-ray series that this patient did not seem to have a systemic lymphoma; CT and MRI were not available at that time. The patient was apparently alive and well without any evidence of recurrence 11 months post-operation. However, a case presented just one year earlier to Currey and Deutsch's description made it evident that a malignant lymphoma of the uveal tract could precede the discovery of a systemic lymphoma.[6] Interestingly, Nevins provided some follow-up information on Currey and Deutsch's patient.[7] He arrived at a hospital dead two years after enucleation. Unfortunately, no autopsy was performed, so it is unknown what the exact cause of death was in the case of this patient.

First Cases of PCNSL with PIOL. As more cases of true PIOL were described in the literature, a characteristic clinical picture of the disease began to develop. Vogel and colleagues from the Armed Forces Institute of Pathology (AFIP) in Washington, D.C., described six cases of patients with eye, brain, or bifocal reticulum cell sarcoma. These patients complained of changes in vision, notably blurred and declining vision.[8] Ophthalmic examination was reminiscent of uveitic processes: some patients were noted to exhibit keratic precipitates and anterior chamber cell and flare; others had retinal hemorrhages. One of Vogel's patients, a 67-year-old Caucasian male, initially had lymphomatous infiltration in the left eye, but later the right eye also developed it. The clinical diagnosis in the left eye was uveitis with secondary glaucoma in addition to malignant melanoma of the ciliary body, while the right eye carried a diagnosis of absolute glaucoma. Pathologic inspection of both enucleated eyes revealed lymphomatous infiltration of the retinas, choroids, ciliary bodies, and irides. When the patient died three years after his initial ocular symptoms, an autopsy revealed that there was a reticulum cell sarcoma of the brain; only the left cerebral hemisphere was affected by the malignancy.

Another of Vogel and colleagues' patients, a 71-year-old Caucasian female, presented with a blind and painful right eye for one year. Slit lamp examination revealed pericorneal injection of a steamy cornea. Visual acuity was questionable light perception. The only finding in the fellow eye was a cataract. The right eye was enucleated and upon microscopic examination, anterior chamber chronic inflammatory cells as well as blood were noted. Many plasma cells and lymphocytes were seen throughout the iris and ciliary body. The vitreous, too, contained many inflammatory cells. The retina was thickened, both focally and diffusely by a neoplastic mononuclear cell infiltrate; some cells were characterized by small fusiform nuclei and others exhibited large hyperchromatic nuclei. The diagnosis given was reticulum cell sarcoma of the retina as well as a diffuse chronic nongranulomatous uveitis.

Nevins and colleagues[7] reported a patient with a primary intraocular reticulum cell sarcoma in 1968. The patient was a 64-year-old Caucasian female who had complained of 18 months of visual problems initiated by blurriness. Her visual acuity was initially recorded as 20/25 and 20/20 in the right and left eyes, respectively, with correction. In 10 months, her vision had declined to hand motion (HM) OD and 20/30 OS. There was a vitreous hemorrhage in the right eye. Her vision continued to decrease, and nearly a year later, her right eye was light perception (LP) and her vision in the left eye had deteriorated to 20/200. There is no mention about the clinical features of this patient prior to her visit to Nevins and colleagues. However, she was put on a regimen of 40 mg of prednisone daily, which seemed to have improved her vision in the left eye to 20/60; the right eye remained LP. Slit lamp examination at this time revealed a distinct absence of any anterior segment inflammation; there were no anterior cell or flare and no keratic precipitates. However, funduscopic examination was more revealing. The vitreous contained vitreous strands and cells. The right fundus exhibited a slightly elevated white zone of peripapillary retinopathy. The left eye also exhibited an elevated white lesion with small dot and flame hemorrhages. Chorioretinal pigmentation was also noted in the peripheral retina. The vitreous, similar to but less intense than that in the right eye, showed vitreous stranding and cells. Vision deteriorated in the left eye to 20/300, and the right eye remained LP. Systemic examinations at that time were normal except for a chest X-ray that showed a healed granuloma in the right lower lobe of the lung and a white blood cell count of 23,000 with normal differential. By then, the right eye was HM and the vision in the left eye had improved to 20/60. Due to Cushingoid features that began to develop in the patient, the intake of prednisone was reduced to 10 mg daily. Subsequently, the patient's vision declined to no light perception (NLP) in the right eye and HM in the left. Attempts at salvaging vision by increasing the prednisone were unsuccessful.

Systemic illness became evident by then as the patient became lethargic, had slowed mentation, and became stuporous. The patient eventually died. Autopsy was performed, and systemic nocardiosis was determined to be the cause of death. Multiple abscesses were found in the brain, lungs (there was also an empyema of the right hemithorax), heart, thyroid, and kidneys. *Nocardia asteroides*, the fungus that causes nocardiosis, is typically found in immunocompromised patients (such as those taking corticosteroids) and characteristically causes cavitations in the lungs allowing it to spread to distant sites such as the CNS to form abscesses. Though systemic nocardiosis was found in this patient, who had been on prednisone therapy for 7 months, no evidence of a systemic lymphomatous process was found. However, ophthalmic pathologic inspection revealed that a primary lymphomatous process had occurred in the eyes. Upon gross inspection, the right eye had vitreous opacities and a peripapillary area of exudation that was green-white. Grossly, the left eye had an area of exudative retinopathy in the paramacular area. Histopathologically, the main findings in the right eye were focal areas in the choroid of perivascular lymphocytic infiltration. Above these areas of infiltration, the RPE was noted to be reactive with areas of chorioretinal adhesions and retinal disorganization marked by gliosis. In addition, there were rare plasma cells in the iris stroma, some containing Russell bodies. Vitreous stranding with some chronic inflammatory cells and macrophages were also found over the vitreous base. The choroid itself was diffusely thickened up to 15 times the normal thickness. The tumor was noted to extend through small lesions in Bruch's membrane to the subretina and overlying retina as well as the optic nerve head. The histopathology of the left eye also showed areas of lymphocytic infiltration, but with very minimal choroidal thickening and no to little overlying retinal involvement. However, there was a subretinal plaque, positively birefringent, overlying the area of the lesion, that disrupted the RPE and minimally elevated the retina. Unlike in the right eye, a neoplastic process was not evident in the left eye. The tumor cells in the right eye were multinucleated. Other nuclear features included hyperchromatism, large size, and being vesicular or oval in shape. Moderate pleomorphism of the cells was also identified in addition to mitotic figures. Both eyes were diagnosed as having a posterior chronic nongranulomatous uveitis. The right eye was diagnosed as "primary, solitary, intraocular reticulum cell sarcoma which probably arose in the choroid." However, Nevins concedes that one cannot discount the possibility that the retina was the primary tissue of origin of the lymphoma. Indeed, this case could be a PIOL.

An interesting case of a uveitis produced from a metastatic cerebral reticulum cell sarcoma to the vitreous was presented by Minckler *et al.*, also from the AFIP.[9] The patient was a 66-year-old female who noted decreased visual acuity in both eyes. Visual acuity was measured as 20/50 and 20/40 in the right and left eyes, respectively. However, just 18 months earlier her visual acuity had been measured as 20/25 bilaterally. Vitreous clouding was noted on examination, which preceded the development of CNS symptoms, including headache and mental status changes. Mild anterior chamber flare and keratic precipitates were also noted during ophthalmic examinations prior to her death three years from her initial presentation. An autopsy was performed upon this patient's death. The examination of the brain revealed a hemorrhagic tumor that was partially necrotic and had replaced the substance of the thalamus and was found to be impinging upon the left lateral ventricle. Microscopic examination showed infiltration by mononuclear cells that are characteristic of reticulum cell sarcoma. The left eye was examined and showed clouding of the vitreous with clumps of gray-white material at the base of the vitreous. Some of this material was noted to be consistent with atypical mononuclear cells having large nuclei and infolded nuclear membranes. The nucleoli were prominent in these cells, and some cells exhibited necrosis as their nuclei showed karyorrhexis and karyolysis. The iris also contained inflammatory cells, but the retina was spared from any infiltration except for a disciform chorioretinal scar located in the region of the macula. Focal collections of chronic inflammatory cells were found in the choroid, and optic nerve atrophy was also exhibited. The right eye also showed inflammatory cells in the anterior vitreous, and this was the only abnormality. The vitreous cells in both eyes were considered to be reticulum cell sarcoma cells.

Modern Clinical Manifestations

Despite advances in imaging and diagnostic modalities, PIOL is still considered to be a masquerade syndrome, often eluding diagnosis for many months.[10–16] Awareness of the demographics, systemic and ocular manifestations, and clinical findings can help guide an ophthalmologist/neurologist/oncologist's differential diagnosis toward PIOL.

Systemic Presentations and Manifestations

B Symptoms. B symptoms, including unexplained and persistent fever and chills, drenching night sweats, fatigue, and weight loss, are often present in patients with malignancy or chronic infection. Though the central nervous system may seem distant and protected from the rest of the body, systemic presentations of lymphomatous processes in the central nervous system are well recognized. While certain systemic signs might suggest a systemic NHL, PIOL can produce some similar systemic signs, especially when it occurs with cerebral disease. Classically, systemic NHL is characterized by B symptoms, including low-grade fevers in excess of 38°C, night sweats, and weight loss in excess of 10% of a patient's body weight, which occurs over six months.[17] Such systemic complaints by a patient should arouse suspicion that a systemic lymphomatous process is occurring. Even when ocular symptoms such as blurred vision and floaters are a complaint of the patient, the occurrence of systemic symptoms requires that a systemic NHL be ruled out. Indeed, in 1951, Cooper and Ricker elicited symptoms such as a 10% weight loss from the first described patient with ocular lymphoma[1] that were evocative of today's B symptoms. Importantly, the presence of B symptoms should be noted in the patient's chart since this can be prognostically useful. Approximately 40% of patients with systemic NHL will present with B symptoms.[17] In cases where B symptoms are present, it is important to inquire about the patient's past medical history (including any past history of cancer, other underlying diseases, and infections), family history of malignancies, history of travel to other countries, recent contacts with the sick, and exposure to toxic and noxious agents in the patient's occupation. When a systemic NHL is present, another systemic complaint or presenting feature can include lymphadenopathy. Patients may complain of a rapidly growing peripheral lymph node or perhaps a lymph node that seems to slowly grow and then regress, only to reappear later. An infectious process should be excluded in cases of lymphadenopathy, and attention should be paid to common sites of lymphadenopathy associated with systemic NHL, including the cervical and supraclavicular lymph nodes.[18] Other lymph nodes that should be assessed during the physical exam include the inguinal and femoral lymph nodes, those located in the tonsils, and those around the liver, spleen, and abdomen. However, since up to 35% of systemic NHLs can present extranodally,[17] the lack of lymphadenopathy should not steer one away from suspecting this disease. Thus, it is important to perform a chest X-ray, thoracic and abdominal CT scans, a bone marrow biopsy, brain MRI, and HIV testing. When systemic findings are found in association with cerebral or ocular lymphomas, metastasis from a systemic NHL to the CNS, systemic metastasis from a PCNSL or PIOL (which is rare with approximately 7% to 10% of PCNSL metastasizing to other systemic extranodal sites[19]), or systemic symptoms produced from lymphomatous process not extending beyond the neuraxis should be considered.

In their histopathologic case series of eight patients with PIOL, Qualman and colleagues described one patient who, unlike their other patients, initially complained of fever and cervical lymphadenopathy.[20] Although the ocular presentation of the tumor in this particular 49-year-old black female was confined mainly to the posterior choroid, there was vitreal involvement. However, in keeping with a metastasis from a systemic NHL, there was lymphomatous involvement of the eyelids and left conjuctivum, sites from which the diagnosis of diffuse large cell lymphoma was made. Autopsy upon the death of the patient, 14 months after initially complaining of systemic symptoms, confirmed the diagnosis of a visceral diffuse large cell lymphoma with ocular involvement. The authors pointed out that this case did not have optic nerve or chiasm involvement nor was the brain involved in this patient's systemic NHL. Another patient in their series had visual complaints, primarily decreased visual acuity in both eyes, and also had systemic symptoms early in the disease course. Though the patient became terminally comatose with primitive reflexes and a left Babinski reflex, in addition to a left ptotic eyelid, the patient's brain at autopsy did not reveal lymphomatous disease. Instead, multiple visceral organs were infiltrated with diffuse large cell lymphoma. Histopathologic analysis of the deceased man's eyes disclosed choroidal infiltration by diffuse large cell lymphoma, but the vitreous also contained lymphomatous cells.

Systemic complaints, especially fever, night sweats, a decrease in weight, or lymphadenopathy, are suggestive of a systemic NHL. When uveitis is a complaint in the presence of systemic symptoms suggestive of NHL, an ophthalmologist must rule out a metastatic seeding from the viscera to the choroid or uvea of the eye.

Systemic Examinations. As noted previously, PIOL can occasionally present with systemic complaints, though systemic findings may be more difficult to uncover. The discovery of systemic findings such as cachexia and lymphadenopathy should cause one to consider systemic tumors. Again, the presence of B symptoms may very well suggest an NHL. Systemic examination can be as simple as examining the skin. This becomes important with cutaneous T cell lymphoma (CTCL), also known as mycosis fungoides.[21,22] Though its association with PIOL is rare, cases of intraocular involvement by cutaneous T cell lymphomata have been reported.[23] Thus, it is important to check the integumentary system, paying attention to the presence of skin rashes or plaques. CTCL most often affects the skin of the legs and torso[24] and can often be confused with the plaque lesion of psoriasis.[25]

PCNSL and PIOL Simulating Systemic Symptoms. Despite B symptoms being associated with systemic lymphomatous disease, their occurrence is not exclusive to systemic NHL. For example, in one particular study, 8% of immunocompetent Canadian patients with PCNSL presented with constitutional B symptoms.[26] Likewise, in a retrospective review of immunocompetent patients from France and Belgium, 7% of the patients showed systemic manifestations prior to being diagnosed with PCNSL.[27] Systemic symptoms included gastrointestinal symptoms, respiratory illness, or fever. Some of the systemic symptoms produced in PIOL and PCNSL have to do with local or global effects on the brain. For example, increased intracranial pressure due to edema of cerebral parenchyma caused by lymphoma can produce headache. Headache in this instance appears to be due to the pain fibers that travel within cranial nerve V within the dural blood vessels. Local or distant mass effects on the reticular formation within the brainstem may produce depressed consciousness, which can be interpreted as malaise. The vomiting center within the medulla can be stimulated as well due to direct mass effect or cerebral edema. While the classical B symptoms have definite criteria, the systemic symptoms produced from PIOL and PCNSL might be more subtle and therefore require an astute clinician's careful inquiry into the patient's history. Rarely, central neurogenic hyperventilation may occur due to lymphoma occurring in the brainstem.[28]

CNS and Ocular Symptoms, and Manifestations

CNS Symptoms. When the CNS is affected by the lymphomatous disease, changes in behavior and mental status usually occur. Like other malignancies that afflict the brain, mass lesion effects that produce focal neurologic symptoms and deficits can suggest the presence of an intracranial tumor. CNS symptoms vary between immunocompetent patients and patients with severe deficits in their immune system, such as AIDS patients.

In 1993, Whitcup *et al.* reported 12 cases of intraocular lymphoma.[29] The majority of cases complained of blurred vision and floaters. However, two patients presented with neurologic symptoms. One patient presented with seizures and the other with diplopia and, interestingly, a hoarse voice. Half of the patients in Whitcup's study had CNS lesions as seen on radiography by the time the diagnosis of PIOL was made. Five other patients eventuated to CNS disease as determined by CSF cytology after PIOL had been diagnosed. One patient refused lumbar puncture for CSF cytology altogether.

When the systemic disease metastasizes to the leptomeninges, cranial nerve, spinal cord, and radicular symptoms can occur.[30] Primary lymphoma of the leptomeninges is less common, but would manifest in much the same way as a metastasis from a systemic source.[31] Thus, visual and auditory deficits might be present, or facial nerve paresthesias or pain might occur. Compression of the spinal cord or dorsal or ventral roots may manifest as incontinence or limb parasthesias, though primary lymphomatous involvement of the spinal cord is quite rare.[32] While immunocompetent patients seem to have focal lesions, AIDS patients can present with multifocal lesions that can be more complex and diffuse neurologic manifestations.[27,33] In Bataille's examination of CNS symptoms manifesting from PCNSL, the most common finding (70% of cases) was a focal neurologic deficit, such as aphasia, ataxia, or a hemiparesis. Psychiatric manifestations, including depression, slowed mentation, and confusion were seen in 43% of the cases upon first presentation. Gastrointestinal symptoms, such as nausea and vomiting, were also common (33% in association with increased intracranial pressure).

Ocular Manifestations, Symptoms, and Complaints. More typically, a patient with PIOL will present with ocular complaints of blurred vision or decreased visual acuity.[11–13,16,29,34–42] The patient may note a new onset of metamorphopsias or "floaters." Photopsias, or "flashes," seems to be described infrequently in the literature. These complaints almost reflexively bring uveitis to the forefront of an ophthalmologist's differential diagnosis. Less often, patients complain of discharge and photophobia. Ocular pain or foreign body sensation is also infrequently a complaint of patients with PIOL, but is not unheard of.[29,43] Occasionally, periorbital swelling may be a complaint.[41.]

Iris involvement has been documented in PIOL. While posterior synechiae may be a common finding in uveitis, such iris lesions are not common in PIOL patients. For example, in Matsuo's case series of 10 consecutive patients with PIOL over a 16-year period, two patients were noted to have posterior synechiae.[44] In Velez and colleagues' review of the previous literature accounting for 163 cases of PIOL, only five cases were noted, on clinical examination, to have posterior synechiae.[45] Likewise, iris infiltration with lymphomatous cells was a rare occurrence, with five cases exhibiting it. Velez and colleagues reported two patients from the National Eye Institute (NEI) who exhibited infiltration of the iris by PIOL.[45] One patient, a 51-year-old Caucasian male, had an eight-year history of decreased vision and floaters bilaterally. Through the years he had been diagnosed as having intermediate uveitis and had bilateral pars plana vitrectomies with scleral buckles. Prior to presentation at the NEI, this patient was noted to have anterior chamber cells in the right eye and cell and flare in the vitreous. Subretinal lesions whitish in color were noted upon funduscopic examination of the right eye. When the patient was examined at the NEI, iris heterochromia of the right eye was noted. The right eye's iris had lost the varied hues of grey and blue that characterized the left eye. Instead, the right eye appeared more uniformly greyish-white, and there were engorged circumcorneal vessels. Findings on slit lamp examination suggestive of iris involvement in PIOL include a thickened cornea, engorged iridal vessels, and iris nodules.[45] Gonioscopy may reveal cellular infiltration as well.[45]

An ophthalmologist must have a high index of suspicion that a uveitic process may be a hint of a lymphomatous process. Etiological factors involved in the production of uveitis serve to point one's clinical suspicions toward a possible PIOL diagnosis or at least a diagnosis of "rule out PIOL."[13] Often in medicine, when a disease follows a pattern or clinical script, the ability to tease out a diagnosis from characteristic clinical nuances can help rule in or rule out certain disease processes. Such is the case with PIOL. When a patient who is middle-aged or older arrives at his or her ophthalmologist's office with complaints of blurred vision and possibly floaters, perhaps two thoughts should spring to the mind of the ophthalmologist: the patient may have a uveitic process occurring, but perhaps a process more sinister, such as PIOL, could potentially, albeit much less frequently, be producing such complaints in the patient. On the basis of a patient's clinical history, slit lamp and dilated fundus examinations, ultrasonographic and photographic (including fluorescein angiography or indocyanine green) examinations, and lab work, such as serologies for infectious or autoimmune markers (e.g. CBC; VDRL; Toxoplasma, Histoplasma, and cat scatch titers; tuberculin skin tests; angiotensin converting enzyme; and HLA-typing), an ophthalmologist can substantiate his or her suspicion about the cause of a patient's uveitis. In addition, chest X-ray or CT scan may help rule out other causes of uveitis, such as sarcoidosis.[46,47] Thus, a patient's clinical history and physical exam findings will help dictate the tests that should be ordered. If PIOL is suspected, brain MRI and lumbar puncture for CSF examination and cytology should be arranged.

Masquerade Syndrome. When PIOL presents as a "uveitis," several key features allow an ophthalmologist to pursue the possibility of this diagnosis further.[11–13,16,29,34–42] PIOL should be considered when an elderly patient presents with chronic uveitis unresponsive to corticosteroid therapy.

As noted previously, inflammatory infiltrates simulating uveitis can make the diagnosis of PIOL elusive. However, the presence of a dense vitritis and intraretinal or subretinal lesions appearing as creamy, yellow-to-white infiltrates may provide convincing evidence that a more malignant process is occurring. Other retinal lesions that may be noted include retinal hemorrhages,[48] birdshot chorioretinopathy,[49] and punctate inner choroidopathy.[43,50]

Ocular Examinations

Slit Lamp Biomicroscopy. The most common findings seen on slit lamp biomicroscopy include anterior chamber cells (simply called "cell") and protein (known as "flare"). Collections of cells that accumulate on the corneal endothelium, known as keratic precipitates (KP), may also be seen on slit lamp examination.[13] Such keratic precipitates may be small or can be larger, forming mutton fat keratic precipitates.[51] Anterior chamber inflammation composed of many PIOL cells may be so pronounced as to simulate a hypopyon (termed pseudohypopyon secondary to the collection of tumor cells, not inflammatory cells).[37–39] Anterior chamber cells may even collect within the canal of Schlem blocking the flow of aqueous humor and resulting in increased intraocular pressure[39] and secondary glaucoma. Velez and colleagues' extensive review of case reports of PIOL showed that 43% of the total 163 patients exhibited anterior chamber cells.[45] Indeed, in the series of nine patients by Char *et al.*, four exhibited minor or no anterior chamber cells,[37] and in Siegel and colleagues' series of 14 patients observed over 10 years, only three exhibited trace to obvious anterior uveitis.[42] Thus, when a patient complains of a blurring of visual acuity, the ophthalmologist should pursue a dilated ophthalmoscopic examination to investigate the lack of anterior chamber cell and flare.

Dilated Fundus Examination. Dilated fundus examination often shows a vitritis (vitreous cells and haze), further suggesting uveitis. This is the most common ocular finding in PIOL. For example, in a review of 163 cases from the literature, 66% of patients were noted to have a vitritis.[45] At times the opacities in the vitreous may be so dense that they preclude a clear view of the fundus.[37] The vitritis can exhibit many cells in sheets and clumps, and there may be haze, but this finding is less common than in uveitis. In our extensive knowledge and experience of the unique clinical characteristics of PIOL, the simple office technique of having a patient with vitreous cells shake his or her head can be very telling. In PIOL, visual acuity can show temporary improvement as the vitreous cells and necrotic debris are dislodged from their position in the vitreous humor and settle toward the bottom of the globe. In uveitis, such a maneuver may not improve visual acuity, especially when vitreous hazing and stranding is a major component of the uveitic process. Despite the vitritis noted on ophthalmoscopic examination, the visual acuity can actually be much better than expected.[11] In a series of 12 patients, Whitcup *et al.* reported eight patients with bilateral involvement. Visual acuities in these patients were good, ranging most frequently from 20/20 to 20/40.[29] There were two eyes in two patients that exhibited HM vision or NLP.

Another important finding during the examination of the fundus is subretinal lesions. Classically, these lesions have been described as being whitish-yellow to slightly orange in color, with a fluffy appearance. In addition, the subretinal infiltrates may have distinct or lobulated borders. As the tumor initially infiltrates the space between the retinal pigment epithelium (RPE) and Bruch's membrane, causing RPE detachments, the tumor mass can sometimes be visualized with marked contrast to the remaining attached RPE.[52,53] The involvement of the retina by the tumor can produce RPE detachments[9,54] in addition to exudative retinal detachments.[53,55] The detachment of the RPE from Bruch's membrane may lead to RPE atrophy in areas associated with tumor infiltration; these areas of atrophy may show scarring.[52] Pigment epithelium not directly involved or detached by the tumor may exhibit foci of hypertrophy. Often, these lesions may be multiple in numbers and begin as round to oval in shape. As they enlarge, the lesions may become confluent[10,11,13] and their borders may become more indistinct and ragged as they extend through the RPE.

Though chorioretinal lesions might be found rarely in patients with PIOL, they may not always be in the orange-yellow-white color recognized as being the characteristic of PIOL. For example, in the series by Vogel *et al.*, one patient had a rather uncharacteristically colored lesion of greyish-white, though the fluffy borders of this lesion were similar to the classically described borders of PIOL subretinal lesions.[8] In a cohort of 10 patients, 60% of patients exhibited sub-RPE infiltrates that were yellowish in color, with the distinguishing fluffy border. In Siegel and colleagues' description of 14 cases of PIOL over 10 years, none were noted to have fluffy subretinal infiltrates of any color.[42] Such lesions may look obscure due to the overlying vitritis.[35] When lesions of the fundus are noted, it is important to document them with photography. This can help to track changes in the size of the tumor. Small punctate retinal lesions may grow over time so that some may actually coalesce forming an even larger lesion. While it is known that tumor infiltrates in such a way that a confluence between the different foci occurs, the rapidity with which this process occurs is difficult to ascertain as there are no studies documenting this with respect to discrete time intervals. In addition, treatment with corticosteroids for presumed uveitis can lead to a reduction in tumor size and some lesions may spontaneously resolve. However, maintaining records using fundus photography and fluorescein angiography (to be discussed in Chapter 6, "Imaging") can help follow the progression of lymphomatous involvement. Tumor infiltration seems to exhibit a spread from the sub-RPE to the retina, with some cases eventuating to the involvement of the optic nerve.

In 1989, Siegel and colleagues presented their experience with 14 patients with primary intraocular lymphoma (the term, "reticulum cell sarcoma" was still being used at the time) over a 10-year period.[42] Ocular findings in their patients at presentation displayed a uveitic picture. Anterior uveitis was noted in three patients, bilaterally in two and unilaterally in one. Vitreous cells were present in all patients, bilaterally in 10 patients and unilaterally in two patients. A 27-year-old female patient, in addition to having bilateral vitreous cells, exhibited RPE atrophy in her left eye. Another patient, a 66-year-old female had bilateral posterior detachments.

A 55-year-old female exhibited a Koeppe nodule (iris nodule at the pupil's border) as well as retinal masses and infiltrates in her right eye. Three other patients had unilateral retinal exudates and another had unilateral subretinal lesions. A 64-year-old female had unilateral cystoid macular edema and retinal exudates. In Char and colleagues' retrospective series of 20 patients,[53] ocular involvement was bilateral in 18 patients. Ophthalmic examination revealed vitreous cells in all patients. Anterior chamber cells were present in 15 patients. Chorioretinal lesions were noted in 16 patients. Two patients had retinal hemorrhages in addition to chorioretinal lesions, and another patient had an exudative retinal detachment. Four patients showed negative results for chorioretinal lesions, while one patient had a fundus that could not be visualized due to very dense media opacities.[53] Chorioretinal lesions displayed areas of RPE hyperplasia, and some cases exhibited the classical diffuse and creamy infiltration. Char *et al.* noted that the time interval between symptoms and diagnosis of PIOL ranged from 0 to 60 months, with 11 patients examined prior to 1980 having a mean interval between symptoms and diagnosis of 24.3 months. Nine patients examined after 1980 had a mean interval of 5.8 months. Asymmetrical cellular involvement (both anterior chamber and vitreous) and chorioretinal lesions were the rule in these cases. PIOL eventuated to CNS disease in 16 of the cases. Three other patients developed systemic lymphoma between one-and-a-half to three years after being diagnosed with PIOL. In the series of 12 cases recorded by Whitcup and colleagues,[29] visual acuity ranged from unilateral NLP and HM in two patients to 20/20 or 20/16 in some. In fact, though dense vitritis and retinal lesions were present, six patients had visual acuities that were 20/40 or better. Some of the retinal lesions are described as multiple and punctate located in the subretina and being yellow in color. Table 5.2 shows that the most common presenting ocular complaint in PIOL is blurred vision or metamorphopsias. Lymphomatous infiltration of the optic nerve can produce optic neuritis, and optic nerve atrophy can also be a manifestation.[43] Acute retinal necrosis (ARN) presentation has also been documented in the case of some patients,[43,56] developing from lymphomatous infiltration of a retinal artery and leading to thrombosis. It is important, however, that ARN due to viral etiologies be ruled out. This may be done by using genotypic profiling via the polymerase chain reaction (PCR) amplification on ocular biopsies to detect viral DNA.[57,58] In addition, using older but important techniques of viral culture and

Table 5.2 Clinical Manifestations in Major Case Series of PIOL in patients without HIV

Author	Year	N[1]	Initial Complaints	Ocular Examinations						
				Slit Lamp				Vitreous	Dilated Fundus	
				Cornea	Anterior Chamber	Iris	Lens		Retina	Optic Nerve
Freeman	1987	32	NS[2]	NS	25% with anterior uveitis (most of these with combined anterior and posterior uveitis)	NS	NS	50% with solely posterior uveitis/vitritis (22% with combined posterior and anterior uveitis)	19% with chorioiditis, chorioretinitis, or sub-RPE infiltrates; 3% with white macular lesions	3% with optic neuropathy
Char	1988	20	13% with decreased/blurred VA[3] and/or floaters; 35% CNS[4] symptoms	NS	25% with anterior uveitis	NS	NS	72% of patients with posterior uveitis/vitritis	19% with chorioiditis, chorioretinitis, or sub-RPE[5] infiltrates; 3% with scattered whitish macular lesions	3% with optic neuropathy
Whitcup	1993	12	92% with floaters and/or blurred VA; 17% with CNS symptoms (1 patient with seizure, 1 patient with diplopia and hoarse voice)	NS	42% anterior uveitis	NS	NS	100% of patients with vitreous cells (often forming into thick sheets) and haze	?50% with retinal lesions (including subretinal infiltrates, punctuate retinal lesions, retinal vasculitis, RPE changes, macular edema, macular star)	NS

(Continued)

Table 5.2 (*Continued*)

Author	Year	N[1]	Initial Complaints	Ocular Examinations						
				Slit Lamp					Dilated Fundus	
				Cornea	Anterior Chamber	Iris	Lens	Vitreous	Retina	Optic Nerve
Peterson	1993	24	83% with ocular symptoms (17 patients with blurred vision, 6 patients with floaters, 2 patients with eye pain or foreign body sensation)	NS	25% with anterior uveitis	NS	NS	87.5% with lymphocytic infiltrate	25% with chorioretinal involvement 1 patient developed ARN6 secondary to retinal artery thrombosis from lymphoma infiltration	1 patient with known PCNSL developed optic neuritis
Akpek	1999	10	70% with decreased vision 10% with floaters only 20% with decreased vision and floaters 50% with CNS symptoms (1 patient with diplopia, 1 patient with confusion, 2 patients with decreased memory and imbalance, 1 patient with limb parasthesias)	NS	NS	NS	NS	NS	60% with fundus lesions including sub-RPE infiltrates, retinoschoroiditis, and vasculitis 10% with dense vitreous clouding 30% with vitritis only consisting of large clumps or sheets of cells or clumps of cells on vitreous strands AND no retinal or vascular involvement	NS

(*Continued*)

Table 5.2 (*Continued*)

Author	Year	N[1]	Initial Complaints	Ocular Examinations							
				Slit Lamp					Dilated Fundus		
				Cornea	Anterior Chamber	Iris	Lens	Vitreous	Retina		Optic Nerve
Cassoux	2000	42	NS	NS	21% with keratic precipitates	2.4% with posterior synechiae	NS		60.5% with RPE changes		3.7% with optic nerve swelling
					2.4% with mutton fat keratic precipitates				33% with punctate retinal infiltrates		
					1.2% with pseudo-hypopyon				8.6% with vasculitis		
					2.4% with glaucoma				3.7% with subretinal mass		
									2.5% with exudative retinal detachment		
									10% with no abnormalities		

(*Continued*)

Table 5.2 (*Continued*)

Author	Year	N[1]	Initial Complaints	Ocular Examinations							
				Slit Lamp				Vitreous	Dilated Fundus		
				Cornea	Anterior Chamber	Iris	Lens		Retina	Optic Nerve	
Hoffman	2003	10	86% (of 14 total patients with PIOL/PCNSL or systemic lymphoma) with blurred vision 43% (of 14 total patients with PIOL/PCNSL or systemic lymphoma) with floaters	NS	30% with anterior uveitis	NS	NS	Vitritis in 90%	30% with choroidal involvement (most consisting of subretinal pale or pigmented areas) 20% with vasculitis/perivascular infiltrates 20% with retinitis 10% with serous detachment 10% with posterior scleritis	10% with optic disc swelling	
Hormigo	2004	31	55% with floaters 39% with blurred vision 29% with visual loss 3% with flashes & floaters	NS	NS	NS	NS	NS	NS	NS	

[1]N = number of patients; [2]NS = not stated; [3]VA = visual acuity; [4]CNS = central nervous system; [5]RPE = retinal pigment epithelium; [6]ARN = acute retinal necrosis

checking titers of antiviral antibodies or using the fluorescent antibody test can be useful in determining whether ARN is due to a virus.

Other fundus findings may include multifocal white lesions having the appearance of being "punched out" or "atrophic." These lesions may also coalesce to form larger, disciform scars. They may also eventuate to pigment epithelial or outer retinal atrophy.[49,59] It is important to distinguish these lesions from similar lesions seen in birdshot retinochoroidopathy.[49]

Summary of Clinical Manifestations and Findings

The fact that a uveitic process is the usual presentation of PIOL makes it a masquerade syndrome that is often difficult to properly diagnose when it is first noticed by an ophthalmologist. Thus, knowledge of the presentations both non-specific and quasi-specific can help an ophthalmologist to diagnose this disorder.

Let us first succinctly review some of the typical non-specific presentations and symptoms that we have just discussed above (Table 5.2). Immunocompetent patients are most frequently in their fifties or sixties.[13,40] The usual complaint is blurred vision, decreased visual acuity, or floaters. Often these symptoms appear to be a normal process of aging. For example, cataractous and presbyopic changes are common in this age group.[60] Patients' description of floaters can seem quite similar to benign floaters described by many normal people.[43] Less typical complaints may include ocular pain or foreign body sensation.[29,41,43]

Slit lamp biomicroscopy can be helpful, but often the findings are non-specific (Table 5.2). For example, keratic precipitates (including the larger, mutton fat variety) may be found adhering to the corneal endothelium.[13] Within the anterior chamber, a uveitic-like process may occur in which inflammatory cells can be found. These cells can be an extension of the inflammatory and neoplastic processes occurring in the vitreous.[13] The inflammation in the anterior chamber is described as cell and flare. Lymphocytic infiltration of the anterior chamber may be significant enough to simulate a "hypopyon" (pseudohypopyon). Other slit lamp findings (for example, involvement of the iris or its angle) may be rarer. The iris may be thickened due to infiltration or there may be discrete foci of tumor appearing as iris nodules. The color of the iris may have changed as well, resulting in heterochromia iridis,[45] though the patient may have not recognized this change himself or herself. However, the simple office technique of comparing the color of the iris in one eye with that in the other can provide subtle hints to an ophthalmologist. Infiltration of the trabecular meshwork or canal of Schlemm by lymphoma cells can produce increased intraocular pressures (IOPs), representing secondary glaucoma. Therefore, it is important to document IOP at each examination. It has been hypothesized that an anterior chamber seeding with lymphoma cells may precede iris involvement.[45] Rubeosis iridis can also infrequently occur.[61]

Since vitritis is the most common finding in patients with PIOL (Table 5.2), dilated ophthalmoscopic examination is essential. The vitritis in PIOL consists of cells and haze, often with the lymphoma cells forming clumps, sheets, or strands.[13,51,62] Vitreous hemorrhage is an infrequent occurrence in PIOL patients.[16] Though vitritis may be marked, visual acuity can be surprisingly good, or at least better than expected.[29]

Fundus lesions may consist of the almost classical creamy, white-to-yellow-to-orange subretinal infiltrates (Table 5.2).[11,13] Such lesions can be single or multiple. They may have fluffy, indistinct borders or perhaps more discrete edges.[61] Lesions may also be somewhat obscure due to haziness produced by the vitritis that is so frequently found. Though the lesions may be multiple, some can coalesce and become more confluent; however, the lesions can also regress. The resolution of these lesions can result in RPE atrophy or subretinal fibrosis.[11,49,59] Less common fundus findings include retinal hemorrhages and vascular sheathing. When an older patient with a posterior "uveitis" is diagnosed, a lack of chorioretinal lesions when a vitritis is present should not dissuade an ophthalmologist from suspecting PIOL.

It should be noted that anterior and posterior segment findings are not typically present at the same time, with posterior segment findings antedating involvement of the anterior chamber,[45] though iridocyclitis and secondary glaucoma have been noted in the literature to be present prior to the detection of fundus lesions.[8,63]

Since uveitis is diagnosed most frequently prior to discovering that PIOL is the actual disease process that is occurring, corticosteroids are usually prescribed to the patient.[40] The lymphomatous process may initially respond to corticosteroid treatment. For example, in Hormigo's series, half of the 31 patients showed an initial response to the steroid treatment.[40] However, the improvement in uveitis is short-lived and may become refractory to treatment. This can often be a useful clue that uveitis is not the disease that is affecting the patient. Unfortunately, steroid treatment can hamper the diagnosis of PIOL because lymphomatous cells may have decreased in number or may have become more fragile and, therefore, more subject to rupture prior to cytologic and immunologic analyses.

Even when all the demographical factors, and clinical signs and symptoms seem to make PIOL highly likely, a definitive diagnosis can still be rather elusive. The reason for this is that lymphoma cells must be identified either from CSF or vitrectomy aspirate. Without these cells, a formal diagnosis of PIOL cannot be made and, thus, treatment cannot resolutely begin.

Differential Diagnoses

Uveitis. One of the most common misdiagnoses for PIOL is uveitis, which may be due to numerous reasons.[64,65] Uveitis may be due to infectious causes (viral, bacterial, or parasitic), inflammatory conditions, or non-inflammatory diseases. Each entity is discussed in detail in the following sections.

Viral Causes of Infectious Uveitis. Acute retinal necrosis due to varicella zoster virus (VZV) or herpes simplex virus (HSV) has been described as manifesting as an acute iridocyclitis, vitritis, necrotizing retinitis, and vasooclusive processes of the retinal vasculature. This, in turn, can lead to a decline in vision and also to retinal detachments.[66–68] West Nile virus has been noted to induce a retinal edema in association with artery occlusions and non-perfusive vasculitis.[69] Other reports of West Nile virus have shown that the infection can also produce retinal hemorrhages, chorioretinal scarring, keratic precipitates, and vitritis — essentially a uveitic picture.[70,71] Cytomegalovirus (CMV) retinitis is associated with AIDS patients having low CD4 counts (less than 50 cells/mL). Often, CMV retinitis can present with a blurred vision and vitritis, a complaint and clinical finding one finds commonly in PIOL. PIOL has also been noted to produce retinal vasculitis and hemorrhage, simulating a viral retinitis.[34,48,72] In such cases, patients may be treated with antiviral medications with no response before the diagnosis of PIOL is made.[72]

Bacterial Causes of Infectious Uveitis. *Treponema pallidum,* the agent that causes syphilis, may present with uveitis or chorioretinitis or retinal vasculitis.[73] Ocular tuberculosis has been noted to worsen when corticosteroids are used, similar to PIOL. Often this disease will present with systemic symptoms, including weight loss, night sweats, and chronic cough.[74–76] Cat scratch disease caused by *Bartonella henseai* can be associated with neuroretinitis and Parinaud's occuloglandular syndrome.[77–79]

Parasitic Causes of Infectious Uveitis. *Toxoplasma gondii* can produce a chorioretinitis with a vitreous cellular infiltrate.[80] Though lesions of the fundus, including pigmented scars, may appear whitish to yellow, they lack the characteristic creamy infiltration of the subretina that can be seen in PIOL.

Non-Infectious Uveitis. Syndromes of ocular uveitis primarily include birdshot choroidopathy and pars planitis (also known as intermediate uveitis). Birdshot choroidopathy is a bilateral posterior uveitis. This disease derives its name from a distinctive form of inflammatory cellular aggregate that looks like birdshot pellet ammunition.[81] These yellow-to-white lesions (one of the white dot syndromes) may resemble the small punctate lesions associated with PIOL.[29,49] Patients may complain of blurry vision, which is a similar complaint of some PIOL patients. Other ocular complaints may include floaters and a loss of color vision. During ophthalmoscopic examination, it is important to pay attention to the pattern of the lesions. In birdshot retinochroidopathy, the lesions can be seen to radiate from the optic nerve and follow the larger choroidal vessels. Women are affected more commonly than men in birdshot retinochoroidopathy and, as in PIOL, they are in their forties and fifties. Other ocular examination findings may include vitritis and an edematous optic disc. Unlike PIOL, birdshot retinochoroidopathy is associated with an HLA phenotype, HLA-A29.[82] In this case, fluorescein angiography, in addition to HLA typing, can provide useful clues in distinguishing which disease process is more likely. PIOL may present with punctate whitish lesions at the location of the pars plana so as to mimic a pars planitis.

Systemic and Ocular Inflammatory Disease. Systemic inflammatory diseases can also produce uveitis. Diseases associated with the human leukocyte antigen B27 phenotype (HLA B27), including the spondy-loarthropathies (e.g. ankylosing spondylitis, reactive arthritis), inflammatory bowel disease, and psoriatic arthritis, though HLA B27 positivity is not found in all cases of these diseases and not requisite for the development of uveitis.

Sarcoidosis, the commonest systemic disease associated with uveitides, can be the presenting feature in this disease.[83] The eye is affected up to 25% of the time in sarcoidosis, and ocular complaints in this disease include blurred vision, dry eyes, red eye, and photophobia. Ophthalmic examination in sarcoidosis may reveal a uveitis, or a conjunctival or lacrimal nodule. The fundus may present with punctate yellow-to-white RPE lesions that can be reminiscent of small punctate subretinal infiltrates in PIOL.[84,85] The presence of extraocular symptoms such as erythema nodosum and pulmonary hilar lymphadenopathy on chest X-ray or CT scan can help differentiate sarcoidosis from PIOL.

Behçet disease is best known for a characteristic clinical triad of oral and genital ulcerations and uveitis.[86] It is not common in the United States and seems to exhibit a racial predilection as areas in the Mediteranean and Asia exhibit a higher prevalence. In Japan, for example, Behçet disease is the second most common cause of uveitis after Vogt-Koyanagi-Harada syndrome. Some ocular manifestations that occur in Behçet disease that can be found in PIOL include posterior and anterior uveitis, iridocyclitis, retinal vasculitis, optic neuritis, and chorioretinitis.[87,88] However, findings such as scleritis, keratitis, and conjunctivitis may steer an ophthalmologist away from PIOL and towards Behçet disease. In addition, answers given by the patient to clinical inquiries such as the existence of oral or genital ulcers or skin lesions ranging from erythema nodosum to ulcerations can be of benefit since these lesions are more common in Behçet disease.

Vogt-Koyanagi-Harada (VKH) syndrome is a bilateral panuveitis, often leading to exudative retinal detachments. In addition, the syndrome is associated with poliosis (whitening of a patch of hair), vitiligo (a condition in which the immune system destroys melanocytes in the skin, producing white patches in the skin), and auditory disturbances.[89–91] Rubsamen and Gass retrospectively reviewed the clinical charts, photographs, and fluorescein angiograms of 21 patients with VKH syndrome during the period from March 1969 through February 1990.[92] All the patients presented with loss of visual acuity in one or both eyes. Unlike in PIOL, a prodromal period was associated with 62% of cases. Prodromal symptoms, which began one week prior to the loss of vision, again unlike PIOL which is not associated with a prodromal phase, included headaches, ocular pain, tinnitus, fevers, and nuchal rigidity. Ninety percent of patients had uveitis or retinal detachments. Upon slit lamp biomicroscopy, 82% of patients had anterior uveitis consisting of cell and flare. Keratic precipitates were noted in 38% of patients, and all patients had vitreous cells. In addition, 43% had hyperemia and swelling of the disc. Multifocal exudative retinal detachments were initially found at presentation or later in 95% of patients. Some patients showed retinal striae due to the exudative retinal detachment. Other patients displayed a "setting sun" fundus. Long-term ocular findings included fundus pigment atrophy in 100% of patients, chronic anterior uveitis in 43%, elevated intraocular pressure in 45%, cataractous change in 36%, Dalen-Fuchs nodules in 44%, iris nodules in 29%, choroidal neovascular membrane (CNVM) in 9%, and optic neuropathy in 2%.[92]

Other Ocular and Systemic Malignant Diseases. Choroidal Extranodal Marginal Zone Lymphoma (EMZL) of Mucosa Associated Lymphoid Tissue (MALT) type (previously known as reactive lymphoid hyperplasia; also known as intraocular pseudotumor),[93] is another entity that can mimic a neoplastic process and has been noted to produce diagnostic challenges, much like PIOL.[94] Cheung and associates at the NEI described a 63-year-old black man with a previous history of controlled open-angle glaucoma and cataract extraction and posterior chamber intraocular lens placement in the right eye.[95] Five months after the extraction of lens, he complained about decreased vision in the right eye. A uveitic-like process was distinctly absent in his eyes: there were no cells in the anterior chamber or vitreous. There was a well-positioned posterior chamber intraocular lens in the right eye and a dense posterior subcapsular cataract (PSC) in the left. Though a uveitis was lacking, ophthalmoscopic examination revealed many subretinal creamy yellow-white lesions scattered about in a diffusely thickened choroid. The lesions (which were one-half to one disk diameter in size) involved the macula, and there was a superotemporal choroidal elevation in the right eye. The left eye was also involved and had scattered lesions in the posterior pole, similar to that of the right. Three months after these findings, there was an increase in the number of yellow-white lesions. Again, there was a distinctive lack of inflammation in both anterior and posterior segments. Previously, primary uveal marginal zone lymphoma, which is an EMZL MALT (known in the past as reactive lymphoid hyperplasia) was thought to represent a hyperplastic rather than neoplastic and malignant process of lymphocytes. It is now known that this process is actually a low-grade B-cell NHL.[93] Like in the case of PIOL, the definitive diagnosis of such a uveal EMZL MALT lymphoma requires a histologic examination of chorioretinal lesions. Fortunately, the prognosis of EMZL of MALT type is quite good. Unfortunately, much of the literature describes the so-called reactive lymphoid hyperplasia being diagnosed only after enucleation of the involved eye. In the case of Cheung and colleagues, a chorioretinal biopsy was considered first rather than enucleation. However, the relative lack in height of choroidal thickening (less than 3 mm) made the extraction of adequate amounts of tissue for histologic analysis difficult. This patient's chorioretinal biopsy proved to yield the diagnosis of "reactive lymphoid hyperplasia." Others have described biopsy of the ciliary body or extraocular tissues in the diagnosis of reactive lymphoid hyperplasia.[96,97] More recently, use of the polymerase chain reaction (PCR) amplification and the detection of a monoclonal spike (positive in most cases) have aided in the diagnosis of EMZL MALT lymphomas.[98]

Neurofibromatosis type I (von Recklinghausen disease), an autosomal dominant disease associated with café-au-lait skin spots, multiple neurofibromas, and pigment iris hamartomas (Lisch nodules), has also been described to be associated with a malignant melanoma of the choroid. In 1978, Wiznia and associates reported a 60-year-old Caucasian female who was noted to have choroidal mass lesions and a secondary retinal detachment in the left eye.[99] A slightly elevated choroidal mass of approximately 5- to 6-disk diameters was noted. Though neurofibromatosis type I is associated with fundal masses, the lack of anterior or posterior uveitis in addition to a paucity of creamy white-yellow chorioretinal lesions would help steer an ophthalmologist away from the diagnosis of PIOL. In addition, when a patient presents with decreased vision in the presence of choroidal melanoma and iris hamartomas with café-au-lait spots and neural tumors, one might think of von Recklinghausen's disease before considering PIOL.

An **astrocytic hamartoma of the retina** may present with retinal lesions reminiscent of PIOL. Reeser and colleagues reported an 11-year-old boy who presented with decreased vision in his left eye.[100] Five years earlier, a hit on the left side of his head with a baseball bat prompted a visit to an ophthalmologist, who noted a yellow-white retinal lesion temporal to the disk in the left eye. He was diagnosed with retinal astrocytoma. The boy did not have tuberous sclerosis. Over the years, the retinal lesion increased with extension to the nasal portion of the optic disk, to above and below the temporal vascular arcades, and into the macula. In addition there were occasional nerve fiber layer hemorrhages.

Other lymphoproliferative conditions should be considered in the differential diagnosis and include systemic lymphoma with secondary (metastatic) ocular involvement and intravascular lymphomatosis (also known as intravascular large B-cell lymphoma).[101,102] Metastatic lymphomas to the eye are often NHL or, less commonly, mycosis fungoides (cutaneous T-cell lymphoma). These tumors tend to invade the uvea. Clinical manifestations include anterior uveitis and choroidal thickening. Intravascular lymphomatosis is an extremely rare malignancy; it is a large-cell lymphoproliferative disorder that seldom involves the eye. It is a widespread intravascular aggregation of large B-cell lymphoma (though rare T-cell,[103–105] histiocytic,[106,107] and NK cell[108] lymphomas have been reported), and the prognosis is rather poor. It mostly affects the skin and CNS producing rather heterogeneous lesions in these tissues.[101,109] Elner and associates reported small, white retinal and choroidal infiltrates and retinal pigmentary alteration secondary to retinal and choroidal vascular occlusion in intravascular lymphomatosis.[110]

Other Ocular Non-Malignant Disease. A flecked appearance of subtle, whitish sub-pigment epithelial lesions in the retina may give the appearance of fundus flavimaculatus (Stargardt's Disease). However, such an appearance was produced, in fact, by systemic NHL that metastasized to the eye (secondary intraocular lymphoma).[111]

References

1. Cooper EL, Ricker JL. (1951) Malignant lymphoma of the uveal tract. *Am J Ophthalmol* **34**: 1153–1158.
2. Currey TA, Deutsch AR. (1965) Reticulum cell sarcoma of the uvea. *Southern Med J* **58**: 919.

3. Zimmerman HM. (1975) Malignant lymphomas of the nervous system. *Acta Neuropathol Suppl (Berl)* **Suppl 6**: 69–74.
4. Barr CC, Green WR, Payne JW, *et al.* (1975) Intraocular reticulum-cell sarcoma: clinico-pathologic study of four cases and review of the literature. *Surv Ophthalmol* **19**(4): 224–239.
5. Wagoner MD, Gonder JR, Albert DM, Canny CL. (1980) Ocular pathology for clinicians: 3. Intraocular reticulum cell sarcoma. *Ophthalmology* **87**(7): 724–727.
6. Marcus HC. (1963) Malignant lymphoma of the uveal tract. *Arch Ophthalmol* **69**: 251–253.
7. Nevins RC, Jr., Frey WW, Elliott JH. (1968) Primary, solitary, intraocular reticulum cell sarcoma (microgliomatosis). (A clinicopathologic case report.) *Trans Am Acad Ophthalmol Otolaryngol* **72**(6): 867–876.
8. Vogel MH, Font RL, Zimmerman LE, Levine RA. (1968) Reticulum cell sarcoma of the retina and uvea. Report of six cases and review of the literature. *Am J Ophthalmol* **66**(2): 205–215.
9. Minckler DS, Font RL, Zimmerman LE. (1975) Uveitis and reticulum cell sarcoma of brain with bilateral neoplastic seeding of vitreous without retinal or uveal involvement. *Am J Ophthalmol* **80**(3 Pt 1): 433–439.
10. Davis JL. (2004) Diagnosis of intraocular lymphoma. *Ocul Immunol Inflamm* **12**(1): 7–16.
11. Chan CC, Wallace DJ. (2004) Intraocular lymphoma: update on diagnosis and management. *Cancer Control* **11**(5): 285–295.
12. Hormigo A, DeAngelis LM. (2003) Primary intraocular lymphoma: Clinical features, diagnosis and treatment. *Clin Lymphoma* **4**(1): 22–29.
13. Levy-Clarke GA, Chan CC, Nussenblatt RB. (2005) Diagnosis and management of primary intraocular lymphoma. *Hematol Oncol Clin North Am* **19**(4): 739–749.
14. Read RW, Zamir E, Rao NA. (2002) Neoplastic masquerade syndromes. *Surv Ophthalmol* **47**(2): 81–124.
15. Rothova A, Ooijman F, Kerkhoff F, *et al.* (2001) Uveitis masquerade syndromes. *Ophthalmology* **108**(2): 386–399.
16. Zaldivar RA, Martin DF, Holden JT, Grossniklaus HE. (2004) Primary intraocular lymphoma: clinical, cytologic, and flow cytometric analysis. *Ophthalmology* **111**(9): 1762–1767.
17. Anderson T, Chabner BA, Young RC, *et al.* (1982) Malignant lymphoma. 1. The histology and staging of 473 patients at the National Cancer Institute. *Cancer* **50**(12): 2699–2707.
18. Shimoyama M, Oyama A, Tajima *et al.* (1993) Differences in clinicopathological characteristics and major prognostic factors between B-lymphoma

and peripheral T-lymphoma excluding adult T-cell leukemia/lymphoma. *Leuk Lymphoma* 10(4–5): 335–342.

19. Herrlinger U. (1999) Primary CNS lymphoma: findings outside the brain. *J Neurooncol* 43(3): 227–230.
20. Qualman SL, Mendelsohn G, Mann RB, Green WR. (1983) Intraocular lymphomas. Natural history based on a clinicopathologic study of eight cases and review of the literature. *Cancer* 52: 878–886.
21. Sander CA, Flaig MJ, Jaffe ES. (2001) Cutaneous manifestations of lymphoma: a clinical guide based on the WHO classification. World Health Organization. *Clin Lymphoma* 2(2): 86–100; discussion 101–102.
22. Siegel RS, Pandolfino T, Guitart J, *et al.* (2000) Primary cutaneous T-cell lymphoma: review and current concepts. *J Clin Oncol* 18(15): 2908–2925.
23. Erny BC, Egbert PR, Peat IM, *et al.* (1991) Intraocular involvement with subretinal pigment epithelium infiltrates by mycosis fungoides. *Br J Ophthalmol* 75(11): 698–701.
24. Stenson S, Ramsay DL. (1981) Ocular findings in mycosis fungoides. *Arch Ophthalmol* 99(2): 272–277.
25. Kazakov DV, Burg G, Kempf W. (2004) Clinicopathological spectrum of mycosis fungoides. *J Eur Acad Dermatol Venereol* 18(4): 397–415.
26. Hao D, DiFrancesco LM, Brasher PM, *et al.* (1999) Is primary CNS lymphoma really becoming more common? A population-based study of incidence, clinicopathological features and outcomes in Alberta from 1975 to 1996. *Ann Oncol* 10(1): 65–70.
27. Bataille B, Delwail V, Menet E, *et al.* (2000) Primary intracerebral malignant lymphoma: report of 248 cases. *J Neurosurg* 92(2): 261–266.
28. Laigle-Donadey F, Iraqi W, *et al.* (2005) Primary central nervous system lymphoma presenting with central neurogenic hyperventilation. A case report and review of the literature. *Rev Neurol (Paris)* 161(10): 940–948.
29. Whitcup SM, de Smet MD, Rubin BI, *et al.* (1993) Intraocular lymphoma. Clinical and histopathologic diagnosis. *Ophthalmology* 100: 1399–1406.
30. Bierman P, Giglio P. (2005) Diagnosis and treatment of central nervous system involvement in non-Hodgkin's lymphoma. *Hematol Oncol Clin North Am* 19(4): 597–609, v.
31. Lachance DH, O'Neill BP, Macdonald DR, *et al.* (1991) Primary leptomeningeal lymphoma: report of 9 cases, diagnosis with immunocytochemical analysis, and review of the literature. *Neurology* 41(1): 95–100.
32. Kawasaki K, Wakabayashi K, Koizumi T, *et al.* (2002) Spinal cord involvement of primary central nervous system lymphomas: histopathological examination of 14 autopsy cases. *Neuropathology* 22(1): 13–18.

33. Fine HA, Mayer RJ. (1993) Primary central nervous system lymphoma. *Ann Intern Med* 119(11): 1093–1104.
34. Akpek EK, Ahmed I, Hochberg FH, *et al.* (1999) Intraocular-central nervous system lymphoma: clinical features, diagnosis, and outcomes. *Ophthalmology* 106(9): 1805–1810.
35. Buggage RR, Chan CC, Nussenblatt RB. (2001) Ocular manifestations of central nervous system lymphoma. *Curr Opin Oncol* 13(3): 137–142.
36. Chan CC. (2003) Molecular pathology of primary intraocular lymphoma. *Trans Am Ophthalmol Soc* 101: 275–292.
37. Char DH, Ljung BM, Miller T, Phillips T. (1988) Primary intraocular lymphoma (ocular reticulum cell sarcoma) diagnosis and management. *Ophthalmology* 95: 625–630.
38. Char DH, Margolis L, Newman AB. (1981) Ocular reticulum cell sarcoma. *Am J Ophthalmol* 91(4): 480–483.
39. Freeman LN, Schachat AP, Knox DL, Michels RG, Green WR. (1987) Clinical features, laboratory investigations, and survival in ocular reticulum cell sarcoma. *Ophthalmology* 94: 1631–1639.
40. Hormigo A, Abrey L, Heinemann MH, DeAngelis LM. (2004) Ocular presentation of primary central nervous system lymphoma: diagnosis and treatment. *Br J Haematol* 126(2): 202–208.
41. Jahnke K, Korfel A, Komm J, *et al.* (2005) Intraocular lymphoma 2000–2005: results of a retrospective multicentre trial. *Graefes Arch Clin Exp Ophthalmol*: 1–7.
42. Siegel MJ, Dalton J, Friedman AH, *et al.* (1989) Ten-year experience with primary ocular 'reticulum cell sarcoma' (large cell non-Hodgkin's lymphoma). *Br J Ophthalmol* 73(5): 342–346.
43. Peterson K, Gordon KB, Heinemann MH, DeAngelis LM. (1993) The clinical spectrum of ocular lymphoma. *Cancer* 72(3): 843–849.
44. Matsuo T, Yamaoka A, Shiraga F, Matsuo N. (1998) Two types of initial ocular manifestations in intraocular-central nervous system lymphoma. *Retina* 18(4): 301–307.
45. Velez G, de Smet MD, Whitcup SM, *et al.* (2000) Iris involvement in primary intraocular lymphoma: report of two cases and review of the literature. *Surv Ophthalmol* 44(6): 518–526.
46. Wegelius C. (1964) Case findings and roentgen diagnostics of pulmonary sarcoidosis. *Acta Med Scand Suppl* 425: 92–95.
47. Szwarcberg JB, Glajchen N, Teirstein AS. (2005) Pleural involvement in chronic sarcoidosis detected by thoracic CT scanning. *Sarcoidosis Vasc Diffuse Lung Dis* 22(1): 58–62.
48. Ridley ME, McDonald HR, Sternberg P, Jr., *et al.* (1992) Retinal manifestations of ocular lymphoma (reticulum cell sarcoma). *Ophthalmology* 99(7): 1153–1160; discussion 1160–1151.

49. Lang GK, Surer JL, Green WR, *et al.* (1985) Ocular reticulum cell sarcoma. Clinicopathologic correlation of a case with multifocal lesions. *Retina* 5(2): 79–86.

50. Buggage RR, Velez G, Myers-Powell B, *et al.* (1999) Primary intraocular lymphoma with a low interleukin 10 to interleukin 6 ratio and heterogeneous IgH gene rearrangement. *Arch Ophthalmol* 117(9): 1239–1242.

51. Cassoux N, Merle-Beral H, Leblond V, *et al.* (2000) Ocular and central nervous system lymphoma: clinical features and diagnosis. *Ocul Immunol Inflamm* 8(4): 243–250.

52. Tuaillon N, Chan CC. (2001) Molecular analysis of primary central nervous system and primary intraocular lymphoma. *Curr Mol Med* 1(2): 259–272.

53. Char DH, Ljung BM, Deschenes J, Miller TR. (1988) Intraocular lymphoma: immunological and cytological analysis. *Br J Ophthalmol* 72(12): 905–911.

54. Gass JD, Sever RJ, Grizzard WS, *et al.* (1984) Multifocal pigment epithelial detachments by reticulum cell sarcoma. A characteristic funduscopic picture. *Retina* 4(3): 135–143.

55. Michelson JB, Michelson PE, Bordin GM, Chisari FV. (1981) Ocular reticulum cell sarcoma. Presentation as retinal detachment with demonstration of monoclonal immunoglobulin light chains on the vitreous cells. *Arch Ophthalmol* 99(8): 1409–1411.

56. Gass JD, Trattler HL. (1991) Retinal artery obstruction and atheromas associated with non-Hodgkin's large cell lymphoma (reticulum cell sarcoma). *Arch Ophthalmol* 109(8): 1134–1139.

57. Madhavan HN, Priya K, Bagyalakshmi R. (2003) Phenotypic and genotypic methods for the detection of herpes simplex virus serotypes. *J Virol Methods* 108(1): 97–102.

58. Madhavan HN, Priya K, Anand AR, Therese KL. (1999) Detection of herpes simplex virus (HSV) genome using polymerase chain reaction (PCR) in clinical samples comparison of PCR with standard laboratory methods for the detection of HSV. *J Clin Virol* 14(2): 145–151.

59. Dean JM, Novak MA, Chan CC, Green WR. (1996) Tumor detachments of the retinal pigment epithelium in ocular/central nervous system lymphoma. *Retina* 16(1): 47–56.

60. Loh KY, Ogle J. (2004) Age related visual impairment in the elderly. *Med J Malaysia* 59(4): 562–568; quiz 569.

61. Coupland SE, Heimann H, Bechrakis NE. (2004) Primary intraocular lymphoma: a review of the clinical, histopathological and molecular biological features. *Graefes Arch Clin Exp Ophthalmol* 242(11): 901–913.

62. Chan CC, Buggage RR, Nussenblatt RB. (2002) Intraocular lymphoma. *Curr Opin Ophthalmol* 13(6): 411–418.

63. Raju VK, Green WR. (1982) Reticulum cell sarcoma of the uvea. *Ann Ophthalmol* **14**(6): 555–560.
64. Henderly DE, Genstler AJ, Smith RE, Rao NA. (1987) Changing patterns of uveitis. *Am J Ophthalmol* **103**(2): 131–136.
65. Rothova A, Buitenhuis HJ, Meenken C, *et al.* (1992) Uveitis and systemic disease. *Br J Ophthalmol* **76**(3): 137–141.
66. Culbertson WW, Blumenkranz MS, Pepose JS, *et al.* (1986) Varicella zoster virus is a cause of the acute retinal necrosis syndrome. *Ophthalmology* **93**(5): 559–569.
67. Garweg J, Bohnke M. (1997) Varicella-zoster virus is strongly associated with atypical necrotizing herpetic retinopathies. *Clin Infect Dis* **24**(4): 603–608.
68. Hellinger WC, Bolling JP, Smith TF, Campbell RJ. (1993) Varicella-zoster virus retinitis in a patient with AIDS-related complex: case report and brief review of the acute retinal necrosis syndrome. *Clin Infect Dis* **16**(2): 208–212.
69. Kaiser PK, Lee MS, Martin DA. (2003) Occlusive vasculitis in a patient with concomitant West Nile virus infection. *Am J Ophthalmol* **136**(5): 928–930.
70. Garg S, Jampol LM. (2005) Systemic and intraocular manifestations of West Nile virus infection. *Surv Ophthalmol* **50**(1): 3–13.
71. Anninger WV, Lomeo MD, Dingle J, *et al.* (2003) West Nile virus-associated optic neuritis and chorioretinitis. *Am J Ophthalmol* **136**(6): 1183–1185.
72. de Smet MD, Nussenblatt RB, Davis JL, Palestine AG. (1990) Large cell lymphoma masquerading as a viral retinitis. *Int Ophthalmol* **14**(5–6): 413–417.
73. Margo CE, Hamed LM. (1992) Ocular syphilis. *Surv Ophthalmol* **37**(3): 203–220.
74. Poulsen A. (1950) Some clinical features of tuberculosis. 1. Incubation period. *Acta Tuberc Scand* **24**(3–4): 311–346.
75. Poulsen A. (1957) Some clinical features of tuberculosis. *Acta Tuberc Scand* **33**(1–2): 37–92; concl.
76. Arango L, Brewin AW, Murray JF. (1973) The spectrum of tuberculosis as currently seen in a metropolitan hospital. *Am Rev Respir Dis* **108**(4): 805–812.
77. Ormerod LD, Dailey JP. (1999) Ocular manifestations of cat-scratch disease. *Curr Opin Ophthalmol* **10**(3): 209–216.
78. Cunningham ET, Koehler JE. (2000) Ocular bartonellosis. *Am J Ophthalmol* **130**(3): 340–349.
79. Bar S, Segal M, Shapira R, Savir H. (1990) Neuroretinitis associated with cat scratch disease. *Am J Ophthalmol* **110**(6): 703–705.
80. Davis JL, Solomon D, Nussenblatt RB, *et al.* (1992) Immunocytochemical staining of vitreous cells. Indications, techniques, and results. *Ophthalmology* **99**(2): 250–256.

81. Priem HA, Oosterhuis JA. (1988) Birdshot chorioretinopathy: clinical characteristics and evolution. *Br J Ophthalmol* 72(9): 646–659.
82. LeHoang P, Ozdemir N, Benhamou A, *et al.* (1992) HLA-A29.2 subtype associated with birdshot retinochoroidopathy. *Am J Ophthalmol* 113(1): 33–35.
83. Rizzato G, Angi M, Fraioli P, *et al.* (1996) Uveitis as a presenting feature of chronic sarcoidosis. *Eur Respir J* 9(6): 1201–1205.
84. Obenauf CD, Shaw HE, Sydnor CF, Klintworth GK. (1978) Sarcoidosis and its ophthalmic manifestations. *Am J Ophthalmol* 86(5): 648–655.
85. James DG. (1986) Ocular sarcoidosis. *Ann N Y Acad Sci* 465: 551–563.
86. Behçet H. (1940) Some observations on clinical picture of the so-called triple symptom complex. *Dermatologica* 81: 73–83.
87. Tugal-Tutkun I, Onal S, Altan-Yaycioglu R, *et al.* (2004) Uveitis in Behcet disease: an analysis of 880 patients. *Am J Ophthalmol* 138(3): 373–380.
88. Haim S. (1968) Contribution of ocular symptoms in the diagnosis of Behcet's disease. Study of 23 cases. *Arch Dermatol* 98(5): 478–480.
89. Harada H. (1926) Beitrag zur klinischen kenntis von nichteitriger Choroiditis (Choroidtis diffusa acuta). *Acta Soc Ophthalmol Jpn* 30: 356–378.
90. Koyanagi Y. (1906) Dysakusis, alopecia und poliosis bei schwerer uveitis nicht traumatischen Ursprungs. *Klin Monatsbl Augenheilkd* 44: 228–242.
91. Vogt A. (1906) Fruhzeitiges Ergrauen der Zilien und Bemerkungen uber den sogenannten plotzlichen Eintritt diser Veranderung. *Klin Monatsbl Augenheilkd* 44: 228–242.
92. Rubsamen PE, Gass JD. (1991) Vogt-Koyanagi-Harada syndrome. Clinical course, therapy, and long-term visual outcome. *Arch Ophthalmol* 109(5): 682–687.
93. Coupland SE, Joussen A, Anastassiou G, Stein H. (2005) Diagnosis of a primary uveal extranodal marginal zone B-cell lymphoma by chorioretinal biopsy: case report. *Graefes Arch Clin Exp Ophthalmol* 243(5): 482–486.
94. Crookes GP, Mullaney J. (1967) Lymphoid hyperplasia of the uveal tract simulating malignant lymphoma. *Am J Ophthalmol* 63(5): 962–967.
95. Cheung MK, Martin DF, Chan CC, *et al.* (1994) Diagnosis of reactive lymphoid hyperplasia by choroidal biopsy. *Am J Ophthalmol* 118(4): 457–462.
96. Ryan SJ, Jr., Frank RN, Green WR. (1971) Bilateral inflammatory pseudotumors of the ciliary body. *Am J Ophthalmol* 72(3): 586–591.
97. Jakobiec FA, Sacks E, Kronish JW, *et al.* (1987) Multifocal static creamy choroidal infiltrates. An early sign of lymphoid neoplasia. *Ophthalmology* 94(4): 397–406.
98. Coupland SE, Anastassiou G, Bornfeld N, *et al.* (2005) Primary intraocular lymphoma of T-cell type: report of a case and review of the literature. *Graefes Arch Clin Exp Ophthalmol* 243(3): 189–197.

99. Wiznia RA, Freedman JK, Mancini AD, Shields JA. (1978) Malignant melanoma of the choroid in neurofibromatosis. *Am J Ophthalmol* **86**(5): 684–687.
100. Reeser FH, Aaberg TM, Van Horn DL. (1978) Astrocytic hamartoma of the retina not associated with tuberous sclerosis. *Am J Ophthalmol* **86**(5): 688–698.
101. Ferreri AJ, Campo E, Seymour JF, *et al.* (2004) Intravascular lymphoma: clinical presentation, natural history, management and prognostic factors in a series of 38 cases, with special emphasis on the 'cutaneous variant'. *Br J Haematol* **127**(2): 173–183.
102. Al-Hazzaa SAF, Green WR, Wann RB. (1993) Uveal involvement in systemic angiotropic large cell lymphoma. *Ophthalmology* **100**(6): 961–965.
103. Domizio P, Hall PA, Cotter F, *et al.* (1989) Angiotropic large cell lymphoma (ALCL): morphological, immunohistochemical and genotypic studies with analysis of previous reports. *Hematol Oncol* **7**(3): 195–206.
104. Ko YH, Han JH, Go JH, *et al.* (1997) Intravascular lymphomatosis: a clinicopathological study of two cases presenting as an interstitial lung disease. *Histopathology* **31**(6): 555–562.
105. Sepp N, Schuler G, Romani N, *et al.* (1990) "Intravascular lymphomatosis" (angioendotheliomatosis): evidence for a T-cell origin in two cases. *Hum Pathol* **21**(10): 1051–1058.
106. O'Grady JT, Shahidullah H, Doherty VR, al-Nafussi A. (1994) Intravascular histiocytosis. *Histopathology* **24**(3): 265–268.
107. Snowden JA, Angel CA, Winfield DA, *et al.* (1997) Angiotropic lymphoma: report of a case with histiocytic features. *J Clin Pathol* **50**(1): 67–70.
108. Wu H, Said JW, Ames ED, *et al.* (2005) First reported cases of intravascular large cell lymphoma of the NK cell type: clinical, histologic, immunophenotypic, and molecular features. *Am J Clin Pathol* **123**(4): 603–611.
109. Chapin JE, Davis LE, Kornfeld M, Mandler RN. (1995) Neurologic manifestations of intravascular lymphomatosis. *Acta Neurol Scand* **91**(6): 494–499.
110. Elner VM, Hidayat AA, Charles NC, *et al.* (1986) Neoplastic angioendotheliomatosis. A variant of malignant lymphoma immunohistochemical and ultrastructural observations of three cases. *Ophthalmology* **93**(9): 1237–1245.
111. Gass JD, Weleber RG, Johnson DR. (1987) Non-Hodgkin's lymphoma causing fundus picture simulating fundus flavimaculatus. *Retina* **7**(4): 209–214.

Chapter 6

Imaging

Imaging is the first step in evaluating diagnostic suspicion of PIOL. A variety of imaging modalities, some absolutely essential and others optional, may be used. These can provide the ophthalmologist with important clues (Table 6.1). As PIOL has a high possibility of involving the CNS, CNS imaging must be included and assessed.

Full Field Fundus Photography

Full field fundus photography is an important step in documenting the ophthalmoscopic features of PIOL. The characteristic lesions of PIOL, the creamy, yellow-white-to-orange sub-RPE infiltrates, can be photographed, giving the ophthalmologist a baseline lesion or lesions to follow. The number, shape, growth, confluence, and extension of these lesions into the sub-retinal space from the sub-RPE location,[1] or even their possible regression, can all be tracked with fundus photography. In addition, fundus photography can provide a record of the existence of retinal vasculitis, retinal edema, and optic nerve head changes, such as, optic disc infiltration and edema. Infiltration of the retina by lymphoma cells can result in retinal thickening. This causes the retina to lose its transparency, and the retina may look gray to white.[2] In a study of five patients with PIOL, initial retinal findings included vascular sheathing (40%), perivascular exudates (40%), deep white spots (60%), retinal thickening (40%), and a grayish-whitish color to the retina (40%).[2] Subsequent examinations showed hemorrhagic retinal infiltrates or necrosis (80%), exudative retinal detachment (60%), and macular scar development (20%).[2] These findings and their progression can easily be followed with fundus photography provided that the cataracts and media opacities, especially those from vitritis, are not severe.

Table 6.1 Imaging Modalities and their Importance

	Full Field Fundus Photography	U/S[1]	FA[2]	ICGA[3]	OCT[4]	Brain MRI[5]	Brain CT[6]	Chest X-Ray	Body CT/MRI
Essential	✓					✓	If MRI contra-indicated		
Often Necessary			✓						
Occasionally Necessary		✓						To rule out systemic disease (e.g., those that cause uveitis) or patients suspicious for systemic NHL (e.g., patients with prior history of systemic NHL)	To rule out systemic disease (e.g., those that cause uveitis) or patients suspicious for systemic NHL (e.g., patients with prior history of systemic NHL)
Optional			✓	✓	✓		✓	✓	✓
Utility not Described				✓	✓				

[1]U/S = ultrasound; [2]FA = fluorescein angiography; [3]ICGA = indocyanine green angiography; [4]OCT = ocular coherence tomography; [5]Brain MRI = Brain magnetic resonance imaging; [6]Brain CT = Brain computed tomography.

Ophthalmoscopic imaging is both necessary and important for evaluating PIOL.

Ultrasound

In cases where vitritis is severe (as when vitreous cells form clumps or sheets that obscure a view of the fundus) or a dense cataract precludes view of the fundus, one simple technique to begin with is B-scan ultrasonography. Ultrasound can help determine whether there are any masses or lesions intraocularly or extraocularly (e.g., associated with ocular adnexa as in extranodal marginal zone lymphoma). Intraocular masses visualized with ultrasonography may represent PIOL or may signal a systemic metastasis, such as a systemic NHL that has affected the eye, usually the choroid.[3,4] In addition, choroidal or subretinal masses may be visualized upon ophthalmoscopic examination and fundus photography, but details of the lesions may be unattainable due to overlying retinal changes, e.g. retinal detachments. Ultrasound can help further characterize these lesions. However, ultrasonography is nonspecific and while it may help in determining whether a process is occurring intra- or extraocularly, other modalities are more often employed to document PIOL. Nevertheless, there are some ultrasonographic features associated with PIOL. Vitreous cells, the most common feature of PIOL, may appear as vitreous debris upon ultrasound. Thickening of the choroid and sclera as well as chorioretinal lesions secondary to reactive inflammatory reaction may rarely be revealed. When significant infiltration by lymphoma cells occurs, exudative, serous, or bullous retinal detachments can occur. The retinal detachment may be partial or may be significant enough to be noted as a funnel retinal detachment on ultrasound. Of course, funnel and serous retinal detachments can occur in other secondary lymphomatous processes as well, such as those that can occur with extranodal marginal zone lymphoma (EMZL) of mucosa-associated lymphoid tissue (MALT) with intraocular involvement.[5,6] Primary uveal EMZL MALT can impart a low to medium reflectivity to a thickened choroid on ultrasound.[7] Ultrasound can help demonstrate how extensive the tumor is. Typically, a lymphomatous lesion will be low-reflective.[8] As the lesion of PIOL is not vascularized, color Doppler imaging would not be expected to show vascularity in this case as compared with cases of systemic metastases.[3] In primary uveal lymphoma, ultrasonographic features may be different than those in

PIOL and can include choroidal changes, such as diffuse thickening of the choroid and serous detachment.[9] However, even in PIOL there can be choroidal or scleral thickening.[1]

A few case series exist on the ultrasonographic features of PIOL. Ursea and colleagues performed both A- and B-scan ultrasonography on 16 eyes in 13 patients with PIOL.[10] Vitreous debris was the most common ultrasonographic finding, with 87.5% of the eyes exhibiting this feature. Vitreous debris was evidenced by low reflective scattered echoes within the vitreous. Half of the eyes studied showed choroidal and scleral thickening and a quarter of the eyes showed a widened optic nerve shadow on ultrasound. Irregular retrobulbar fat, an elevated lesion, retinal detachment, and Tenon capsule accentuation were each found in 18.7% of the eyes. Posterior vitreous detachment was found in 12.5% of the eyes, and a vitreous membrane was found in one eye (6.2%).

While ultrasound is a useful tool that can help the ophthalmologist view the extent of lesions or disease not viewed during slit lamp or ophthalmoscopic examination, many of its findings, such as, vitreous debris and choroidal thickening are non-specific. For example, vitreous debris can certainly be due to uveitis of myriad etiologies and choroidal thickening can be due to other tumors. Therefore, other imaging techniques are more commonly employed, including fluorescein angiography and magnetic resonance imaging (MRI). Nevertheless, ultrasound can help an ophthalmologist consider whether a lymphomatous process is likely affecting the eye and, importantly, it can be used to document response to treatment.

While definitely useful in some instances, ultrasound is an optional imaging test in PIOL and is not routinely obtained when this diagnosis is pursued.

Fluorescein Angiography

Often when no retinal lesions are identified during direct or indirect ophthalmoscopic exam, fluorescein angiography may provide useful clues. Fluorescein angiography (FA) is widely used in retinal vascular diseases, such as diabetic retinopathy, choroidal neovascularization, and retinal vasculitis. Even when obvious retinal lesions are present, such as the characteristic creamy yellow-whitish sub-RPE infiltrates, FA is an important tool in confirming an ophthalmologist's suspicion of a malignant lymphoid process. FA in PIOL seems to have a characteristic appearance. Commonly, RPE disturbances are noted and include granularity, mottling, and late staining patterns.[11,12] "Leopard spot" patterns have also been described,[13] although this term has been used to describe the hyperfluorescent spots in ocular syphilis.[14,15] Blockage of fluorescence at the level of the RPE, termed mottling, due to tumor infiltration can correspond to the deep retinal or subretinal creamy colored lesions noted on fundus photography. Early staining of the subretinal infiltrates may show nonfluorescence[1] as viable tumor cells are not easily penetrated by fluorescein dye because their cell membranes remain intact.[16] Late staining may show some weak staining of the borders of the lesions or incomplete staining of the lesions, imparting a hypofluorescent appearance. Late staining may also occur near the macula or outside the macula.[1,2,17,18] FA is also used to confirm the location of the lesions as being at the level of the RPE.[2] In areas where tumor infiltration has caused detachment of the overlying RPE and retina, blocked fluorescence will be noted and there may be staining at the detachment's borders.[19] There may also be small hyperfluorescent lesions representing window defects from RPE atrophy.[2] The combination of blocked fluorescence and hyperfluorescence produces a pattern of granularity.[2,12] Small branch artery occlusions, which have been noted to occasionally occur in PIOL,[20] can be documented with FA.[2] In a study of five patients with PIOL, Ridley *et al.* found FA to be important in documenting retinal changes over time.[2] For example, in some patients there was vascular sheathing with little perivascular exudate and leakage on initial FA. When FA was performed at a later stage, vascular leakage had increased. However, others have reported that vascular leakage is less common in PIOL compared with inflammatory conditions.[12] Velez *et al.* analyzed the angiographic findings of 31 eyes in 17 patients at the National Eye Institute (NEI).[12] The most common angiographic finding was disturbance of the RPE in 65% of the eyes. RPE disturbances included granularity, late staining at the level of the RPE, and blockage of fluorescence. Unlike viable tumor, nonviable tumor cells will take up fluorescein dye and can appear hyperfluorescent. FA has been shown to reveal RPE changes when none were noted upon ophthalmoscopic examination in patients with vitritis.[12] Importantly, although FA is a valuable tool in the diagnosis of PIOL, occasionally no abnormalities are noted in patients with PIOL. For example, in the study by Velez *et al.* 14% of the eyes with histopathologically proven PIOL had no abnormalities noted on FA, although vitritis was noted on fundsocopic examination.[12] In France, Cassoux and colleagues reported on various features of patients with PIOL and PCNSL, including FA findings in 44 patients.[11] The most common FA findings were window defects and round, hypofluorescent lesions in 54.5% of the patients. Round hyperfluorescent lesions were the second most common angiographic finding, seen in 34% of the patients. Retinal vasculiitis was found in 13.63% of the patients, with half of this group having occlusive vasculitis. Papilledema and cystoid macular edema were the least common features, being seen in 3.70% and 2.46% of the patients, respectively. FA showed utility in uncovering retinal lesions in 5% of the patients who had no lesions noted on ophthalmoscopic examination.

Therefore, while FA is not an essential imaging test in PIOL, it may be helpful to determine the extent of tumor infiltration and magnitude of RPE atrophy. Table 6.2 summarizes three large series of PIOL with FA.[11,12,21]

Indocyanine Green Fluorescein Angiography

Indocyanine green angiography (ICG) is an excellent tool for visualizing the choroidal vasculature. ICG is typically used in evaluating subretinal and choroidal disease processes, but the use of ICG for PIOL has not been well described to our knowledge nor has its use in this lymphomatous lesion been determined. In other diseases, especially the posterior uveitides that can mimic some of the findings in PIOL, however, ICG can be a useful adjunctive study.[22] For example, ICG has been shown in some cases to reveal lesions in ocular syphilis, which can mimic PIOL, when none were found in FA.[15] Abnormalities revealed by ICG include hyperfluorescent spots and hyperfluorescence of retinal vessels, and the resolution of these lesions can be followed with ICG.[15] It is used in the diagnosis of Behçet disease, another clinical entity that can have similar manifestations as PIOL. Hyperfluorescent spots and hypofluorescent plaques, filling defects of and leakage from the choroid, and irregular filling of the choriocapillaris have been described.[23,24] However, the ICG findings in Behçet disease are nonspecific. Ocular tuberculosis may be evaluated using ICG,[25,26] although, again, the lesions and fluorescence patterns revealed are not specific to this disease. In Vogt-Koyanagi-Harada (VKH) disease, ICG can be

Table 6.2 Fluorescein Angiogram Findings from Larger Case Series

Author	# Pts	FA Findings	Subclinical Lesions	No Lesions
Whitcup[21]	7	Punctate hyperfluorescent window defects in posterior pole at level of RPE Hypo- and hyperfluorescent lesions in some patients 1 patient with lesions showing blocked fluorescence during early phase of FA progressing to hyperfluorescence during late phase Macular edema in 3 patients (43%)Retinal vasculitis in 1 patient (14%)	Yes, number not specified	Not stated
Cassoux[11]	44	Round hyperfluorescent window defects in 24 patients (54.5%) Round hypofluorescent lesions in 15 patients (34%) Vasculitis in 6 patients (13.63%), which was occlusive in 3 Papilledema in 3 patients (3.70%) Cystoid macular edema (2.46%)	Yes, in 4 patients (5%)	Yes, in 4 patients (5%)
Velez[12]	17	RPE disturbances • Granularity in 19 eyes (61%) • Blockage of fluorescence in 17 eyes (55%) • Late staining in 14 eyes (45%) Optic nerve staining/leakage in 14 eyes (45%) Peripheral punctate hyperfluorescent lesions in 8 eyes (8%) Pigment epithelial detachments appearing either hyper- or hypofluorescent in 6 eyes (19%) Cystoid macular edema in 6 eyes (19%) Perivascular staining/leakage in 2 eyes (6%)	Yes, in 3 patients [4 eyes (13%)]	Yes, in 4 patients [4 eyes (13%)]

used to follow new or recurrent disease[27,28] and has also been used in sarcoidosis to reveal lesions not found in FA.[29] A characteristic ICG pattern consisting of hypofluorescent dark spots in both active and chronic, treated disease has been described.[30,31] In choroidal tumors, ICG can help in making the diagnosis,[32] perhaps differentiating these lesions from those of PIOL, which occur sub-RPE rather than choroidally.

Although ICG can offer an insight into understanding chorioretinal diseases, one systematic review of the literature on the use of ICG in chorioretinal diseases noted that no clinical trials have shown any benefit of ICG in diagnosing, managing, or treating any specific chorioretinal disease. There have yet to be reports examining any ICG features in PIOL. Considering that some lesions in other chorioretinal processes were exposed in ICG when they were subclinical during ophthalmoscopic examination and absent during FA, perhaps ICG may also uncover subclinical lesions in PIOL.

Ocular Coherence Tomography

To our knowledge, no case series exists on ocular coherence tomography (OCT) findings in PIOL. However, there are case reports on the use of this imaging modality. Interestingly, one report deals with a pediatric patient, 15 years of age.[33] Prior to initiation of corticosteroid and radiation therapy, OCT was taken of each eye. This showed RPE elevation and sub-RPE fluid. The OCT also revealed a relatively normal retinal architecture, save for the fact that it was detached due to the underlying fluid. It should be noted that B-scan ultrasonography showed similar findings, although with less detail of the retinal architecture than the OCT. After radiation therapy, OCT showed resolution of the subretinal fluid and neurosensory detachment. Because PIOL characteristically occurs in the sub-RPE space, OCT would also be expected to reveal a mass in this region, while systemic metastases would be expected to be found as optically dense masses in the choroid. However, there are reports of systemic metastases localizing only to the retina. They appear as optically dense lesions within the retina and with a distinct absence of tumor in the subretinal space and choroid.[34]

Astrocytic hamartomas, which could possibly be a differential diagnosis for PIOL (see Chapter 5 — Clinical Manifestations of PIOL), appear to have a characteristic appearance. An optically dense mound is noted with the anterior retinal surface appearing thickened and homogeneous, while the posterior surface appears "moth eaten."[35] When calcification has occurred within the astrocytic hamartoma, there will be high reflectivity of the mass.[35] Although the lesion of PIOL may resemble the lesion of an astrocytic hamartoma on casual observation of an OCT study, close inspection should enable the ophthalmologist to differentiate between these two lesions.

OCT enables one to analyze the cross sectional area of a retinal lesion, but the utility of OCT as an adjunctive test in PIOL has not been determined. Due to its higher cost compared with ultrasound, when a patient has media opacities that preclude adequate view of retinal, subretinal, or choroidal lesions, ultrasound can be performed as a first line imaging modality. When other tumors are high on the differential, an OCT may be considered to analyze the retinal architecture.

Brain Imaging

When PIOL is suspected, it is imperative to determine if there is cerebral involvement. As about 20% of PCNSL cases eventually have ocular involvement and 80% of PIOL cases eventuate to cerebral involvement, it is imperative that there is no occurrence of disease outside of the eyes as treatment modalities and prognosis will then be affected (see Chapter 10 — Management and Treatment). Computed tomographic (CT) scan or magnetic resonance imaging (MRI) are two imaging techniques that can help to identify lesions both in the CNS and the eye (whether intraocular or retrobulbar). Generally, gadolinium-enhanced MRI is recommended over CT.[36] Patients with CNS disease may have either a single lesion or multiple lesions that either have discrete or more diffuse borders.[37] The lesions may have well demarcated borders, but borders can be indistinct.[38]

Immunocompetent patients frequently have solitary lesions,[39] especially on first imaging. Later, multiple lesions may develop. By contrast, the PCNSL lesions found upon first imaging in AIDS patients can be either solitary or multiple, with multiplicity being more common in this population than in the immunocompetent group.[40,41] CNS disease in AIDS patients can produce a diagnostic dilemma as lesions can appear heterogeneous and as ring enhancing lesions. This makes it impossible to differentiate them from lesions of toxoplasmosis, an opportunistic infection that commonly afflicts this group of patients.[37,42,43] In such cases, positron emission tomography (PET),[44] proton magnetic resonance spectroscopy (MRS),[45] and/or perfusion (MR perfusion), and thallium 201 single photon-computed tomography (SPECT)[46] can be used to further differentiate between the two disease processes. In both immunocompetent and immuno-compromised patients, the cerebral lesions in PIOL are usually located supratentorally and periventricularly.[39,47] Major brain structures that are affected by lymphomatous infiltration include the basal ganglia, thalamus, and corpus callosum, with some suggesting that involvement of the corpus callosum is highly suggestive of PCNSL.[39] There is typically a lack of necrosis, calcification, and moderate to absent peritumoral edema.[48,49] Infratentorial structures that may be affected by PCNSL include the cerebellum.

CT Imaging. It is recommended that if CT is used, contrast be administered. Only 10% of lesions are detected on noncontrast CT.[50,51] The lesions of PIOL typically are isodense or hyperdense on CT with contrast administration. When intravenous contrast agent is used, the lesions enhance homogeneously. In a study of 20 patients with PCNSL, single enhancing lesions were the most common finding, with the frontal lobe being the most commonly affected.[52] However, MRI revealed that involvement was actually more extensive than noted on CT scan in two of the cases.

MRI Imaging. PIOL lesions appear hypointense on T1-weighted MRI and isointesnse or hyperintense on T2-weighted imaging. The use of gadolinium enhances the intensity of the lesions,[53,54] and the lesions typically enhance homogeneously. Some T2-weighted lesions do stain hypointense, and there may be a peritumorous area of hyperintensity representing a small amount of parenchymal edema. Aside from exposing parenchymal involvement of the brain, MRI is also a good imaging technique to reveal PIOL in the eyes, leptomeninges, and spinal cord.

MRI, then, is absolutely essential in PIOL and PCNSL. This imaging modality provides the ophthalmologist with information as to whether the disease is located solely intraocularly or has affected other parts of the CNS as well. This is critical because if the brain, cerebellum, and/or spinal cord are affected, the ophthalmologist will definitely need to coordinate treatment of the patient with a neuro-oncologist.

Systemic Imaging

In cases where systemic lymphoma with metastasis to the eye is suspected or in patients with a prior history of systemic lymphoma, systemic imaging may be pursued to detect visceral disease. Obtaining images of systemic organs is generally not necessary for cases of suspected PIOL or PCNSL, and this practice is not highly recommended.[55-58]

When there is good reason to suspect a systemic lymphoma, systemic imaging should begin with a chest X-ray in addition to standard tests, such as, complete blood cell count, erythrocyte sedimentation rate, blood chemistries and bone marrow evaluation.[59] Further imaging studies might include body CT, but clinical history and physical examination will help direct the imaging of the organ or organs that are likely be involved in systemic disease.

References

1. Gass JD, Sever RJ, Grizzard WS, *et al.* (1984) Multifocal pigment epithelial detachments by reticulum cell sarcoma. A characteristic funduscopic picture. *Retina* 4(3): 135–143.
2. Ridley ME, McDonald HR, Sternberg P, Jr, *et al.* (1992) Retinal manifestations of ocular lymphoma (reticulum cell sarcoma). *Ophthalmology* 99(7): 1153–1160; discussion 1160–1151.
3. Apte RS A-AN, Green WR, Schachat AP, *et al.* (2005) Systemic non-Hodgkin B-cell lymphoma encountered as a vanishing choroidal mass. *Arch Ophthalmol* 123(1): 105–109.
4. Read RW, Zamir E, Rao NA. (2002) Neoplastic masquerade syndromes. *Surv Ophthalmol* 47(2): 81–124.
5. Sarraf D, Jain A, Dubovy S, *et al.* (2005) Mucosa-associated lymphoid tissue lymphoma with intraocular involvement. *Retina* 25(1): 94–98.
6. Coupland SE, Joussen A, Anastassiou G, Stein H. (2005) Diagnosis of a primary uveal extranodal marginal zone B-cell lymphoma by chorioretinal biopsy: case report. *Graefes Arch Clin Exp Ophthalmol* 243(5): 482–486.
7. Jakobiec FA, Sacks E, Kronish JW, *et al.* (1987) Multifocal static creamy choroidal infiltrates. An early sign of lymphoid neoplasia. *Ophthalmology* 94(4): 397–406.

8. Coupland SE, Anastassiou G, Bornfeld N, *et al.* (2005) Primary intraocular lymphoma of T-cell type: report of a case and review of the literature. *Graefes Arch Clin Exp Ophthalmol* 243(3): 189–197.

9. Cheung MK, Martin DF, Chan CC, *et al.* (1994) Diagnosis of reactive lymphoid hyperplasia by choroidal biopsy. *Am J Ophthalmol* 118(4): 457–462.

10. Ursea R, Heinemann MH, Silverman RH, *et al.* (1997) Ophthalmic, ultrasonographic findings in primary central nervous system lymphoma with ocular involvement. *Retina* 17(2): 118–123.

11. Cassoux N, Merle-Beral H, Leblond V, *et al.* (2000) Ocular and central nervous system lymphoma: clinical features and diagnosis. *Ocul Immunol Inflamm* 8(4): 243–250.

12. Velez G, Chan CC, Csaky KG. (2002) Fluorescein angiographic findings in primary intraocular lymphoma. *Retina* 22(1): 37–43.

13. Fahim DK, Bucher R, Johnson MW. (2005) The elusive nature of primary intraocular lymphoma. *J Neuroophthalmol* 25(1): 33–36.

14. Gass JD, Braunstein RA, Chenoweth RG. (1990) Acute syphilitic posterior placoid chorioretinitis. *Ophthalmology* 97(10): 1288–1297.

15. Mora P, Borruat FX, Guex-Crosier Y. (2005) Indocyanine green angiography anomalies in ocular syphilis. *Retina* 25(2): 171–181.

16. Gass JD. (1972) Fluorescein angiography. An aid in the differential diagnosis of intraocular tumors. *Int Ophthalmol Clin* 12(1): 85–120.

17. Peterson K, Gordon KB, Heinemann MH, DeAngelis LM. (1993) The clinical spectrum of ocular lymphoma. *Cancer* 72(3): 843–849.

18. Kirmani MH, Thomas EL, Rao NA, Laborde RP. (1987) Intraocular reticulum cell sarcoma: diagnosis by choroidal biopsy. *Br J Ophthalmol* 71(10): 748–752.

19. Dean JM, Novak MA, Chan CC, Green WR. (1996) Tumor detachments of the retinal pigment epithelium in ocular/ central nervous system lymphoma. *Retina* 16(1): 47–56.

20. Gass JD, Trattler HL. (1991) Retinal artery obstruction and atheromas associated with non-Hodgkin's large cell lymphoma (reticulum cell sarcoma). *Arch Ophthalmol* 109(8): 1134–1139.

21. Whitcup SM, de Smet MD, Rubin BI, *et al.* (1993) Intraocular lymphoma. Clinical and histopathologic diagnosis. *Ophthalmology* 100: 1399–1406.

22. Garcia-Saenz MC, Gili Manzanaro P, Banuelos Banuelos J, *et al.* (2003) [Indocyanine green angiography in chorioretinal inflammatory diseases]. *Arch Soc Esp Oftalmol* 78(12): 675–683.

23. Gedik S, Akova Y, Yilmaz G, Bozbeyoglu S. (2005) Indocyanine green and fundus fluorescein angiographic findings in patients with active ocular Behcet's disease. *Ocul Immunol Inflamm* 13(1): 51–58.

24. Atmaca LS, Sonmez PA. (2003) Fluorescein and indocyanine green angiography findings in Behcet's disease. *Br J Ophthalmol* 87(12): 1466–1468.
25. Tayanc E, Akova Y, Yilmaz G. (2004) Indocyanine green angiography in ocular tuberculosis. *Ocul Immunol Inflamm* 12(4): 317–322.
26. Wolfensberger TJ, Piguet B, Herbort CP. (1999) Indocyanine green angiographic features in tuberculous chorioretinitis. *Am J Ophthalmol* 127(3): 350–353.
27. Bouchenaki N, Herbort CP. (2001) The contribution of indocyanine green angiography to the appraisal and management of Vogt-Koyanagi-Harada disease. *Ophthalmology* 108(1): 54–64.
28. Oshima Y, Harino S, Hara Y, Tano Y. (1996) Indocyanine green angiographic findings in Vogt-Koyanagi-Harada disease. *Am J Ophthalmol* 122(1): 58–66.
29. Matsuo T, Itami M, Shiraga F. (2000) Choroidopathy in patients with sarcoidosis observed by simultaneous indocyanine green and fluorescein angiography. *Retina* 20(1): 16–21.
30. Fardeau C, Herbort CP, Kullmann N, *et al.* (1999) Indocyanine green angiography in birdshot chorioretinopathy. *Ophthalmology* 106(10): 1928–1934.
31. Howe LJ, Stanford MR, Graham EM, Marshall J. (1997) Choroidal abnormalities in birdshot chorioretinopathy: an indocyanine green angiography study. *Eye* 11 (**Pt 4**): 554–559.
32. Kubicka-Trzaska A, Starzycka M, Romanowska-Dixon B. (2002) Indocyanine green angiography in the diagnosis of small choroidal tumours. *Ophthalmologica* 216(5): 316–319.
33. Sobrin L, Dubovy SR, Davis JL, Murray TG. (2005) Isolated, bilateral intraocular lymphoma in a 15-year-old girl. *Retina* 25(3): 370–373.
34. Truong SN, Fern CM, Costa DL, Spaide RF. (2002) Metastatic breast carcinoma to the retina: optical coherence tomography findings. *Retina* 22(6): 813–815.
35. Shields CL, Materin MA, Shields JA. (2005) Review of optical coherence tomography for intraocular tumors. *Curr Opin Ophthalmol* 16(3): 141–154.
36. Bierman P, Giglio P. (2005) Diagnosis and treatment of central nervous system involvement in non-Hodgkin's lymphoma. *Hematol Oncol Clin North Am* 19(4): 597–609, v.
37. Fitzsimmons A, Upchurch K, Batchelor T. (2005) Clinical features and diagnosis of primary central nervous system lymphoma. *Hematol Oncol Clin North Am* 19(4): 689–703.
38. Braus DF, Schwechheimer K, Muller-Hermelink HK, *et al.* (1992) Primary cerebral malignant non-Hodgkin's lymphomas: a retrospective clinical study. *J Neurol* 239(3): 117–124.

39. Bataille B, Delwail V, Menet E, *et al.* (2000) Primary intracerebral malignant lymphoma: report of 248 cases. *J Neurosurg* 92(2): 261–266.
40. Hochberg FH, Miller DC. (1988) Primary central nervous system lymphoma. *J Neurosurg* 68(6): 835–853.
41. Fine HA, Mayer RJ. (1993) Primary central nervous system lymphoma. *Ann Intern Med* 119(11): 1093–1104.
42. Chang L, Cornford ME, Chiang FL, *et al.* (1995) Radiologic-pathologic correlation. Cerebral toxoplasmosis and lymphoma in AIDS. *AJNR Am J Neuroradiol* 16(8): 1653–1663.
43. Ernst TM, Chang L, Witt MD, *et al.* (1998) Cerebral toxoplasmosis and lymphoma in AIDS: perfusion MR imaging experience in 13 patients. *Radiology* 208(3): 663–669.
44. Hoffman JM, Waskin HA, Schifter T, *et al.* (1993) FDG-PET in differentiating lymphoma from nonmalignant central nervous system lesions in patients with AIDS. *J Nucl Med* 34(4): 567–575.
45. Chinn RJ, Wilkinson ID, Hall-Craggs MA, *et al.* (1995) Toxoplasmosis and primary central nervous system lymphoma in HIV infection: diagnosis with MR spectroscopy. *Radiology* 197(3): 649–654.
46. Lorberboym M, Estok L, Machac J, *et al.* (1996) Rapid differential diagnosis of cerebral toxoplasmosis and primary central nervous system lymphoma by thallium-201 SPECT. *J Nucl Med* 37(7): 1150–1154.
47. Blay JY, Conroy T, Chevreau C, *et al.* (1998) High-dose methotrexate for the treatment of primary cerebral lymphomas: analysis of survival and late neurologic toxicity in a retrospective series. *J Clin Oncol* 16(3): 864–871.
48. Korfel A, Finke J, Schmidt-Wolf I, Thiel E. (2001) 5. Report on workshop: primary CNS lymphoma. *Ann Hematol* 80 Suppl 3: B20–23.
49. Jellinger KA, Paulus W. (1992) Primary central nervous system lymphomas — an update. *J Cancer Res Clin Oncol* 119(1): 7–27.
50. Thomas M, MacPherson P. (1982) Computed tomography of intracranial lymphoma. *Clin Radiol* 33(3): 331–336.
51. Cellerier P, Chiras J, Gray F, *et al.* (1984) Computed tomography in primary lymphoma of the brain. *Neuroradiology* 26(6): 485–492.
52. Grote TH, Grosh WW, List AF, *et al.* (1989) Primary lymphoma of the central nervous system. A report of 20 cases and a review of the literature. *Am J Clin Oncol* 12(2): 93–100.
53. Buhring U, Herrlinger U, Krings T, *et al.* (2001) MRI features of primary central nervous system lymphomas at presentation. *Neurology* 57(3): 393–396.
54. Gliemroth J, Kehler U, Gaebel C, *et al.* (2003) Neuroradiological findings in primary cerebral lymphomas of non-AIDS patients. *Clin Neurol Neurosurg* 105(2): 78–86.

55. Freeman LN, Schachat AP, Knox DL, *et al.* (1987) Clinical features, laboratory investigations, and survival in ocular reticulum cell sarcoma. *Ophthalmology* **94**: 1631–1639.

56. Nasir S, DeAngelis LM. (2000) Update on the management of primary CNS lymphoma. *Oncology (Huntingt)* **14**(2): 228–234; discussion 237–242, 244.

57. Schabet M. (1999) Epidemiology of primary CNS lymphoma. *J Neurooncol* **43**(3): 199–201.

58. Levy-Clarke GA, Chan CC, Nussenblatt RB. (2005) Diagnosis and management of primary intraocular lymphoma. *Hematol Oncol Clin North Am* **19**(4): 739–749.

59. Buggage RR, Chan CC, Nussenblatt RB. (2001) Ocular manifestations of central nervous system lymphoma. *Curr Opin Oncol* **13**(3): 137–142.

Chapter 7

Pathology

Today, many tests are available to us to determine the pathologic nature of a cell (e.g., expression of oncogenic signals), but one of the primary modes of identifying neoplastic cells is by conventional pathological (cytological or histological) examination. This literally means looking at the cell for features of neoplasia under light microscopy. In fact, diagnosing PIOL requires histologic diagnosis of the existence of lymphoma cells.

Cytology

The cytology of vitreous or CSF is often required for the diagnosis of PIOL or PCNSL. The neoplastic cells that comprise PCNSL and PIOL have a characteristic appearance. The cells of PCNSL and PIOL are atypical lymphocytes. These cells are large and may be twice the size and up to five times the diameter of a small lymphocyte. Using Giemsa or Diff Quick staining, the nucleus is large such that there is scant basophilic cytoplasm (high nucleus-to-cytoplasm ratio).[1,2] The nucleus can be round to oval in shape and often has in-foldings. Using Papanicolaou staining, some have described the nuclear in-foldings as producing a "nose-like" appearance,[3] and some nuclei indeed look like a bulbous nose viewed in profile or are reminiscent of a shape more cerebriform. These lymphoma cells may also have segmented nuclei, and this can produce a clover leaf appearance.[4,5] Rather than consisting solely of euchromatin or heterochromatin, the nuclear chromatin is heterogeneous and coarse; unevenly distributed granules can be found throughout the nucleus. Frequently, multiple, irregular nucleoli are prominently identified.[3,6] Indeed, these four features are used as cytologic criteria to diagnose PIOL by pathologists and ophthalmologists.[4,6–14] Mitotic figures are occasionally seen.[2,15–17] However, the demonstration of the "owl-eye" or "popcorn" cell, characteristic of the Reed-Sternberg cell of Hodgkin's lymphoma, should prompt a hunt for Hodgkin's disease elsewhere in the body.

In vitrectomy (vitreous) or lumbar puncture (CSF) samples, inflammatory cells are often seen. Macrophages may be intermixed with the lymphoma cells. The macrophage, which is also large and approximately the same size as or larger than the lymphoma cell, can be identified because it has much more abundant cytoplasm than the lymphoma cell. In addition, the cytoplasm of the macrophage is vesicular, giving the cytoplasm a foamy appearance. Reactive lymphocytes are present; they vary from small to large proliferative lymphocytes, most of which are T-cells. Another prominent feature is the presence of necrosis of the lymphoma cells among the viable PIOL cells.

While the identification of lymphoma cells may seem relatively simple, making a confident diagnosis of PCNSL or PIOL is hampered by the dearth of lymphoma cells or necrosis. In addition, necrotic debris may represent the main component of the specimen, making it difficult for the histopathologist to identify PCNSL or PIOL cells.[2,18–20] The lymphoma cells of PIOL and PCNSL are very fragile, and if systemic corticosteroids have been used to treat a presumed "uveitis," the lymphoma cells may be even more fragile. In many cases, necrotic debris characterizes the CSF or vitrectomy sample, although less necrotic debris is found in CSF samples.[4] Cells undergoing apoptosis are frequently found. In addition, karryorhectic cells may be seen. Smaller, round lymphocytes (reactive lymphocytes), macrophages, and polymorphonuclear lymphocytes may also be present as a reactive inflammatory infiltrate.[21] However, despite this "muddy" picture, a small number of lymphoma cells may still be identified, sealing the diagnosis of PCNSL/PIOL. Identification of lymphoma cells obviously requires an experienced histocytologist.

Further testing of lymphoma cells can include immunohistochemistry and flow cytometry to identify the B- or T-cell (rare) lineage monoclonality of the lymphomatous cells. B-PIOL cells are frequently monoclonal, bearing either kappa or lambda light chain. T-cell PIOL produces additional diagnostic difficulties because the neoplastic cells in this process can range in size from small to large and present a picture not unlike a reactive inflammation; however, they bare monoclonal T-cell receptor (TCR) on their surface.[22]

Vitrectomy specimens from cases of uveitis may share some similarities with those of PIOL, but reactive inflammatory cells will predominate and there will be an absence of malignant cells. Indeed, Char noted that in PIOL vitrectomy specimens, there was not a large inflammatory infiltrate.[7,8] Non-granulomatous uveitic cases will have a lymphohistiocytic infiltrate, while uveitic cases of a granulomatous nature will have in addition epithelioid histiocytes (macrophages) and multinucleated giant cells. In Zaldivar's cytologic evaluation of three cases of uveitis and seven cases of PIOL/PCNSL, the distinct difference between the two disease processes was the existence of pleomorphic cells with large nuclei and very little cytoplasm in the PIOL/PCNSL cases.[18] Clinical history and examination should provide helpful hints for the diagnosis.

Ocular Pathology

Macroscopic Inspection. The majority of findings upon gross inspection of the eye with PIOL are concentrated in the subretina and retina. The subretinal space may be thickened and identified with an infiltrating white mass. The retina itself may have thinned due to underlying tumor destruction, and retinal pigment epithelium (RPE) detachments may be noted.[23] In areas where lymphomatous lesions have resolved, RPE atrophy or disciform scarring may be noted. Lymphomatous cells may infiltrate the retina, causing a thickened appearance and can also be found perivascularly.[24] In addition, tumor infiltration may be found in the vitreous and optic nerve.[1] Necrosis is present inside the large foci of PIOL.

Choroidal and scleral involvement is extremely rare in PIOL, but has been described. For example, Cummings described a 57-year-old woman who noted the onset of floaters in her left eye.[25] After moving between diagnoses of macular degeneration and uveitis (with topical corticosteroid treatment), pars plana vitrectomy (PPV) revealed a T-cell reactive process, while a later fine-needle aspiration of a subretinal infiltrate revealed some rare atypical cells. However, the eye became blind and enucleation was performed to enable pathologic inspection. It was found that the tumor had not only infiltrated the choroid, but had invaded through this structure and showed a number of foci that had penetrated the inner sclera.

The iris, another structure that is extremely rarely involved in PIOL, may show stromal thickening and nodularity in areas of tumor infiltration.[13]

Velez and colleagues described two cases of rare iridal involvement at the National Eye Institute.[13] One PIOL case had an iris biopsy performed that revealed stromal infiltration with lymphoma cells; these lymphoma cells were also noted to locate perivascularly around the iridal vessels. In the second PIOL case, a patient displayed a thickened, heterochromic iris of the right eye in association with PIOL. Similar to the first case, the iris biopsy showed diffuse iris stromal infiltration with large pleomorphic cells. Reactive inflammatory cells were also present. These cases underscore the importance of iris biopsy to make the diagnosis of PIOL in suspect cases, where previous PPV failed to yield a diagnosis.

In other exceptional cases, there may be involvement of only the vitreous with atypical lymphocytes distinctly absent in the subretinal space and the retina.[26-28]

Microscopic Inspection. Light microscopic examination reveals a uniform population of atypical lymphoid cells exhibiting a characteristic localization and often found tightly packed in the sub-RPE space between the RPE and Bruch's membrane.[1,2,14,29] As PIOL is most often a diffuse large B-cell lymphoma (DLBCL), the morphology that PIOL lesions take is much the same. The tumor is composed of a diffusely infiltrating population of large, mature, atypical lymphomatous cells that exhibit a diffuse growth pattern, replacing the normal architecture of the stroma that it affects. The cells are high-grade lymphoma cells and exhibit a variable number of mitoses, from numerous to occasional. These atypical cells may also be found in the vitreous, retina, optic nerve head, optic nerve, and sheath. This suggests that PIOL cells home to this particular location possibly by the use of cellular signaling (discussed in Chapter 12). The localization of tumor cells in the sub-RPE space can lead to alterations in the overlying RPE and retina, such as RPE atrophy and detachments, retinal detachments, and retinal necrosis.[27,30,31] In more advanced lesions, necrosis of the upper regions of the tumor mound that are farther away from the choroid can be seen.

Although sub-RPE infiltration by lymphoma cells is the most typical finding in PIOL, PIOL cells often invade the retina, vitreous, and optic nerve. Occasionally, iris involvement has been described.[13] In these cases, lymphoma cells may surround iridal vessels or be located within the stroma of the iris, replacing the normal stromal cells.[13]

Reactive lymphocytes are another component frequently noted in microscopic examination. These lymphocytes are usually smaller than the PIOL/PCNSL cells. They are mostly T-lymphocytes, while the PIOL cells are mostly B-cell in origin. However, while tumor infiltrates the sub-RPE space, retina, and vitreous, reactive lymphocytes are mostly located in the choroid.

Immunohistochemistry reveals that these PIOL cells express B-cell markers, such as, CD19, CD20, CD22, and surface immunoglobulin (sIg). Germinal center markers are also expressed, including BCL6 and CD10. Infrequently, the PIOL cells are T-cell and express CD3 T-cell marker.

Brain Pathology

Macroscopic Inspection. Tumors composed of dense cellularity may appear with distinct to ill-defined borders and have been noted to appear similar to gliomas.[32] The tumor itself is soft, and cut surfaces are described as being granular, homogeneous yellow-white in color[33] or perhaps gray, but can also be more variegated. Within the lesion there may be foci of hemorrhagic necrosis, which may be rather prevalent in lesions found in AIDS patients. Perivascular infiltration of the parenchyma is noted. Lesions may be found subependymally and can even break through into the ventricles. Lesions in immunocompetent patients are often solitary, while in immunocompromised patients they are more often multiple. However, even in immunocompetent patients, lesions can progress to multiplicity and seems to be the natural course of the disease.[33,34] Lesions are typically located supratentorally, but in Hochberg and Miller's study of 56 patients, 21 patients had infratentorial lesions and 12 had both supra- and infratentorial lesions.[33] Remick and colleagues reported on the locations of lesions in 13 immunocompetent patients.[35] Most of the lesions were in the frontal, parietal, or frontoparietal regions (46%); three were in the corpus callosum (23%); and one in the cerebellum (8%).

Microscopic Inspection. PCNSL, like PIOL, is most frequently a DLBCL and as such it exhibits a diffuse growth pattern. Histologically, this is a high grade, typically atypical B-cell proliferation of large cells. They are either centroblasts (large, non-cleaved cells) or immunoblasts and exhibit a variable number of mitoses (from occasional to frequent). Endothelial proliferation by PCNSL is scant. Sheets of cells characterize the hub of the lymphomatous lesions, while infiltrating edges may abut edematous areas of non-infiltrated brain parenchyma. Upon microscopic inspection, the tumor may actually be noted to infiltrate a wider area than is noted on macroscopic assessment. The tumor lesions occupy two areas in the brain: perivascularly (called perivascular cuffing, from which it infiltrates the parenchyma, and similar to that seen in PIOL) and submeningeally. These locations are important because lesions located within the parenchyma, away from vascular sites, are exposed to lower doses of cytotoxic pharmacologics by virtue of the blood-brain barrier. This sets the stage for local disease recurrence (see Chapter 11 — Prognosis).

Immunohistochemistry shows the same picture as that for PIOL. As the majority of PCNSL cells are B-cells, they stain for CD19, CD20, and surface immunoglobulin (sIg).[36] Just as in PIOL and other DLBCLs, the germinal center markers BCL6 and CD10 are also expressed. Typically, mature B-cells will not express terminal deoxynucleotidyltransferase (TdT), an enzyme that catalyzes the addition of deoxynucleotides and which is usually expressed in lymphoblasts.[37,38] Aside from its usual expression in normal lymphoblasts, TdT is also found in the blast cells of certain leukemias. Interestingly, a report of a 9-year-old child with PCNSL diagnosed by CSF cytology revealed TdT expression, and the cells were characteristic of a precursor B-cell lymphoblastic lymphoma.[39] In the case of the rare T-cell PCNSL, immunohistochemistry will show that the neoplastic cells bear T-cell markers, such as, CD3, CD4, and CD5, in addition to a rearranged TCR gene, revealing its monoclonality.

Molecular Pathology

Gene Rearrangements. During the maturation process of B-lymphocytes, somatic recombination of the gene segments that make up the immunoglobulin heavy or light chains occurs. A similar process occurs in T-lymphocytes and their *TCR* genes. One of the most telling molecular signs that cells are neoplastic is the finding that the atypical cells are all derived from the same progenitor. The polymerase chain reaction (PCR) amplification has been used since the early 1990s to detect monoclonality and, therefore, neoplasticity of B-cell lymphomas. Initially, in the case of PCNSL, PCR was used on fresh samples of tissue[40] and later using tissue samples that had been embedded in paraffin wax.[41] Today, when checking for the monoclonality of B-cell lymphomas, primers are typically used for the CDR3 region with FR3A, FR2A, and/or CDR3 primers for the VDJ region or some other region. The monoclonality is evidenced when distinct banding (which represents the amplified DNA product) occurs in a particular lane in the gel during electrophoresis. In polyclonal cases, for example, in reactive lymphadenopathy due to an infection, there will be a broad smear (multiple overlapping bands) of polyclonal amplified DNA. In cases where immunoglobulin regions are not expressed at all, for example, in T-cell lymphomas, there will be no banding in a particular lane showing *IgH* gene rearrangement.

PCNSLs have been shown to be monoclonal. For example, *IgH* gene rearrangements in PCNSLs have garnered much attention recently. In one study of monoclonality of 10 cases of PCNSL,[42] five were shown to have clonal gene rearrangements in the V_H4–34 region. All of the cases that used the V_H4–34 region (known as the V_H4 family) had the same mutation in the first codon of CDR1. The other five PCNSL cases used the V_H3 family (e.g., two with rearrangement of the V_H3–23 region).

Monoclonality has been demonstrated in PIOL by showing that the lymphoma cells contain the same *immunoglobulin heavy (IgH) chain* gene or light chain (either κ or λ) restriction. The *IgH* gene is located on chromosome 14. Our laboratory demonstrated this feature of monoclonality in PIOL cells in 1998.[11,43] We microdissected PIOL cells from frozen or paraffin-embedded tissues obtained from two immunocompetent patients and two patients with AIDS and subjected the extracted DNA to the PCR. We demonstrated that there was rearrangement of the third framework region (FR3) in the variable region (V_H) of the *IgH* gene in all the four cases. Subsequently, we reported *IgH* gene rearrangements in 57 PIOL cases.[44] To date, we have recorded a total of 85 cases in which *IgH* gene rearrangements were detected (unpublished data).

Some of the gene rearrangements exhibited by PIOL cells suggest that PIOL and PCNSL are related. Coupland and colleagues extracted DNA from PIOL cells obtained from vitrectomy specimens in 16 patients.[45] PCR was performed on the *IgH* gene, and all PIOL cells from each patient exhibited monoclonality. PCR products were then sequenced in eight cases for the V_H region, from the *IgH* gene segments. Usage of the V_H4–34 gene segment was revealed in four cases (50%), V_H3–23 in two (25%), V_H3–7 in one (12.5%), and V_H3–30 in one (12.5%). Somatic mutations within the second complementarity determining region (CDR2) and FR3 from the *IgH* were also analyzed and were found to show a high frequency (14.5%) of somatic mutations. The majority of Coupland's PIOL cases using the V4–34 gene segments correlated well with that of PCNSL, providing evidence that both lymphomatous processes share a common lineage. Interestingly, Coupland showed that the same B-cell clone was found in three cases that had both PCNSL and PIOL.[45]

Baehring and colleagues analyzed the vitrectomy specimens from 17 patients.[46] Nine of these specimens demonstrated a monoclonal pattern using CDR3 consensus primers. Cytopathology was positive for intraocular lymphoma in five cases and all of these cases (except for one) had positive monoclonal IgH patterns. In two patients, cytopathology was positive for PIOL and monoclonality was seen on first vitrectomy. Subsequent vitrectomy in each of these patients, however, failed to reveal lymphoma cells on cytopathologic evaluation, and PCR for *IgH* gene was not done in either case. Eleven specimens were negative based on cytopathology, but four of these exhibited monoclonality based on PCR (one patient had negative vitrectomy specimens on two separate occasions, but monoclonality via PCR was found on these two occasions). Baehring reported a specificity of 1 (95% CI, 0.854–1.0) and a sensitivity of 0.64 (95% CI, 0.351–0.872); sensitivity is very much affected by the amount of intact lymphoma cells that are obtained within the vitreous specimen. It should be noted that Baehring used both undiluted and diluted vitreous specimens for cytopathology and PCR. Sensitivity could have been increased on microdissected samples, and Baehring points this out. Indeed, samples may be obtained that consist of relatively little lymphoma cells and an overwhelming number of outnumbering ocular resident cells or inflammatory cells that could hide any monoclonality of the lymphomatous cells. Microdissection could select for only those atypical cells that are suspicious for PIOL.[43] It is important to analyze at least 15 cells as monoclonality is based on the identification of a group (not a single cell) of genetically identical cells (clone).

Gene rearrangement pointing to monoclonality has also been described for the rarer T-cell PIOL. Coupland and associates discussed a 50-year-old woman who presented to their clinic with suspected PIOL.[22] A chorioretinal specimen was used for PCR, and a monoclonal *TCR-γ* spike via GeneScan was discovered; no monoclonal B-cell population was found.

Chan performed microdissection in 50 patients with PIOL at the NEI.[44] Chan noted that in all the 50 samples in which microdissection of atypical lymphoid cells was performed, monoclonality of the *IgH* gene was demonstrated at the CDR3 site.[44]

Do we see monoclonal proliferations in ocular disease not associated with PIOL? Indeed, there are such proliferations in diseases like Sjogren's and benign or low-grade (e.g. primary uveal extranodal marginal zone lymphoma) lymphoproliferations. However, in these cases, clinical history and examination will help guide the ophthalmologist to determine which disease entity is most probable. In addition, monoclonality in these entities occurs infrequently.

Translocations. Bcl-2 is an anti-apoptotic molecule whose gene is located on chromosome 18.[47] The immunoglobulin heavy chain (*IgH*) gene is located on chromosome 14. The *bcl-2* t(14;18) translocation brings the *bcl-2* gene under the control of the *IgH* enhancer, resulting in deregulated BCL-2 expression.[48,49] The majority of translocations (60%) occur at the major breakpoint region (Mbr) located within exon 3, while 10–25% of translocations occur at the minor cluster region (mcr) located 20 kb downstream of the Mbr.[50] The frequency of t(14;18), specifically in diffuse large cell lymphomas (the majority of which are B-cell), has been reported as 16%; 13% of DLBCLs exhibit this cytogenetic abnormality at the Mbr, while about 2% of DLBCLs exhibit the translocation at the mcr.[51]

Shen and colleagues at the NEI found that in their sample of four microdissected PIOL cases (two immunocompetent cases and two cases with AIDS) that had undergone PCR, translocation of *bcl-2* had occurred in two immunocompetent patients and one patient with AIDS.[11] Others have also shown that there has been translocation of the *bcl-2* gene.[52] The gene *bcl-2* in on chromosome 18, and translocation of this gene onto chromosome 14 (which contains the *IgH* gene) t(14;18) leads to the production of the BCL-2 mitochondria outer membrane integral membrane protein. This blocks cell death of the lymphocyte and immortalizes it. While not all DLBCLs, of which most PCNSLs and PIOLs are subsets, express translocations involving the *bcl-2* gene, most follicular lymphomas do.[47] This suggests that DLBCLs and its subtypes express heterogeneity in pathogenesis, and some may share certain pathogenic features with follicular lymphomas. In Larocca's study of both immunocompetent and AIDS cases of PCNSL, no translocations of the *bcl-2* gene were found.[53] PIOL has a unique molecular pattern involving *bcl-2.* We at the National Eye Institute (NEI) recently found that 40 of 72 (55%) PIOL patients expressed the *bcl-2* t(14;18) translocation at the Mbr and 15 of 68 (22%) expressed the translocation at the mcr.[54] An analysis of clinical outcome in 23 patients revealed no significant association between *bcl-2* translocation and the survival or relapse. However, patients with the translocation were significantly younger. This finding is important because younger PCNSL/PIOL patients often survive longer than older patients (see Chapter 11 — Prognosis).

Molecular Signals. An interesting gene *bcl-6,* which encodes for a transcriptional repressor, has been shown to be associated with some PCNSLs.[53] Bcl-6, whose gene is located on chromosome 3q27, is a zinc finger transcriptional repressor and is involved in apoptosis and cell growth and differentiation. The BCL-6 trascription repressor protein is expressed mainly by mature B-cells, especially those within the germinal centers of lymphoid organs or those that have traversed these sites. Therefore, the protein expressed by *bcl-6* is an important marker of the derivation of a lymphocyte from a germinal center.[55–57] In a study of histologically proven PCNSL, BCL-6 expression was noted in all 22 of the non-AIDS cases. However, this protein was not noted in AIDS-related PCNSL cases that expressed the latent membrane protein (LMP)-1 antigen encoded by EBV.[53] Mutations in the *bcl-6* gene were noted in 24 of 48 cases (11 of 26 AIDS cases and 13 of 22 non-AIDS cases), suggesting that the neoplastic B-cell progenitor for each of these particular cases had transited through the germinal center. BCL-2 was expressed by two of 14 non-AIDS cases. For AIDS cases, there seemed to be two phenotypes: BCL-6+/LMP-1−/BCL-2− and BCL-6−/LMP-1+/BCL-2+.

The tumor suppressor gene, *p53,* and the oncogene, *c-myc,* have also been implicated in PCNSL. For example, some have found that patients with PCNSLs, who express these two genes or *bcl-6,* have a poorer prognosis than those not expressing these genes,[58] and these results were similar with respect to *c-myc* and *p53* expression in an earlier study on non-PCNSL DLBCL.[59] These findings underscore the heterogeneity within the DLBCL group.

In 20 cases of PCNSL examined by Cobbers and colleagues, 11 cases had weak or no signals of *cyclin-dependent kinase inhibitor 2A (CDKN2A)* mRNA, which encodes for the protein p16. This protein is an inhibitor of cyclin-dependent kinase (CDK), a protein involved in the G1 phase of cell growth. Therefore, *p16* is a tumor suppressor gene and a lack of mRNA expression could allow for immortalization.[60]

Some proteins that have been noted to be expressed by B-cell PIOL include BCL-2, BCL-6, and multiple myeloma protein 1, MUM1.[31] Coupland and colleagues reported that in 50 cases of definite PIOL, seven expressed BCL-2, BCL-6, and 45/50 MUM1.[31] Later, they showed that in eight cases of PIOL and 42 cases of PCNSL,[61] there was high positivity (ranging from 98%–100% of combined cases) for the B-cell transcription factor, BSAP (encoded by *Pax5* gene),[62,63] the B-cell-restricted transcription coactivator, BOB.1/OBF.1.[64,65] the B-cell transcription factor Oct.2,[66,67] and MUM1.[61] Multiple myeloma oncogene 1 (MUM1), now more commonly known as interferon regulator factor 4 (IRF4), functions as a transcription factor regulator.[68,69] It has been hypothesized that the aberrant expression of this protein can be a marker for some types of non-Hodgkin's lymphomas.[70] Coupland *et al.* noted that the transcriptional repressor, BCL-6, was expressed in 86% of their 58 PIOL/PCNSL cases.[61] Recently, in a small study (four cases), we at the NEI detected a high frequency (100%) of *bcl-6* gene expression in four PIOL cases.[54] Coupland and associates[61] also noted that 50 cases of peripheral DLBCLs had similarly high frequencies of BSAP, BOB.1/OBF.2, Oct.2, and MUM1 compared to their 50 PIOL/PCNSL cases, but only 10% of PIOL/PCNSL cases as compared with 45% of peripheral DLBCL cases expressed PU.1, a transcription factor involved in hematopoiesis.[71,72] These data help support the idea that there exists important diversity even within the DLBCL groups.

Infectious DNA. Various infectious agents have been shown to cause malignancy in humans. Viral etiologies have been noted in cancers, such as Kaposi sarcoma (human herpes virus 8 (HHV-8));[73,74] cervical cancer (human papilloma virus (HPV));[75,76] adult T-cell leukemia/lymphoma (human T-lymphotropic virus-1 (HTLV-1));[77] and PCNSL due to latent EBV infection in AIDS patients.[78–80] Sequence analysis of DLBCLs, including of PCNSL and PIOL,[45] immunoglobulins not only identifies their monoclonality, but also suggests that these cells may have been subjected to the germinal center reaction.[1] This provides evidence for distinct molecular subtypes of DLBCLs[81] and suggests that some lymphomas may be influenced by infectious causes. These recent molecular findings have piqued the interest of ophthalmologists to determine whether infectious agents might be at play in ocular tumors.

At the NEI, Chan and associates sought out to determine if EBV and HHV-8 could possibly be associated with PIOL in immunocompetent patients.[82] In a study of 50 patients with PIOL,[44] 32 cases were selected at random for detection of infectious DNA. *HHV-8* DNA was detected in six cases (two cases had AIDS), and *EBV* DNA was detected in two out of 21 randomly chosen cases (one case had AIDS). Interestingly, one AIDS case demonstrated DNA from both *HHV-8* and *EBV*. We also detected *Toxoplasma gondii* DNA in PIOL.[83] In two of the 10 PIOL cases, *T. gondii*, not *HHV-8* or *EBV*, DNA was discovered in the lymphoma but not in normal cells. These two cases resembled ocular toxoplasmosis clinically, and one had high serum titer against *T. gondii*.

While it is known that EBV plays a role in the development of lymphoma in AIDS (post-transplant) and other immunocompetent patients as well as in Burkitt's lymphoma, this infectious DNA does not seem to play a major role in immunocompetent patients with PCNSL/PIOL.

Bacterial infection has also been shown to be associated with the development of cancers. For example, *Helicobacter pylori* (*H. pylori*) is not only the agent associated the majority of duodenal ulcers,[84,85] but it has been shown to cause gastric MALT lymphomas as well.[86-88] This discovery is especially exciting because antibiotics can be used as a potential cure.[89,90] Ocular adnexal tissue MALT lymphomas may be associated with infectious agents. In a study of five patients with conjunctival MALT lymphoma, Chan and colleagues found that microdissected MALT lymphoma cells monotypically expressed either κ or λ light chains and all exhibited *IgH* gene rearrangements of the CDR3 region and, thus, were monoclonal.[91] In four of the cases *H. pylori* DNA was present. Importantly, no *H. pylori* DNA was detected in the conjunctival stromal cells, the normal lymphocytes from a conjunctivitis case, or the orbital MALT lymphoma cells. Recently, small case reports have identified *Chlamydia* associated with ocular adnexal MALT lymphoma and noted regression or reduction in ocular MALT lymphomas with antibiotic therapy.[92-94] The association between bacteria and cancer has prompted others to determine if bacteria might be involved in PCNSL/PIOL.

While infectious agents seem a plausible explanation in the development of some ocular tumors, perhaps even PIOL, more studies are needed to establish a causative role.

References

1. Tuaillon N, Chan CC. (2001) Molecular analysis of primary central nervous system and primary intraocular lymphoma. *Curr Mol Med* 1(2): 259–272.
2. Chan CC, Wallace DJ. (2004) Intraocular lymphoma: update on diagnosis and management. *Cancer Control* 11(5): 285–295.
3. Michels RG, Knox DL, Erozan YS, Green WR. (1975) Intraocular reticulum cell sarcoma. Diagnosis by pars plana vitrectomy. *Arch Ophthalmol* 93(12): 1331–1335.
4. Whitcup SM, de Smet MD, Rubin BI, *et al.* (1993) Intraocular lymphoma. Clinical and histopathologic diagnosis. *Ophthalmology* 100: 1399–1406.
5. Chan CC, Buggage RR, Nussenblatt RB. (2002) Intraocular lymphoma. *Curr Opin Ophthalmol* 13(6): 411–418.
6. Scroggs MW, Johnston WW, Klintworth GK. (1990) Intraocular tumors. A cytopathologic study. *Acta Cytol* 34(3): 401–408.
7. Char DH, Ljung BM, Deschenes J, Miller TR. (1988) Intraocular lymphoma: immunological and cytological analysis. *Br J Ophthalmol* 72(12): 905–911.
8. Char DH, Ljung BM, Miller T, Phillips T. (1988) Primary intraocular lymphoma (ocular reticulum cell sarcoma) diagnosis and management. *Ophthalmology* 95: 625–630.
9. Ridley ME, McDonald HR, Sternberg P, Jr., *et al.* (1992) Retinal manifestations of ocular lymphoma (reticulum cell sarcoma). *Ophthalmology* 99(7): 1153–1160; discussion 1160–1151.
10. Davis JL, Solomon D, Nussenblatt RB, *et al.* (1992) Immunocytochemical staining of vitreous cells. Indications, techniques, and results. *Ophthalmology* 99(2): 250–256.
11. Shen DF, Zhuang Z, LeHoang P, *et al.* (1998) Utility of microdissection and polymerase chain reaction for the detection of immunoglobulin gene rearrangement and translocation in primary intraocular lymphoma [In Process Citation]. *Ophthalmology* 105(9): 1664–1669.
12. Akpek EK, Ahmed I, Hochberg FH, *et al.* (1999) Intraocular-central nervous system lymphoma: clinical features, diagnosis, and outcomes. *Ophthalmology* 106(9): 1805–1810.
13. Velez G, de Smet MD, Whitcup SM, *et al.* (2000) Iris involvement in primary intraocular lymphoma: report of two cases and review of the literature. *Surv Ophthalmol* 44(6): 518–526.

14. Buggage RR, Chan CC, Nussenblatt RB. (2001) Ocular manifestations of central nervous system lymphoma. *Curr Opin Oncol* 13(3): 137–142.
15. Vogel MH, Font RL, Zimmerman LE, Levine RA. (1968) Reticulum cell sarcoma of the retina and uvea. Report of six cases and review of the literature. *Am J Ophthalmol* 66(2): 205–215.
16. Currey TA, Deutsch AR. (1965) Reticulum cell sarcoma of the uvea. *Southern Med J* 58: 919.
17. Nevins RC, Jr., Frey WW, Elliott JH. (1968) Primary, solitary, intraocular reticulum cell sarcoma (microgliomatosis). (A clinicopathologic case report). *Trans Am Acad Ophthalmol Otolaryngol* 72(6): 867–876.
18. Zaldivar RA, Martin DF, Holden JT, Grossniklaus HE. (2004) Primary intraocular lymphoma: clinical, cytologic, and flow cytometric analysis. *Ophthalmology* 111(9): 1762–1767.
19. Green WR. (1984) Diagnostic cytopathology of ocular fluid specimens. *Opthalmology* 91: 726–749.
20. Palexas GN. (1995) Diagnostic pars plana vitrectomy report of a 21-year retrospective study. *Trans Am Ophthalmol Soc* 93: 281–308.
21. Coupland SE, Heimann H, Bechrakis NE. (2004) Primary intraocular lymphoma: a review of the clinical, histopathological and molecular biological features. *Graefes Arch Clin Exp Ophthalmol* 242(11): 901–913.
22. Coupland SE, Anastassiou G, Bornfeld N, *et al.* (2005) Primary intraocular lymphoma of T-cell type: report of a case and review of the literature. *Graefes Arch Clin Exp Ophthalmol* 243(3): 189–197.
23. Dean JM, Novak MA, Chan CC, Green WR. (1996) Tumor detachments of the retinal pigment epithelium in ocular/central nervous system lymphoma. *Retina* 16(1): 47–56.
24. Klingele TG, Hogan MJ. (1975) Ocular reticulum cell sarcoma. *Am J Ophthalmol* 79(1): 39–47.
25. Cummings TJ, Stenzel TT, Klintworth G, Jaffe GJ. (2005) Primary intraocular T-cell-rich large B-cell lymphoma. *Arch Pathol Lab Med* 129(8): 1050–1053.
26. Minckler DS, Font RL, Zimmerman LE. (1975) Uveitis and reticulum cell sarcoma of brain with bilateral neoplastic seeding of vitreous without retinal or uveal involvement. *Am J Ophthalmol* 80(3 Pt 1): 433–439.
27. Parver LM, Font RL. (1979) Malignant lymphoma of the retina and brain. Initial diagnosis by cytologic examination of vitreous aspirate. *Arch Ophthalmol* 97(8): 1505–1507.
28. Zhou M, Chen Q, Wang W. (2003) [Two cases of primary intraocular lymphoma]. *Zhonghua Yan Ke Za Zhi* 39(7): 442–444.
29. Barr CC, Green WR, Payne JW, *et al.* (1975) Intraocular reticulum-cell sarcoma: clinico-pathologic study of four cases and review of the literature. *Surv Ophthalmol* 19(4): 224–239.

30. Gass JD, Sever RJ, Grizzard WS, *et al.* (1984) Multifocal pigment epithelial detachments by reticulum cell sarcoma. A characteristic funduscopic picture. *Retina* 4(3): 135–143.
31. Coupland SE, Bechrakis NE, Anastassiou G, *et al.* (2003) Evaluation of vitrectomy specimens and chorioretinal biopsies in the diagnosis of primary intraocular lymphoma in patients with Masquerade syndrome. *Graefes Arch Clin Exp Ophthalmol* 241(10): 860–870.
32. Stefanko S, Moffe D. (1975) Primary reticulum-cell-sarcoma of the brain. A clinical-pathological study. *Clin Neurol Neurosurg* 77(2): 96–109.
33. Hochberg FH, Miller DC. (1988) Primary central nervous system lymphoma. *J Neurosurg* 68(6): 835–853.
34. Henry JM, Heffner RR, Jr., Dillard SH, *et al.* (1974) Primary malignant lymphomas of the central nervous system. *Cancer* 34(4): 1293–1302.
35. Remick SC, Diamond C, Migliozzi JA, *et al.* (1990) Primary central nervous system lymphoma in patients with and without the acquired immune deficiency syndrome. A retrospective analysis and review of the literature. *Medicine (Baltimore)* 69(6): 345–360.
36. Kumanishi T, Washiyama K, Saito T, *et al.* (1986) Primary malignant lymphoma of the brain: an immunohistochemical study of eight cases using a panel of monoclonal and heterologous antibodies. *Acta Neuropathol (Berl)* 71(3–4): 190–196.
37. Barr RD, Sarin PS, Perry SM. (1976) Terminal transferase in human bonemarrow lymphocytes. *Lancet* 1(7958): 508–509.
38. Goldschneider I, Gregoire KE, Barton RW, Bollum FJ. (1977) Demonstration of terminal deoxynucleotidyl transferase in thymocytes by immunofluorescence. *Proc Natl Acad Sci USA* 74(2): 734–738.
39. Shiozawa Y, Kiyokawa N, Fujimura J, *et al.* (2005) Primary malignant lymphoma of the central nervous system in an immunocompetent child: a case report. *J Pediatr Hematol Oncol* 27(10): 561–564.
40. Trainor KJ, Brisco MJ, Story CJ, Morley AA. (1990) Monoclonality in B-lymphoproliferative disorders detected at the DNA level. *Blood* 75(11): 2220–2222.
41. Wan JH. (1990) Use of polymerase chain reaction (PCR) to detect monoclonality of B-lymphoproliferative disorders at DNA level. *Zhonghua Zhong Liu Za Zhi* 12(4): 242–245.
42. Montesinos-Rongen M, Kuppers R, Schluter D, *et al.* (1999) Primary central nervous system lymphomas are derived from germinal- center B cells and show a preferential usage of the V4–34 gene segment. *Am J Pathol* 155(6): 2077–2086.
43. Chan CC, Shen D, Nussenblatt RB, *et al.* (1998) Detection of molecular changes in primary intraocular lymphoma by microdissection and polymerase chain reaction [letter] [In Process Citation]. *Diagn Mol Pathol* 7(1): 63–64.

44. Chan CC. (2003) Molecular pathology of primary intraocular lymphoma. *Trans Am Ophthalmol Soc* **101**: 275–292.
45. Coupland SE, Hummel M, Muller HH, Stein H. (2005) Molecular analysis of immunoglobulin genes in primary intraocular lymphoma. *Invest Ophthalmol Vis Sci* **46**(10): 3507–3514.
46. Baehring JM, Androudi S, Longtine JJ, *et al.* (2005) Analysis of clonal immunoglobulin heavy chain rearrangements in ocular lymphoma. *Cancer* **104**(3): 591–597.
47. Tsujimoto Y, Croce CM. (1986) Analysis of the structure, transcripts, and protein products of bcl-2, the gene involved in human follicular lymphoma. *Proc Natl Acad Sci USA* **83**(14): 5214–5218.
48. Tsujimoto Y, Finger LR, Yunis J, *et al.* (1984) Cloning of the chromosome breakpoint of neoplastic B cells with the t(14;18) chromosome translocation. *Science* **226**(4678): 1097–1099.
49. Ngan BY, Chen-Levy Z, Weiss LM, *et al.* (1988) Expression in non-Hodgkin's lymphoma of the bcl-2 protein associated with the t(14;18) chromosomal translocation. *N Engl J Med* **318**(25): 1638–1644.
50. Weiss LM, Warnke RA, Sklar J, Cleary ML. (1987) Molecular analysis of the t(14;18) chromosomal translocation in malignant lymphoma. *N Engl J Med* **317**: 1185–1189.
51. Meijerink JP. (1997) t(14;18), a journey to eternity. *Leukemia* **11**(12): 2175–2187.
52. White L, Trickett A, Norris MD, *et al.* (1990) Heterotransplantation of human lymphoid neoplasms using a nude mouse intraocular xenograft model. *Cancer Res* **50**(10): 3078–3086.
53. Larocca LM, Capello D, Rinelli A, *et al.* (1998) The molecular and phenotypic profile of primary central nervous system lymphoma identifies distinct categories of the disease and is consistent with histogenetic derivation from germinal center-related B cells. *Blood* **92**(3): 1011–1019.
54. Wallace DJ, Shen D, Reed GF, *et al.* (2006) Detection of the *bcl-2*t(14;18) translocation and proto-oncogene expression in primary intraocular lymphoma. *Invest Ophthalmol Vis Sci* **47**(7): 2750–2756.
55. Ye BH, Lista F, Lo Coco F, *et al.* (1993) Alterations of a zinc finger-encoding gene, BCL-6, in diffuse large-cell lymphoma. *Science* **262**(5134): 747–750.
56. Ye BH, Rao PH, Chaganti RS, Dalla-Favera R. (1993) Cloning of bcl-6, the locus involved in chromosome translocations affecting band 3q27 in B-cell lymphoma. *Cancer Res* **53**(12): 2732–2735.
57. Cattoretti G, Chang CC, Cechova K, *et al.* (1995) BCL-6 protein is expressed in germinal-center B cells. *Blood* **86**(1): 45–53.

58. Chang CC, Kampalath B, Schultz C, *et al.* (2003) Expression of p53, c-Myc, or Bcl-6 suggests a poor prognosis in primary central nervous system diffuse large B-cell lymphoma among immunocompetent individuals. *Arch Pathol Lab Med* **127**(2): 208–212.

59. Chang CC, Liu YC, Cleveland RP, Perkins SL. (2000) Expression of c-Myc and p53 correlates with clinical outcome in diffuse large B-cell lymphomas. *Am J Clin Pathol* **113**(4): 512–518.

60. Cobbers JM, Wolter M, Reifenberger J, *et al.* (1998) Frequent inactivation of CDKN2A and rare mutation of TP53 in PCNSL. *Brain Pathol* **8**(2): 263–276.

61. Coupland SE, Loddenkemper C, Smith JR, *et al.* (2005) Expression of immunoglobulin transcription factors in primary intraocular lymphoma and primary central nervous system lymphoma. *Invest Ophthalmol Vis Sci* **46**(11): 3957–3964.

62. Busslinger M, Urbanek P. (1995) The role of BSAP (Pax-5) in B-cell development. *Curr Opin Genet Dev* **5**(5): 595–601.

63. Nutt SL, Morrison AM, Dorfler P, *et al.* (1998) Identification of BSAP (Pax-5) target genes in early B-cell development by loss- and gain-of-function experiments. *Embo J* **17**(8): 2319–2333.

64. Gstaiger M, Georgiev O, van Leeuwen H, *et al.* (1996) The B cell coactivator Bob1 shows DNA sequence-dependent complex formation with Oct-1/Oct-2 factors, leading to differential promoter activation. *Embo J* **15**(11): 2781–2790.

65. Luo Y, Roeder RG. (1995) Cloning, functional characterization, and mechanism of action of the B-cell-specific transcriptional coactivator OCA-B. *Mol Cell Biol* **15**(8): 4115–4124.

66. Clerc RG, Corcoran LM, LeBowitz JH, *et al.* (1988) The B-cell-specific Oct-2 protein contains POU box- and homeo box-type domains. *Genes Dev* **2**(12A): 1570–1581.

67. Staudt LM, Clerc RG, Singh H, *et al.* (1988) Cloning of a lymphoid-specific cDNA encoding a protein binding the regulatory octamer DNA motif. *Science* **241**(4865): 577–580.

68. Brass AL, Kehrli E, Eisenbeis CF, *et al.* (1996) Pip, a lymphoid-restricted IRF, contains a regulatory domain that is important for autoinhibition and ternary complex formation with the Ets factor PU.1. *Genes Dev* **10**(18): 2335–2347.

69. Eisenbeis CF, Singh H, Storb U. (1995) Pip, a novel IRF family member, is a lymphoid-specific, PU.1–dependent transcriptional activator. *Genes Dev* **9**(11): 1377–1387.

70. Tsuboi K, Iida S, Inagaki H, *et al.* (2000) MUM1/IRF4 expression as a frequent event in mature lymphoid malignancies. *Leukemia* **14**(3): 449–456.

71. Scott EW, Simon MC, Anastasi J, Singh H. (1994) Requirement of transcription factor PU.1 in the development of multiple hematopoietic lineages. *Science* **265**(5178): 1573–1577.

72. Scott EW, Fisher RC, Olson MC, *et al.* (1997) PU.1 functions in a cell-autonomous manner to control the differentiation of multipotential lymphoid-myeloid progenitors. *Immunity* **6**(4): 437–447.

73. Moore PS, Chang Y. (1995) Detection of herpesvirus-like DNA sequences in Kaposi's sarcoma in patients with and without HIV infection. *N Engl J Med* **332**(18): 1181–1185.

74. Chuck S, Grant RM, Katongole-Mbidde E, *et al.* (1996) Frequent presence of a novel herpesvirus genome in lesions of human immunodeficiency virus-negative Kaposi's sarcoma. *J Infect Dis* **173**(1): 248–251.

75. Walboomers JM, Jacobs MV, Manos MM, *et al.* (1999) Human papillomavirus is a necessary cause of invasive cervical cancer worldwide. *J Pathol* **189**(1): 12–19.

76. Zielinski GD, Snijders PJ, Rozendaal L, *et al.* (2001) HPV presence precedes abnormal cytology in women developing cervical cancer and signals false negative smears. *Br J Cancer* **85**(3): 398–404.

77. Kondo T, Kono H, Miyamoto N, *et al.* (1989) Age- and sex-specific cumulative rate and risk of ATLL for HTLV-I carriers. *Int J Cancer* **43**(6): 1061–1064.

78. De Luca A, Antinori A, Cingolani A, *et al.* (1995) Evaluation of cerebrospinal fluid EBV-DNA and IL-10 as markers for in vivo diagnosis of AIDS-related primary central nervous system lymphoma [published erratum appears in Br J Haematol 1995 Dec;91(4):1035]. *Br J Haematol* **90**(4): 844–849.

79. MacMahon EM, Glass JD, Hayward SD, *et al.* (1991) Epstein-Barr virus in AIDS-related primary central nervous system lymphoma. *Lancet* **338**(8773): 969–973.

80. Cinque P, Brytting M, Vago L, *et al.* (1993) Epstein-Barr virus DNA in cerebrospinal fluid from patients with AIDS- related primary lymphoma of the central nervous system. *Lancet* **342**(8868): 398–401.

81. Alizadeh AA, Eisen MB, Davis RE, *et al.* (2000) Distinct types of diffuse large B-cell lymphoma identified by gene expression profiling. *Nature* **403**(6769): 503–511.

82. Chan CC, Shen DF, Whitcup SM, *et al.* (1999) Detection of human herpesvirus-8 and Epstein-Barr virus DNA in primary intraocular lymphoma. *Blood* **93**(8): 2749–2751.

83. Shen DF, Herbort CP, Tuaillon N, *et al.* (2001) Detection of toxoplasma gondii DNA in primary intraocular b-cell lymphoma. *Mod Pathol* **14**(10): 995–999.

84. Tytgat GN, Rauws EA. (1990) Campylobacter pylori and its role in peptic ulcer disease. *Gastroenterol Clin North Am* 19(1): 183–196.
85. Borody TJ, George LL, Brandl S, *et al.* (1991) Helicobacter pylori-negative duodenal ulcer. *Am J Gastroenterol* 86(9): 1154–1157.
86. Wotherspoon AC, Ortiz-Hidalgo C, Falzon MR, Isaacson PG. (1991) Helicobacter pylori-associated gastritis and primary B-cell gastric lymphoma. *Lancet* 338(8776): 1175–1176.
87. Parsonnet J, Hansen S, Rodriguez L, *et al.* (1994) Helicobacter pylori infection and gastric lymphoma. *N Engl J Med* 330(18): 1267–1271.
88. Isaacson PG. (1999) Mucosa-associated lymphoid tissue lymphoma. *Semin Hematol* 36(2): 139–147.
89. Wotherspoon AC, Doglioni C, Diss TC, *et al.* (1993) Regression of primary low-grade B-cell gastric lymphoma of mucosa-associated lymphoid tissue type after eradication of Helicobacter pylori. *Lancet* 342(8871): 575–577.
90. Hopkins RJ, Girardi LS, Turney EA. (1996) Relationship between Helicobacter pylori eradication and reduced duodenal and gastric ulcer recurrence: a review. *Gastroenterology* 110(4): 1244–1252.
91. Chan CC, Smith JA, Shen DF, *et al.* (2004) Helicobacter pylori (H. pylori) molecular signature in conjunctival mucosa-associated lymphoid tissue (MALT) lymphoma. *Histol Histopathol* 19(4): 1219–1226.
92. Abramson DH, Rollins I, Coleman M. (2005) Periocular mucosa-associated lymphoid/low grade lymphomas: treatment with antibiotics. *Am J Ophthalmol* 140(4): 729–730.
93. Ferreri AJ, Guidoboni M, Ponzoni M, *et al.* (2004) Evidence for an association between *Chlamydia psittaci* and ocular adnexal lymphomas. *J Natl Cancer Inst* 96(8):586–594.
94. Shen D, Yuen HKL, Galita DA, *et al.* (2006) Detection of *Chlamydia pneumoniae* in a bilateral orbital mucosa-associated lymphoid tissue lymphoma. *Am J Ophthalmol* 141(6):1162–1163.

Chapter 8

Immunology of PIOL

We now know the immunogenetics of PCNSL and PIOL, but in the early days of these lymphomas and lymphomas in general, the cell of origin was not always so certain. The majority of PIOLs are B-cell (and rarely T-cell) in origin, and these malignant cells are involved in a complex network of cellular signaling. If this signaling goes awry, it can lead to the development of lymphoma in the eye.

The Role of T-cells in PIOL

The cellular composition of the tumor microenvironment plays a role in tumorigenesis and progression, although its precise relevance is still not well understood and varies among different types of tumors. There are two main subtypes of T-cells, and each seems to play a role in the establishment and maintenance of PIOL cells. T-cells bearing the antigen CD4 are also known as "helper" T-cells because they mediate the normal transformation of B-cells into plasma cells capable of producing immunoglobulins against microbes. Indeed, patients who have thymic aplasia or hypoplasia and, therefore, who have impaired production of T-cells, such as those with the DiGeorge anomaly, may have B-cells that are unable to attain full functionality. This is because these cells lack stimulation from T-cells.[1,2] However, B-cells are able to mature in the absence of T-cells.[3] Such patients are quite susceptible to infections. T-cells bearing the antigen CD8 are also known as "suppressor/cytotoxic" cells because some of these cells recognize foreign antigen presented to them by infected cells. They also bring about the formation of perforin. This punctures holes into the infected cell's plasma membrane and enables apoptotic inducing proteins (granzymes) to enter the target cell, thereby killing it and the infectious agent within.[4,5] In addition, some other CD8 cells suppress the action of CD4 cells and, therefore, also B-cells (which require CD4 cells for their further differentiation). As the vast majority of PIOLs are of B-cell lineage, like lymphomas in general, there are infiltrating lymphocytes in the tumor. The role of T-cells in PIOL is similar to that inside other tumors.

Previous histopathologic studies of PCNSL tissues found populations of lymphoid cells smaller than the neoplastic lymphoma cells. Nishiyama and associates helped to characterize the lineage of these smaller cells as reactive T-cells in seven cases of B-cell PCNSL.[6] While these reactive cells displayed pan-T-cell markers (Leu-1 (now known as CD5) and OKT-11 (now CD2)), a heterogeneous mixture was noted when these T-cells were immunohistochemically sub-typed. Cytotoxic or suppressor T-cells, staining positive for Leu-2a (now CD8) were intermingled with helper or inducer T-cells that stained positive for Leu-3a (now CD4). In all but one case, were the ratios of CD4 to CD8 T-cells less than one; overall, there were more cytotoxic/suppressor T-cells compared with helper/inducer T-cells. Later, Hochberg's group reported T-cell infiltration in 13 B-cell PCNSL cases (six with AIDS).[7] They observed that 10.82% and 4.88% of total cells were CD3 T-cells in non-AIDS and AIDS PCNSL, respectively. Most of the T-cells were CD4 cells, although the AIDS PCNSLs had a significantly higher CD8 cell infiltration compared with non-AIDS PCNSLs.

We have learned from immunohistochemical studies that there can be distinct locations for various cell populations in PIOL. Studies at the National Eye Institute (NEI) helped to immunohistochemically characterize the compartmentalization of the cells involved in PIOL.[8] For example, PIOL cells are characteristically located below the retinal pigment epithelium (RPE) as well as in the retina, vitreous, and optic nerve head/optic nerve.[9–12] Reactive T lymphocytes, on the other hand, are typically and often located in the choroid; the subretinal lymphomatous infiltration may stimulate this secondary inflammatory response. Immunohistochemical staining revealed choroidal staining for the pan-T-cell CD3 antigen, and there was a 2:1 ratio of CD4 (helper T-cells) to CD8 (suppressor T-cells).[8] It was shown that more CD8 T-cells were found adjacent to Bruch's membrane, while CD4 T-cells were found disseminated evenly throughout the choroid.[8] Could this characteristic distribution of T-cells have something to do with preventing the lymphoma cells from entering the choroid towards the sclera, in effect, acting as a barrier against metastasis? Perhaps, it is the lack of T-cells within or around tumor foci that actually promote or allow the lesions to progress. It will be helpful to briefly review some of the features of CD4 and CD8 T-cells for some clues as to their involvement in PIOL.

The Role of CD4 T-cells. Cancer specific immunity elicited with vaccines has traditionally focused on the activation of the CD8 cytolytic T lymphocyte (CTL). This often involves direct stimulation of immunity using HLA-class I binding peptide epitopes.[13–16] Recently, it has become clear that activation of the CTL immune effector arm alone is insufficient to mediate an anticancer response. A major problem is that CD8 T cells cannot be sustained alone without the concomitant activation of CD4 T helper (Th) cells. In fact, it is now widely recognized that the Th cell regulates nearly all aspects of the adaptive immune response.[17] In addition, Th cells can recruit the innate immune system during immune augmentation. Therefore, the focus of the immune response in cancer has shifted away from activating CTL immunity alone to activating Th cell immunity alone or concurrently with CTL. Evidence suggests that activating the Th cell is sufficient to achieve a complete adaptive immune response because once activated, the Th cell will elicit endogenous CD8 T cell and humoral immunity.[17–21]

The Role of CD8 T-cells. CD8 T-cells make up less of the reactive cellular infiltrate of lymphomas compared with CD4 T-cells. However, they seem to play a significant role in the disease outcome as reported in a recent microarray analysis of 267 Hodgkin's lymphoma cases.[22] Interestingly, higher amounts of infiltrating CTLs were correlated with poorer overall survivals and, therefore, held prognostic significance.[22] Besides being the majority of cells noted to be adjacent to Bruch's membrane,[8] it has been shown that the T-cells surrounding tumor cells also consist mainly of CD8-positive cells.[23] Perhaps, the CD4 cells stimulate cytotoxic functions of CD8 cells near the tumor.

A study at the NEI attempted to characterize the cellular infiltrates from vitrectomy specimens of 14 patients with PIOL, uveitis (sterile intraocular inflammation), and infectious ocular diseases.[24] In infectious uveitic cases (e.g., those caused by fungi and viruses), helper T-cells were the predominant cell type (representing about 70 to 95% of the vitreous cellular infiltrate). Cytotoxic T-cells were also present, but much less so (ranging from 5 to 25% of the vitreous cellular infiltrate). B-cells seemed to be less frequently observed in the cellular infiltrate of bacterial cases. The exception to this was for a vitreous specimen obtained from a patient with *Proprionibacteria acnes* in which the helper T-cell represented 10% of the vitreous cellular infiltrate and macrophages represented 90%.[24] Sterile intraocular inflammation was characterized by similarly high helper-to-cytotoxic T-cell ratios (up to 18 times more helper T-cells than cytotoxic T-cells in intermediate uveitis; up to 17 times more helper T-cells in sarcoidosis; and 45 times more in Vogt-Koyanagi-Harada syndrome). Four patients had PIOL, and immunohistochemical staining of the vitreous cells was performed in two cases. One case had 8% of cells being CD4-helper T-cells and an unsatisfactory number of cytotoxic T-cells to make an estimate. However, B-cells, including the PIOL cells with B-lymphocyte lineage, were much more prominent in the vitreous, comprising 85% of the vitreous cellular infiltrate. In the other case, helper and cytotoxic T-cells made up 1 and 2% of the vitreous cellular infiltrates, respectively. Again, B-cells, including the B-PIOL cells, were the predominant cell type, making up 80% of the vitreous cellular infiltrate.[24]

The Role of Macrophages in PIOL

While most tumors do not express MHC class II molecules,[25] the activation of Th cells rests upon tumor antigen presentation by an important antigen presenting cell (APC), the macrophage. Macrophages have been shown to surround tumor cells and later present tumor antigen loaded onto MHC class II molecules to Th cells.[26] This interaction activates macrophages and enables them to suppress tumor cell growth.[26] Macrophages are often a component in the vitreous or CSF samples of PCNSL/PIOL patients.[11] While macrophages are known to secrete pro-inflammatory cytokines, such as, TNF-α and GM-CSF, in the presence of high numbers of B-cell PIOL-produced IL-10, the macrophages may not be fully activated. This leads to their inability to activate Th cells. Therefore, while macrophages may typically be associated with immune surveillance and destruction of tumorigenic cells, PIOL may be able to dismantle this process by secreting high amounts of macrophage-inactivating IL-10.

The Role of the Dendritic Cell in PIOL

Dendritic cells are unique antigen-presenting cells that play a central role in the initiation and direction of immune responses. Dendritic cells link the innate and adaptive immune systems together by their interactions with effector cells of the immune system, including T and B cells and natural killer (NK) cells.[27] They are distinguished from other antigen-presenting cells, such as B cells, macrophages, and monocytes, as being the only cells capable of inducing naïve T-cell responses. Heterogeneity and functional plasticity are major characteristics of dendritic cells. The combination of their subsets, their migration, and their specific environmental stimuli endow dendritic cells with diverse capacities. Their function may be site-specific, and depending on their environmental experience they may drive different types of specific and non-specific responses or induce tolerance. Dendritic cells have been shown to play an important role in tumor suppression and rejection by presenting tumor antigens to CD4 Th-cells.[28,29] This ability can be tampered with by high IL-10 levels,[30] such as those seen in PIOL.[31,32] Dendritic cells loaded *ex vivo* with tumor-associated antigens and administered as a vaccine have shown promise in early clinical trials for a number of malignancies and lymphoproliferative disorders, including follicular lymphoma, multiple myeloma, and chronic lymphocytic leukemia. However, the need for improvement is widely accepted.[33] Recently, several investigators have reported encouraging results using autologous stem cell (containing a high number of dendritic cells) transplantation in conjunction with chemotherapy for PCNSL,[34–36] some with ocular involvement. A greater number of patients and longer follow-up periods are needed to confirm these data.

Cytokines and Chemokines

Cytokine profiling can help distinguish between uveitis and PIOL. In the early- to mid-1990s, there was mounting evidence that IL-10 was secreted by non-Hodgkin's lymphomas (NHLs)[37,38] and could provide a clue for the existence of PIOL.[31,39,40]

IL-10. IL-10 is produced by many cells, including B-cells and in notoriously high amounts by B-cell PIOL cells.[41] IL-10 is produced to a lesser extent by Th2 cells and macrophages[42,43] In B-cell PIOL, we see very high levels of IL-10 compared with uveitis, which consists of an infiltrate composed mostly of macrophages and T-cells. IL-10 functions to inhibit lymphocyte and macrophage activation.[44] By inhibiting macrophagic IL-12 production, differentiation of naïve CD4-positive cells into a Th1 phenotype is restricted.[45] In addition, IL-10 downregulates the expression of MHC class II molecules on the surface of macrophages and other antigen presenting cells.[46] It has been shown in some tumors that IL-10 also downregulates MHC class I molecules, and this can lead to tumors escaping immune surveillance.[47] The interaction between MHC class II molecules and CD4-positive T-cells is necessary for the production of inflammatory cytokine, IFN-γ, by Th1 cells.[46,48] In fact, IL-10 inhibits lymphocytic production of IFN-γ.[45] Indeed, the powerful immunosuppressive actions of IL-10 are evident in animal models of diseases, such as chronic renal disease, where IL-10 suppresses the expression of chemokines like CCL2 and CCL5 and cytokines like IFN-γ. This attenuates the infiltration of renal parenchyma by inflammatory cells and decreases the amount of inflammation and fibrosis in these tissues.[49] Similarly, in a murine model of colitis, recombinant IL-10 administration prevented colonic inflammation.[50] The ability of IL-10 to inhibit inflammation and act as an immunosuppressive could be a potential mechanism used by tumors to defy the immune system's surveillance and destruction of malignancy.[47,51]

Blay and colleagues examined serum IL-10 levels in EBV- and HIV-negative patients and found that in 47 of 101 patients with active NHL, there were detectable serum levels of IL-10 compared with 60 NHL-free patients, none of whom had detectable IL-10 levels.[37] In addition, in 70 patients with high- or intermediate-grade NHL, those with detectable levels of IL-10 had statistically significant shorter overall and progression-free survivals. In patients achieving either complete or partial remission, IL-10 levels were undetectable. Blay noted that patients with the same stage IV disease would have 0% probability of surviving five years with detectable levels of IL-10 versus 85% probability with undetectable levels of IL-10. Therefore, IL-10 seems to be secreted by B-cell lymphomas in an autocrine fashion to promote tumor growth and perhaps gives one an indication about the activity level of the tumor. In other words, active, more aggressive tumors will produce higher levels of IL-10, while tumors that are less active and less aggressive will produce lower, even undetectable levels of this tumor growth-enhancing cytokine. Blay points out, however, that IL-10 levels are not associated with tumor burden and that different histologic and immunologic classes of NHL tumors may be associated with detectable levels of IL-10. While IL-10 may not be a perfect marker for lymphomas, it is undeniable that IL-10 plays an important role in the development of aberrant B lymphocytes and can inhibit anti-tumor responses by inflammatory cells, a key occurrence in lymphomagenesis.

B-cell lymphomas studied from patients with AIDS showed that such EBV-positive cell lines produced high amounts of IL-10.[52] Benjamin *et al.* found that Burkitt's lymphoma lines obtained from patients with AIDS were EBV-positive, and these tumors also expressed IL-10.[52] Burkitt's lymphoma lines obtained from non-AIDS patients, but were EBV-positive, also produced IL-10. Indeed, others showed similar induction of IL-10 production in EBV-infected B cells. In a simple, yet elegant experiment, human B cells were obtained from tonsilar tissue and then infected with EBV.[53] It was shown that these infected B-cells began producing IL-10, peaking at the same time EBV nuclear antigen was expressed. However, in AIDS patients with PCNSL, although EBV DNA was detected in the CSF, IL-10 levels did not seem to be a specific marker for the disease. This was because other cerebral diseases involved in AIDS, including toxoplasmosis and cryptococcus were associated with similarly elevated levels of IL-10.[54] Animal models of lymphoma also corroborated the findings that IL-10 was involved in tumorigenesis. From profiling of the cytokinic mRNA from four murine B lymphocytic lines (two mature lymphoma lines, a plasmacytoma, and a pre-B lymphoma), it was found that both IL-6 and IL-10 mRNA were expressed in all the lines (whether grown *in situ* (intraperitoneal) or *in vitro*).[38] Although IL-10 to IL-6 ratios were not directly measured, IL-10 levels in culture media and ascitic fluid were measured. It was found that IL-10 levels were higher in ascitic fluid than in culture supernatant, suggesting that *in situ* factors influence cytokine expression. Other cytokines, including TGF-β and TNF-α, were also expressed by the lymphocytic lines. Interestingly, it was found that IL-2 mRNA expression was distinctly absent from all the lines, save one *in situ* tumor. This suggested that the lymphoma lines studied were capable of limiting T-cell anti-tumor responses.[38]

In a study of CSF and serum samples from 11 immunocompetent patients with PCNSL, 10 immunocompetent patients without disease, and

11 immunocompetent patients with other CNS tumors, increased levels of IL-10 were found in the PCNSL patients, but not in disease-free patients or those with other types of CNS tumors.[55] In fact, increased IL-10 levels were correlated with radiographic worsening of brain lesions in the PCNSL patients. Considering that EBV DNA is rarely found in immunocompetent patients with PCNSL, IL-10 may be a marker for PCNSL in immunocompetent patients who have a suspicious clinical history and exam.

The association of high levels of IL-10 with NHLs, including PCNSLs, provided the impetus for us, as early as in 1995, to determine whether IL-10 levels were elevated in PIOL cases. At the NEI, we had analyzed the levels of various interleukins in the vitreous samples of three patients with PIOL and five patients with uveitis.[31] Patients with PIOL had high levels of vitreal IL-10, while uveitic patients had no detectable IL-10, except for one patient with sarcoidosis who had detectable IL-10 in the core vitreous. Interestingly, one PIOL patient had seven vitrectomies performed over a period of seven months, and the number of malignant cells correlated with the level of IL-10 detected. In general, a greater amount of malignant cells in a vitrectomy specimen resulted in a greater vitreal IL-10 level. This patient was also the only one among the three PIOL patients who had detectable IL-6 levels, a classical uveitic cytokine which was detected in all but one uveitis patient. Further studies conducted at our laboratories confirmed the association of high levels of IL-10 with PIOL.

Later, we examined IL-10 to IL-6 ratios by obtaining the vitreous specimens from five PIOL/PCNSL and 11 uveitis patients.[39] In addition, we examined CSF samples for the same ratio provided by 11 PCNSL patients. We found that in all the PIOL/PCNSL vitrectomy specimens there were detectable levels of IL-10, while only four (31%) of the patients with uveitis had detectable IL-10 levels.[39] Notably, the vitreal IL-10 levels were significantly higher in the PIOL patients compared to the patients with uveitis. IL-6 levels were detected in the vitreous of two patients with PIOL/PCNSL and eight (62%) with uveitis; there was no significant difference in the levels of this cytokine between the two disease groups. When we compared IL-10 levels to the levels of IL-6 for each disease group, we found that the vitreous specimens of all the PIOL/PCNSL patients had higher levels of IL-10 than IL-6. This was not the case for any of the uveitis specimens. As for the CSF samples, we found that in the 11 cases where malignant cells could be identified, IL-10 levels exceeded

IL-6 levels in six (55%) cases. Of the 53 CSF samples in which we could not identify malignant cells, IL-10 levels exceeded IL-6 levels in seven (13%) cases. The estimated risk of having increased IL-10 to IL-6 ratio was nearly eight times (and at least 1.5 times) higher in patients having IL-10 levels than IL-6 in the CSF.[39]

Further association of high IL-10 levels with PIOL was provided by our laboratory in 2003.[40] We examined vitreal cytokine levels in 35 PIOL and 64 uveitis (infectious and noninfectious) patients seen at the NEI between 1993 and 2001.[40] In each vitreous specimen, the IL-10 to IL-6 ratio (logarithmic scale) was calculated and revealed a significant difference between the two disease processes; the mean IL-10 to IL-6 ratio was 5.23 for the PIOL vitrectomy specimens and that of the uveitis vitrectomy specimens was 0.23. Correctly classifying PIOL based on an IL-10/IL-6 ratio greater than 1.0 was accomplished 74.7% of the time, and the sensitivity and specificity for the cutoff rule was 74.3% and 75.0%, respectively.[40] It is important to note that as PIOL and uveitis are complementary disease groups, a reversal in sensitivity and specificity was observed. Thus, uveitis had a sensitivity of 75.0% and a specificity of 74.3%.[40]

Further evidence that IL-10 levels can provide a clue in the diagnosis of PIOL came from a study in France by Merle-Beràl and colleagues.[32] Vitrectomy specimens from 36 patients with PIOL were analyzed for IL-10 levels using enzyme immunoassay. This group had previously developed cut-off values of 150 pg/ml and 50 pg/ml for undiluted and diluted vitreous specimens, respectively, based on previously unpublished comparisons made with intraocular inflammatory conditions. Out of 23 pure and 12 diluted vitreous samples, 20 (87%) pure and all diluted had IL-10 levels above their respective cut-off values. One patient's pure vitreous sample had a low IL-10 level (8 pg/mL), and this patient was later found to have a T-cell lymphoma. Overall, IL-10 levels for all the vitreous samples were high with a mean value of 2518 pg/mL. Use of vitreal IL-10/IL-6 ratios has helped us make diagnoses of PIOL in Japan as well.[56]

IL-6. This pleiotropic cytokine has functions that are mediated through association with either its membrane-bound cognate receptor (IL-6R) found on hepatocytes and leukocytes or its soluble receptor sIL-6R. IL-6 has been shown to promote differentiation of T- and B-cells and is important for terminal differentiation of B-cells. In response to various stimuli (i.e., infection or injury) IL-6 is released by macrophages, endothelial cells, and fibroblasts, and this cytokine seems to be involved in promoting a Th1 phenotype and opposing a Th2 phenotype.[57] Some have shown that IL-6 has pro-apoptotic effects on B lymphocytes.[58] Therefore, as we will discuss in this chapter, removing such constraints on B lymphocytes can leave the door open for deviant processes, notably the development of lymphoma within the CNS and the eye. In general, IL-6 is considered a pro-inflammatory cytokine with many of its functions carried out through the activation of protein kinases and transcription proteins.[57,59] Some of the functions of IL-6 include the production of acute phase proteins and the differentiation of T-cells into cytotoxic T-cells.[60] IL-6 also leads to the recruitment of monocytes to sites of inflammation[61,62] and, therefore, is important for the maintenance of inflammation.[59] Indeed, in IL-6 deficient mice, acute-phase inflammation and the fever response are reduced[63,64] and can be restored with the administration of recombinant IL-6.[64] Increased levels of IL-6 in the eye have been associated with autoimmunity and inflammation. Therefore, IL-6 is classically thought of as being an inflammatory cytokine released by inflammatory cells, including T-cells. In humans, high levels of IL-6 in the aqueous humor have been associated with uveitic conditions. For example, Murray and colleagues showed that for Fuch's heterochromic cyclitis (a non-infectious form of uveitis) and infectious uveitis caused by *Toxoplasma gondii* there were high levels of IL-6 in the aqueous in most patients (63% of patients for both types of uveitides) as compared with patients without uveitis.[65] In addition, the high levels of IL-6 detected in the eye were independent of serum levels of IL-6, which were normal to low.

IL-10/IL-6 Ratio. Vitreal IL-10 levels have been shown to be elevated in PIOL, while IL-6 levels are increased in uveitis, and IL-10/IL-6 ratios greater than 1.0 suggest an intraocular malignancy. This useful tool is by no means meant to be diagnostic for the disease.[39,66] However, in the majority of B-cell PIOL cases, IL-10/IL-6 ratio is greater than one. Only a few exceptions were reported. For example, a 40-year-old gentleman with a history of recurrent bilateral panuveitis (despite treatment with corticosteroids and acyclovir) and retinal detachment in the left eye was evaluated at the NEI.[67] While both eyes exhibited diffuse, atrophic and pigmented chorioretinal scarring and cystoid macular edema in the right eye, the left eye tellingly had creamy subretinal infiltrates. A chorioretinal biopsy revealed atypical subretinal cells that stained positively for CD20 (B-cell marker), and PCR showed *IgH* gene rearrangements in the third complementarity determining region (CDR3). However, despite the presence of this B-cell PIOL, the vitreal IL-10 to IL-6 ratio was less than 1.0. Early disease stage might help explain this low ratio as upon histopathologic inspection, the tumor was noted to be located primarily subretinally with a lack of retinal infiltration. Certainly, diagnosis of PIOL remains dependent upon the identification of malignant cells in CSF or vitrectomy specimens.[39] Nonetheless, in cases where there is a high clinical suspicion for PIOL and where CSF and vitrectomy specimens have failed to reveal lymphoma cells, an IL-10/IL-6 ratio greater than 1.0 can provide evidence that PIOL is possible.[40,68,69] It can also convey the need to pursue this diagnosis by performing further vitrectomies or perhaps even a chorioretinal biopsy.

Chemokines and their Receptors. Chemokines are important molecules (molecular weight of 8–10 kDa) involved in cell recruitment to various tissue sites within the body. Previously, chemokines were known by a variety of names, usually due to associated functions on cellular targets. Today, a systematic nomenclature exists, which relates the basic cysteine motif common to all chemokines.[70] The chemokines are named for the first two cysteines (all chemokines except for one containing four cysteine residues) found in each one's respective motif. Chemokines with the two cysteines next to each other are called "CC." Those with one non-cysteine amino acid between the two cysteines are called "CXC," where "X" represents the non-cysteine amino acid. If there is only one cysteine (which is preceded by a non-cysteine amino acid), the chemokine is simply called "XC." Finally, if three non-cysteine residues exist between the first two cysteines, the chemokine is known as "CX3C." An "R" follows this nomenclature to represent a receptor and an "L" represents the ligand.[70]

Chemokines are important cellular chemotactic proteins that act through their respective chemokine receptors to elicit cell trafficking, an essential property, especially in the immune system. However, aberrant chemokine-chemokine receptor interactions can lead to undesired immune cell trafficking and be a possible path leading to disease. Chemokines and their receptors are involved in disease processes, such as rheumatoid arthritis,[71] inflammatory bowel disease,[72] and multiple sclerosis.[73] Evidence also exists on the involvement of chemokines and their receptors in cancer, including breast cancer metastasis,[74] chronic lymphocytic leukemia,[75] and B-cell NHL.[76]

Two chemokines involved in B-cell chemoattraction include CXCL12 (also known as SDF-1 (stromal derived factor-1, which binds to CXCR4 receptor on B-cells)) and CXCL13 (also known as BCA-1/BLC (B-cell specific chemokine, which binds to CXCR5 receptor on B-cells)). The interaction of CXCL13 with its receptor, CXCR5 on B-cells is necessary for the formation of germinal centers[77] and for the germinal center B-cells to undergo somatic hypermutation and subsequent affinity maturation. After activation, these B-cells seem to become more responsive to CXCL12, thereby chemoattracting the B-cells out of the germinal center as these B-cells also express the receptor for CXCL12, CXCR4.

As the CNS, including the eye, is an immunologically privileged site, it remains an enigma as to why a lymphoma should involve this location. Chemokines and their receptors might provide some insights into the pathogenesis of PCNSL/PIOL. The expression of chemokine receptors on various tumor cells has been shown to be involved in their localization to certain sites.[74,78] Similarly, chemokines have been shown to be involved in PCNSL and PIOL. At the NEI, we have shown that B-cell-attractive chemokines are expressed in the retinal tissues of patients with PIOL.[79] Tissue provided from two enucleated eyes and one chorioretinal biopsy, all containing PIOL, and one normal autopsy eye were analyzed. Microdissection was performed on frozen sections of the ocular tissues to obtain either PIOL cells or retinal pigment epithelium (RPE). Reverse transcriptase (RT)-PCR was performed on the extracted RNA for PIOL cells as well as RPE cells that were adjacent to the PIOL cells and RPE cells that were located away from the tumor. PIOL cells were shown to express both B-cell chemokine receptors, CXCR5 and CXCR4, while adjacent RPE cells expressed CXCL13 and CXCL12. RPE tissue distant from tumor invasion also showed expression of *CXCL13* mRNA that was more abundant than tumor-adjacent RPE tissue; distant RPE did not express mRNA for *CXCL12*. The more abundant expression of mRNA by distant RPE cells was of interest to us and could possibly be explained by three mechanisms. First, there could be downregulation of CXCL12 and CXCL13 in the tumor-adjacent RPE cells, perhaps after interaction with their respective chemokine receptors on the infiltrating lymphoma cells. Second, RPE cells adjacent to tumor are damaged or destroyed, while more distant RPE is intact. Finally, reactive inflammatory cells (T lymphocytes and macrophages) can also be admixed in the area of tumor infiltration. The RPE from the normal autopsy eye did not show mRNA expression of either *CXCL12* or *CXCL13*. Therefore, deviant expression of chemokines by PIOL-susceptible RPE could be a means for the recruitment of malignant B-cells as well as their infiltration of areas with increased expression of such chemokines.

In a study of biopsy specimens from 24 patients with PCNSL (17 HIV-negative, three HIV-positive, and four with unknown HIV status), immunostaining for CXCL13 revealed that all the samples were positive for expression of the chemokine.[80] Double immunostaining for CD20 (B-cell antigen) and CD31 (vascular endothelial antigen) on five biopsy specimens revealed that CXCL13 was expressed by the lymphoma and the vascular endothelial cells. There was no staining of normal, non-infiltrated brain tissue. Furthermore, immunostaining for CXCR5, CXCL13's receptor, resulted in staining of the membranes of the lymphoma cells. More recently, Jahnke and colleagues showed that in 29 biopsy specimens from PCNSL patients, CXCR4, CXCR5, and CCR7 were expressed only in the cytoplasm or nucleus, but not on the membrane of lymphoma cells.[81] This was in contrast to lymphoma cells from peripheral-NHL biopsy specimens. These data could offer an explanation as to why PCNSL so rarely metastasizes.

There is a complex interaction between cells, their receptors, and signals (interleukins and chemokines), and this is involved not only in the homing of lymphomas to specific sites in the CNS (both cerebral and ocular), but also in their restriction to these sites and lack of metastasis. Although we do not understand precisely how chemokine and cytokine profiles are involved in the pathogenesis of all PCNSL/PIOLs, we are making progress in elucidating some of the mechanisms by which PIOL is able to make its home in the eye. We are currently examining murine PIOL models[82] (see Chapter 13 – Animal Models of PIOL). Furthermore, we can attempt to interfere with these mechanisms to direct future therapeutic interventions.

References

1. Schubert MS, Moss RB. (1992) Selective polysaccharide antibody deficiency in familial DiGeorge syndrome. *Ann Allergy* **69**(3): 231–238.
2. Smith CA, Driscoll DA, Emanuel BS, *et al.* (1998) Increased prevalence of immunoglobulin A deficiency in patients with the chromosome 22q11.2 deletion syndrome (DiGeorge syndrome/velocardiofacial syndrome). *Clin Diagn Lab Immunol* **5**(3): 415–417.
3. Sullivan KE, Jawad AF, Randall P, *et al.* (1998) Lack of correlation between impaired T cell production, immunodeficiency, and other phenotypic features in chromosome 22q11.2 deletion syndromes. *Clin Immunol Immunopathol* **86**(2): 141–146.
4. Trapani JA, Sutton VR. (2003) Granzyme B: pro-apoptotic, antiviral and antitumor functions. *Curr Opin Immunol* **15**(5): 533–543.
5. Ashton-Rickardt PG. (2005) The granule pathway of programmed cell death. *Crit Rev Immunol* **25**(3): 161–182.
6. Nishiyama A, Saito T, Abe S, Kumanishi T. (1989) An immunohistochemical analysis of T cells in primary B cell malignant lymphoma of the brain. *Acta Neuropathol (Berl)* **79**(1): 27–29.
7. Bashir R, Chamberlain M, Ruby E, Hochberg FH. (1996) T-cell infiltration of primary CNS lymphoma. *Neurology* **46**(2): 440–444.
8. Lopez JS, Chan CC, Burnier M, *et al.* (1991) Immunohistochemistry findings in primary intraocular lymphoma. *Am J Ophthalmol* **112**(4): 472–474.
9. Char DH, Margolis L, Newman AB. (1981) Ocular reticulum cell sarcoma. *Am J Ophthalmol* **91**(4): 480–483.
10. Tuaillon N, Chan CC. (2001) Molecular analysis of primary central nervous system and primary intraocular lymphoma. *Curr Mol Med* **1**(2): 259–272.
11. Coupland SE, Heimann H, Bechrakis NE. (2004) Primary intraocular lymphoma: a review of the clinical, histopathological and molecular biological features. *Graefes Arch Clin Exp Ophthalmol* **242**(11): 901–913.
12. Chan CC, Wallace DJ. (2004) Intraocular lymphoma: update on diagnosis and management. *Cancer Control* **11**(5): 285–295.
13. Rosenberg SA, Terry WD. (1977) Passive immunotherapy of cancer in animals and man. *Adv Cancer Res* **25**: 323–388.
14. Kedar E, Weiss DW. (1983) The in vitro generation of effector lymphocytes and their employment in tumor immunotherapy. *Adv Cancer Res* **38**: 171–287.
15. Kawakami Y, Eliyahu S, Sakaguchi K, *et al.* (1994) Identification of the immunodominant peptides of the MART-1 human melanoma antigen recognized by the majority of HLA-A2–restricted tumor infiltrating lymphocytes. *J Exp Med* **180**(1): 347–352.

16. Yang D, Nakao M, Shichijo S, *et al.* (1999) Identification of a gene coding for a protein possessing shared tumor epitopes capable of inducing HLA-A24-restricted cytotoxic T lymphocytes in cancer patients. *Cancer Res* 59(16): 4056–4063.
17. Del Prete G. (1998) The concept of type-1 and type-2 helper T cells and their cytokines in humans. *Int Rev Immunol,* 16(3–4): 427–455.
18. Del Prete GF, De Carli M, Ricci M, Romagnani S. (1991) Helper activity for immunoglobulin synthesis of T helper type 1 (Th1) and Th2 human T cell clones: the help of Th1 clones is limited by their cytolytic capacity. *J Exp Med* 174(4): 809–813.
19. Fallarino F, Grohmann U, Bianchi R, *et al.* (2000) Th1 and Th2 cell clones to a poorly immunogenic tumor antigen initiate CD8+ T cell-dependent tumor eradication in vivo. *J Immunol* 165(10): 5495–5501.
20. Knutson KL, Disis ML. (2005) Tumor antigen-specific T helper cells in cancer immunity and immunotherapy. *Cancer Immunol Immunother* 54(8): 721–728.
21. Knutson KL, Disis ML. (2005) Augmenting T helper cell immunity in cancer. *Curr Drug Targets Immune Endocr Metabol Disord* 5(4): 365–371.
22. Alvaro-Naranjo T, Lejeune M, Salvado-Usach MT, *et al.* (2005) Tumor-infiltrating cells as a prognostic factor in Hodgkin's lymphoma: a quantitative tissue microarray study in a large retrospective cohort of 267 patients. *Leuk Lymphoma* 46(11): 1581–1591.
23. Whitcup SM, de Smet MD, Rubin BI, *et al.* (1993) Intraocular lymphoma. Clinical and histopathologic diagnosis. *Ophthalmology* 100: 1399–1406.
24. Davis JL, Solomon D, Nussenblatt RB, *et al.* (1992) Immunocytochemical staining of vitreous cells: Indications, techniques, and results. *Ophthalmology* 99(2): 250–256.
25. Zou W. (2005) Immunosuppressive networks in the tumour environment and their therapeutic relevance. *Nat Rev Cancer* 5(4): 263–274.
26. Corthay A, Skovseth DK, Lundin KU, *et al.* (2005) Primary antitumor immune response mediated by CD4+ T cells. *Immunity* 22(3): 371–383.
27. Steinman RM. (1991) The dendritic cell system and its role in immunogenicity. *Annu Rev Immunol* 9: 271–296.
28. Chiodoni C, Paglia P, Stoppacciaro A, *et al.* (1999) Dendritic cells infiltrating tumors cotransduced with granulocyte/macrophage colony-stimulating factor (GM-CSF) and CD40 ligand genes take up and present endogenous tumor-associated antigens, and prime naive mice for a cytotoxic T lymphocyte response. *J Exp Med* 190(1): 125–133.
29. Preynat-Seauve O, Schuler P, Contassot E, *et al.* (2006) Tumor-infiltrating dendritic cells are potent antigen-presenting cells able to activate T cells and mediate tumor rejection. *J Immunol* 176(1): 61–67.

30. Steinbrink K, Wolfl M, Jonuleit H, *et al.* (1997) Induction of tolerance by IL-10-treated dendritic cells. *J Immunol* **159**(10): 4772–4780.
31. Chan CC, Whitcup SM, Solomon D, Nussenblatt RB. (1995) Interleukin-10 in the vitreous of primary intraocular lymphoma. *Am J Ophthalmol* **120**(5): 671–673.
32. Merle-Beral H, Davi F, Cassoux N, *et al.* (2004) Biological diagnosis of primary intraocular lymphoma. *Br J Haematol* **124**(4): 469–473.
33. Radford KJ, Vari F, Hart DN. (2005) Vaccine strategies to treat lymphoproliferative disorders. *Pathology* **37**(6): 534–550.
34. Soussain C, Hoang-Xuan K, Levy V. (2004) Results of intensive chemotherapy followed by hematopoietic stem-cell rescue in 22 patients with refractory or recurrent primary CNS lymphoma or intraocular lymphoma. *Bull Cancer* **91**(2): 189–192.
35. Brevet M, Garidi R, Gruson B, *et al.* (2005) First-line autologous stem cell transplantation in primary CNS lymphoma. *Eur J Haematol* **75**(4): 288–292.
36. Lotze C, Schuler F, Kruger WH, *et al.* (2005) Combined immunoradiotherapy induces long-term remission of CNS relapse of peripheral, diffuse, large-cell lymphoma after allogeneic stem cell transplantation: case study. *Neuro-oncol* **7**(4): 508–510.
37. Blay JY, Burdin N, Rousset F, *et al.* (1993) Serum interleukin-10 in non-Hodgkin's lymphoma: a prognostic factor. *Blood* **82**(7): 2169–2174.
38. Bost KL, Bieligk SC, Jaffe BM. (1995) Lymphokine mRNA expression by transplantable murine B lymphocytic malignancies. Tumor-derived IL-10 as a possible mechanism for modulating the anti-tumor response. *J Immunol* **154**(2): 718–729.
39. Whitcup SM, Stark Vancs V, Wittes RE, *et al.* (1997) Association of interleukin-10 in the vitreous and cerebral spinal fluid and primary central nervous system lymphoma. *Arch Ophthalmol* **115**: 1157–1160.
40. Wolf LA, Reed GF, Buggage RR, *et al.* (2003) Vitreous cytokine levels. *Ophthalmology* **110**(8): 1671–1672.
41. Chan CC, Shen DF. (1999) Newer methodologies in immunohistochemistry and diagnosis. In BenEzra, D. (ed), *Uveitis Update*, pp. 1–13, Karger, Basel.
42. Tilg H, Atkins MB, Dinarello CA, Mier JW. (1995) Induction of circulating interleukin 10 by interleukin 1 and interleukin 2, but not interleukin 6 immunotherapy. *Cytokine* **7**(7): 734–739.
43. Daftarian PM, Kumar A, Kryworuchko M, Diaz-Mitoma F. (1996) IL-10 production is enhanced in human T cells by IL-12 and IL-6 and in monocytes by tumor necrosis factor-alpha. *J Immunol* **157**(1): 12–20.
44. Bogdan C, Vodovotz Y, Nathan C. (1991) Macrophage deactivation by interleukin 10. *J Exp Med* **174**(6): 1549–1555.

45. D'Andrea A, Aste-Amezaga M, Valiante NM, *et al.* (1993) Interleukin 10 (IL-10) inhibits human lymphocyte interferon gamma-production by suppressing natural killer cell stimulatory factor/IL-12 synthesis in accessory cells. *J Exp Med* **178**(3): 1041–1048.
46. de Waal Malefyt R, Haanen J, Spits H, *et al.* (1991) Interleukin 10 (IL-10) and viral IL-10 strongly reduce antigen-specific human T cell proliferation by diminishing the antigen-presenting capacity of monocytes via downregulation of class II major histocompatibility complex expression. *J Exp Med* **174**(4): 915–924.
47. Petersson M, Charo J, Salazar-Onfray F, *et al.* (1998) Constitutive IL-10 production accounts for the high NK sensitivity, low MHC class I expression, and poor transporter associated with antigen processing (TAP)-1/2 function in the prototype NK target YAC-1. *J Immunol* **161**(5): 2099–2105.
48. Howard M, O'Garra A, Ishida H, *et al.* (1992) Biological properties of interleukin 10. *J Clin Immunol* **12**(4): 239–247.
49. Mu W, Ouyang X, Agarwal A, *et al.* (2005) IL-10 suppresses chemokines, inflammation, and fibrosis in a model of chronic renal disease. *J Am Soc Nephrol* **16**(12): 3651–3660.
50. Duchmann R, Schmitt E, Knolle P, *et al.* (1996) Tolerance towards resident intestinal flora in mice is abrogated in experimental colitis and restored by treatment with interleukin-10 or antibodies to interleukin-12. *Eur J Immunol* **26**(4): 934–938.
51. Matsuda M, Salazar F, Petersson M, *et al.* (1994) Interleukin 10 pretreatment protects target cells from tumor- and allo-specific cytotoxic T cells and downregulates HLA class I expression. *J Exp Med* **180**(6): 2371–2376.
52. Benjamin D, Knobloch TJ, Dayton MA. (1992) Human B-cell interleukin-10: B-cell lines derived from patients with acquired immunodeficiency syndrome and Burkitt's lymphoma constitutively secrete large quantities of interleukin-10. *Blood* **80**(5): 1289–1298.
53. Burdin N, Peronne C, Banchereau J, Rousset F. (1993) Epstein-Barr virus transformation induces B lymphocytes to produce human interleukin 10. *J Exp Med* **177**(2): 295–304.
54. De Luca A, Antinori A, Cingolani A, *et al.* (1995) Evaluation of cerebrospinal fluid EBV-DNA and IL-10 as markers for in vivo diagnosis of AIDS-related primary central nervous system lymphoma [published erratum appears in *Br J Haematol* 1995 Dec; **91**(4): 1035]. *Br J Haematol* **90**(4): 844–849.
55. Salmaggi A, Eoli M, Corsini E, *et al.* (2000) Cerebrospinal fluid interleukin-10 levels in primary central nervous system lymphoma: a possible marker of response to treatment? *Ann Neurol* **47**(1): 137–138.

56. Yokota M, Takase H, Imai Y, *et al.* (2003) A case of intraocular malignant lymphoma diagnosed by immunoglobulin gene rearrangement and translocation, and IL-10/IL-6 ratio in the vitreous fluid. *Nippon Ganka Gakkai Zasshi* 107(5): 287–291.

57. Horn F, Henze C, Heidrich K. (2000) Interleukin-6 signal transduction and lymphocyte function. *Immunobiology* 202(2): 151–167.

58. Morse L, Chen D, Franklin D, *et al.* (1997) Induction of cell cycle arrest and B cell terminal differentiation by CDK inhibitor p18(INK4c) and IL-6. *Immunity* 6(1): 47–56.

59. Hodge DR, Hurt EM, Farrar WL. (2005) The role of IL-6 and STAT3 in inflammation and cancer. *Eur J Cancer* 41(16): 2502–2512.

60. Simpson RJ, Hammacher A, Smith DK, *et al.* (1997) Interleukin-6: structure-function relationships. *Protein Sci* 6(5): 929–955.

61. Romano M, Sironi M, Toniatti C, *et al.* (1997) Role of IL-6 and its soluble receptor in induction of chemokines and leukocyte recruitment. *Immunity* 6(3): 315–325.

62. Hurst SM, Wilkinson TS, McLoughlin RM, *et al.* (2001) Il-6 and its soluble receptor orchestrate a temporal switch in the pattern of leukocyte recruitment seen during acute inflammation. *Immunity* 14(6): 705–714.

63. Kopf M, Baumann H, Freer G, *et al.* (1994) Impaired immune and acute-phase responses in interleukin-6–deficient mice. *Nature* 368(6469): 339–342.

64. Chai Z, Gatti S, Toniatti C, *et al.* (1996) Interleukin (IL)-6 gene expression in the central nervous system is necessary for fever response to lipopolysaccharide or IL-1 beta: a study on IL-6–deficient mice. *J Exp Med* 183(1): 311–316.

65. Murray PI, Hoekzema R, van Haren MA, *et al.* (1990) Aqueous humor interleukin-6 levels in uveitis. *Invest Ophthalmol Vis Sci* 31(5): 917–920.

66. Akpek EK, Maca SM, Christen WG, Foster CS. (1999) Elevated vitreous interleukin-10 level is not diagnostic of intraocular-central nervous system lymphoma. *Ophthalmology* 106(12): 2291–2295.

67. Buggage RR, Velez G, Myers-Powell B, *et al.* (1999) Primary intraocular lymphoma with a low interleukin 10 to interleukin 6 ratio and heterogeneous *IgH* gene rearrangement. *Arch Opthalmol* 117(9): 1239–1242.

68. Cassoux N, Merle-Beral H, Leblond V, *et al.* (2000) Ocular and central nervous system lymphoma: clinical features and diagnosis. *Ocul Immunol Inflamm* 8(4): 243–250.

69. Velez G, Buggage R. (2001) Interleukin-10 and intraocular-central nervous system lymphoma. *Ophthalmology* 108(3): 427–428.

70. Zlotnik A, Yoshie O. (2000) Chemokines: a new classification system and their role in immunity. *Immunity* 12(2): 121–127.

71. Koch AE, Kunkel SL, Harlow LA, *et al.* (1994) Macrophage inflammatory protein-1 alpha. A novel chemotactic cytokine for macrophages in rheumatoid arthritis. *J Clin Invest* 93(3): 921–928.

72. Danese S, Gasbarrini A. (2005) Chemokines in inflammatory bowel disease. *J Clin Pathol* 58(10): 1025–1027.

73. Sorensen TL, Tani M, Jensen J, *et al.* (1999) Expression of specific chemokines and chemokine receptors in the central nervous system of multiple sclerosis patients. *J Clin Invest* 103(6): 807–815.

74. Muller A, Homey B, Soto H, *et al.* (2001) Involvement of chemokine receptors in breast cancer metastasis. *Nature* 410(6824): 50–56.

75. Mohle R, Failenschmid C, Bautz F, Kanz L. (1999) Overexpression of the chemokine receptor CXCR4 in B cell chronic lymphocytic leukemia is associated with increased functional response to stromal cell-derived factor-1 (SDF-1). *Leukemia* 13(12): 1954–1959.

76. Arai J, Yasukawa M, Yakushijin Y, *et al.* (2000) Stromal cells in lymph nodes attract B-lymphoma cells via production of stromal cell-derived factor-1. *Eur J Haematol* 64(5): 323–332.

77. Forster R, Mattis AE, Kremmer E, *et al.* (1996) A putative chemokine receptor, BLR1, directs B cell migration to defined lymphoid organs and specific anatomic compartments of the spleen. *Cell* 87(6): 1037–1047.

78. Mashino K, Sadanaga N, Yamaguchi H, *et al.* (2002) Expression of chemokine receptor CCR7 is associated with lymph node metastasis of gastric carcinoma. *Cancer Res* 62(10): 2937–2941.

79. Chan CC, Shen D, Hackett JJ, *et al.* (2003) Expression of chemokine receptors, CXCR4 and CXCR5, and chemokines, BLC and SDF-1, in the eyes of patients with primary intraocular lymphoma. *Ophthalmology* 110(2): 421–426.

80. Smith JR, Braziel RM, Paoletti S, *et al.* (2003) Expression of B-cell-attracting chemokine 1 (CXCL13) by malignant lymphocytes and vascular endothelium in primary central nervous system lymphoma. *Blood* 101(3): 815–821.

81. Jahnke K, Coupland SE, Na IK, *et al.* (2005) Expression of the chemokine receptors CXCR4, CXCR5, and CCR7 in primary central nervous system lymphoma. *Blood* 106(1): 384–385.

82. Chan CC, Fischette M, Shen D, *et al.* (2005) Murine model of primary intraocular lymphoma. *Invest Ophthalmol Vis Sci* 46(2): 415–419.

Chapter 9

Diagnostic Approaches

We have already examined the clinical features found in PIOL as well as the imaging techniques that can be employed to help the ophthalmologist and oncologist to pursue a diagnosis of PIOL. While a strong clinical suspicion may exist that a patient has PIOL and a clinical examination helps confirm this suspicion, PIOL can be diagnosed only upon the identification of malignant lymphoid cells in the eye. In this chapter we explore the diagnostic approaches, both historical and current, for PIOL.

Historical Diagnostic Approaches

Early Analyses of the CSF in Malignancy. In 1904, Dufour was the first to describe the evaluation of cerebrospinal fluid (CSF) in malignancy.[1] A 64-year-old male had presented with complaints of weakness in the legs, difficulty in urinating, cachexia, and memory difficulties. The right eye became red as in conjunctivitis and the cornea turned cloudy. The patient received lumbar puncture twice and each time showed yellow CSF with lymphocytosis and fibrin material. When the patient succumbed to his condition, massive infiltration of the spinal cord and roots as well as invasion of the marrow, consistent with a sarcoma, were found at autopsy. Subsequently, others began to value the utility of CSF examination in CNS malignancies, whether primary or secondary.

Marks and Marrack described 17 cases of CSF examinations revealing "abnormal cells, considered to be neoplastic."[2] None of the patients described by Marks and Marrack had PCNSL/PIOL or, as it would have been known during the 1960s, reticulum cell sarcoma. Three patients had histologically proven astrocytomas, two had histologically proven medulloblastomas (one questionably), six had metastatic cancer to the CNS, and four patients did not have biopsies performed, but two were noted to have suprasellar masses on air encephalography. Finally, one patient who had neoplastic-appearing cells within the CSF was determined to have non-specific leptomeningitis, and this case's CSF examination was considered a false positive. Marks and Marrack conceded that while it was possible in suspected cases of CNS malignancy to identify cells suspicious of being neoplastic, "it is impossible, as yet, always to recognize the smeared cells as neoplastic by the methods currently employed."[2] Indeed, even today when we are "lucky" enough to get well-preserved cells in the CSF, there can be some difficulty in determining whether they are truly neoplastic. Difficulty arises from cells that are suggestively, but perhaps not blatantly, atypical.

In another rather large study of the CSF, Kline examined 1,669 CSF specimens.[3] Histologically proven CNS tumors occurred in 96 cases, and 39 (41%) of these exhibited neoplastic cells in the CSF. Metastatic carcinomas and astrocytomas (including glioblastoma multiforme) made up the bulk of the histologically proven cases. There were three cases of Hodgkin's lymphoma involving the CNS, but none of these exhibited neoplastic cells in their respective CSF samples. There were no cases of reticulum cell sarcoma in Kline's study.

The issue of identifying neoplastic cells within the CSF was and still is of concern. However, some pathologists have noted that increasing cognizance amongst clinicians and pathologists of the fact that tumor cells could indeed be found in the CSF, could help uncover these cells more frequently.[4]

Enucleation. Prior to the development of pars plana vitrectomy (PPV) surgery in the 1970s, enucleation was the only way to establish a diagnosis of primary intraocular reticulum cell sarcoma (RCS), now known as PIOL.[5–7] Indeed, enucleation provided unequivocal evidence of neoplastic processes by providing the pathologist with the whole eye and being able to make both macroscopic and microscopic observations of involved ocular tissues. Enucleation was often performed in patients whose eyes no longer had vision or were painful.[5] Enucleation was also performed in patients who had died from their sarcomas (whether primarily or secondarily affecting the CNS) to confirm clinical suspicion of RCS.

The Vitreous: A Glimpse into the Eye. Vitreous comes from the Latin word *vitre-us*, meaning "of glass, glassy, bright" to denote a nature or composition like that of glass.[8] Similarly, the vitreous humor that fills the posterior segment of the eye is usually a transparent, gelatinous substance. The volume is about 4 ml and the weight is roughly 4 grams. Imperfections in glass can make it appear opaque or give it varied hues. Likewise, certain processes in the eye can bring about vitreous changes, often suggesting that a pathologic process is occurring. The vitreous is normally a viscous solution that is 99% water. Within this solution is a meshwork of collagen fibrils and fibers[9] and other structural proteins,[10,11] glycosaminoglycans,[12,13] macrophages, and hyalocytes[4] as well as other molecules such as amino acids, proteins,[15,16] lipids, and ions.[17] Vitreous involvement in the form of inflammatory cells producing a uveitis had been noted to occur in ocular and CNS reticulum cell sarcoma,[18] but was not considered a suggestive feature commonly seen in ocular and cerebral RCS that could be an important clue to its existence until the late 1960s and early 1970s.[19,20]

Some had already described the involvement of the vitreous with neoplastic cells, but these reports dealt with eyes that had undergone enucleation and histopathologic examination.[6,7,21,22] For example, Minckler, Font, and Zimmerman at the Armed Forces Institute of Pathology (AFIP) in Washington, D.C. described an autopsy case involving RCS of the brain and eyes.[21] The patient had been a 65-year-old Caucasian female who had noted decreasing vision bilaterally. Over a period of three years she declined both visually and mentally and succumbed to her progressive illness, which, until her death, had no clinically satisfactory diagnosis. A complete autopsy was performed revealing RCS of the brain; no visceral malignancy was found. Both eyes were sent to the AFIP for histopathologic examination and revealed numerous, atypical cells with large nuclei, so characteristic of RCS, in the vitreous. The retina and optic nerve were relatively normal, except for a disciform chorioretinal scar in the macula (although this could have represented an area of previous retinal pigment epithelium detachment due to lymphomatous infiltration[23] that subsequently resolved). The choroid exhibited the typical reactive inflammatory infiltrate.[21] The right eye also exhibited RCS cells in the vitreous, while the retina and optic nerve were normal. The authors pointed out that this case was unique because only the vitreous showed involvement with neoplastic cells, while the retina was free of infiltration in both eyes. Barr reviewed four cases of RCS the eye, all with neoplastic cells found in the vitreous during pathologic inspection of the enucleated globes.[22]

Vitreous Sampling. Prior to the development of pars plana vitreous surgery by Machemer[24–29] in 1970, there was no adequate way to enter the vitreous cavity for posterior segment surgeries that seem common today. Making certain diagnoses required that the entire eye be removed lest a clinical diagnosis could not be obtained. Indeed, the only way to make a diagnosis of primary intraocular RCS prior to the development of pars plana vitrectomy (PPV) was by performing an enucleation.[22,30] Obviously, a significant amount of morbidity was associated with this procedure, and it was not the most ideal situation for patients.

Klingele and Hogan,[31] and Michels[30] *et al.* were the first to report cases in which the initial diagnosis of PIOL was established by cytologic examination of the vitreous specimen. Klingele and Hogan described eight patients with ocular RCS, two being diagnosed and subsequently treated based on the vitreous sample cytology. One patient, a 65-year-old female had complained of blurred vision in both eyes. Ophthalmic examination revealed 2+ anterior chamber cell and flare and 3+ vitreous haze unresponsive to corticosteroid treatment. Although multiple yellow retinal infiltrates were seen in the right eye, MRI and CSF inspection were normal. However, upon cytologic study of a vitreous aspirate, there were large lymphoblastic cells characteristic of ocular RCS. For this reason, radiation treatment was provided for the eyes. This resulted in resolution of the retinal lesions in the right and improvement in the bilateral uveitis. The second vitrectomy-diagnosed patient described by Klingele and Hogan was a 64-year-old male who had a year-long history of blurred vision in the right eye.[31] He had vitreous haze in both eyes and retinal infiltrates in the right. He had a biopsy performed on a lipoma from the anterior abdominal wall, which showed an angiolipoma with perivascular malignant reticulocytes. The vitreous cytology showed lymphoblastic cells with large, granular nuclei and vesicular cytoplasm. The vitreous cytology, in addition to the abdominal biopsy, helped diagnose this patient's RCS (which seemed to have involved the eye secondarily, judging by the existence of the peripheral lesion) and was a reason for starting ocular radiotherapy.[31]

Michels and associates also performed vitreous biopsy to diagnose ocular reticulum cell sarcoma.[30] Two cases were described, one involving a 61-year-old male who had noted "spots" in his vision, first in the left eye and later in the right. Slit lamp examinations revealed keratic precipitates in the anterior chamber, and ophthalmoscopic examinations revealed vitreous sheets, clumps of debris, and small cells. Peripheral examinations and tests failed to reveal a systemic malignancy, although a bone marrow aspirate showed hypercellularity and increased immature myeloid forms. PPV was done to improve vision, and the vitreous was analyzed. This analysis revealed a number of neoplastic cells consistent with RCS. Because of the tumor cells found in the vitreous, radiation therapy was provided for both eyes. The second patient described by Michels *et al.* was a 71-year-old female who had noted a decline in the vision of the left eye (which went on to develop a non-clearing vitreous hemorrhage) and later blurred vision in the right.[30] Both eyes were recalcitrant to topical corticosteroid treatment. Slit lamp examination showed 1+ flare and few cells bilaterally, and the right anterior vitreous was noted to have many cells and debris. Dense vitreal blood was noted posterior to the lens. Ophthalmoscopic examination revealed RPE atrophic lesions and cystoid macular edema in the right eye. Dense vitreous hemorrhage in the left eye precluded examination of the fundus. Chest X-ray and CT showed a right, solid 2 cm hilar mass. A PPV was performed, and the left fundus was noted to have similar, but more extensive atrophic lesions than those in the right eye. A sample of vitreous was examined, and this disclosed many tumor cells that generated a diagnosis of RCS. Due to the yield of tumor cells in the vitreous, care was coordinated with oncology services and a lumbar puncture was performed. However, CSF examination did not reveal atypical cells. Radiation therapy was initiated for this patient.

Later, Parver and Font also made a diagnosis of RCS based on the cytologic analysis of a vitreous sample.[32] A 42-year-old female noticed bilateral blurred vision. She was treated with oral corticosteroids for supposed uveitis, but vision failed to improve and the patient developed mental status changes. Two lumbar punctures failed to reveal any abnormalities, and a month after admission to hospital the patient was noted to have bilateral vitreous haze and round, fluffy white lesions located in the temporal retina. CT scan showed the existence of two frontal lobe lesions that were highly vascularized. A PPV of the right eye was performed, which disclosed atypical lymphocytes consistent with RCS. Before any treatment could be initiated, the patient succumbed to her condition and died. A histopathologic inspection of the brain and eyes confirmed the diagnosis of RCS.[32]

Use of cytologic analysis of the vitreous to make a diagnosis of reticulum cell sarcoma has also been important in the immunocompromised population, patients highly at risk for the development of PCNSL/PIOL.[33-36] Ziemianski and colleagues described a 42-year-old Caucasian male who presented with bilateral decreased vision after renal transplantation one year earlier.[37] A biopsy of the right parietal lobe, prompted by neurologic symptoms, showed a malignant lymphoma. Treatment was initiated using a combination of radiotherapy, cyclophosphamide, and prednisone. Ophthalmic examination revealed 2+ cell and flare in the anterior chambers of the eyes. Funduscopic examination showed 2+ vitreous haze and a secondary detachment of the superior retina. The left eye had 2+ vitreous haze and a secondary detachment of the inferior retina. Despite treatment with subtenon injection, systemic, and topical corticosteroids, the vitritis was refractory to treatment and worsened to 4+ vitreous haze bilaterally, precluding any view of the fundi. As the differential diagnosis for this patient's ocular findings included infectious and malignant causes, a diagnostic PPV was performed. Cytology revealed the atypical lymphocytes so characteristic of PIOL/ PCNSL, and radiotherapy was administered.[37]

These cases relating some of the first employments of PPV to obtain vitreous for cytologic analysis, illustrate the importance of making a diagnosis of PIOL/PCNSL rapidly, so that treatment may be instituted. Indeed, today when there is even the slightest hint that PIOL is present, PPV and LP are important diagnostic tools that are used to determine whether or not to begin treatment or to look for other causes of pathology. Parver and Font stated in 1975, "(t)he fact that ocular involvement can be an early manifestation of RCS should alert the ophthalmologist and neurologist to consider the diagnosis of RCS [especially in middle-to-older patients with recalcitrant uveitis]…" and "(i)f standard investigations [such as LP, CT scan (prior to the development of MRI)] for RCS yield negative results and there is a high index of suspicion, cytologic examination of the vitreous may prove diagnostic in this life-threatening disease."[32] Even today we follow these important recommendations to make life-extending and saving diagnoses. As diagnosis of PIOL or PCNSL is dependent upon the demonstration of neoplastic lymphocytes in the vitreous or the CSF, respectively, it is essential that a vitrectomy (or LP) be performed; there is no other way to obtain these cells. Cytology, then, remains the benchmark for the diagnosis of PIOL.

Diagnostic Tools. Initially, when CSF samples were obtained, cellular material was obtained by centrifugation in a conical tube. The supernatant was removed, the tube was inverted to remove any excess fluid, and the cellular contents at the bottom of the tube were scraped onto a glass slide.[4] However, some noted that this method could produce much stress on the cells yielding debris. The development of membrane techniques, such as, the Millipore (Millipore Corporation) and Nuclepore (General Electric Company) filters, helped increase the amount of tumor cells collected from various body fluids, including the CSF.[38–40] However, these membranes were noted to clog, which could decrease the amount of cells captured.[41] The cells caught in the filter membranes will not be available for further immunophenotyping and molecular analysis. Indeed, the use of the Cytocentrifuge (developed by Shandon Scientific Company Limited in London, England) is an important tool that has allowed us to preserve cellular material in the CSF and vitreous samples.[41] Especially in PIOL and PCNSL where the diagnosis rests on the identification of atypical cells, the acquisition of as many cells as possible with minimal to no distortion is essential. The use of the Cytocentrifuge, however, does not occur at all centers. Some of the mechanics of the Cytocentrifuge will be discussed below under "Modern Diagnostic Tools".

Modern Diagnostic Approaches

Vitrectomy with Cytologic Analysis. A vitreous biopsy should be performed if LP is negative upon repeat. Cytologic examination of vitreous samples is a mainstay in the diagnosis of PIOL.

Modern vitrectomy technique has tremendously decreased adverse effects. While vitrectomy is an important diagnostic procedure, it is not without imperfections. Vitreous specimens may not always contain neoplastic cells, and this might especially be the case if there is minimal vitreal involvement by the PIOL cells. Blumenkranz and colleagues reported about four cases, all suspect for PIOL, in which vitrectomies were performed. These revealed reactive/inflammatory cells, but no malignant lymphocytes.[42] Three of these patients who had presented with ocular symptoms went on to develop cerebral lesions as revealed by computerized tomography (CT) scan. The fourth patient, who presented with elevated whitish-yellow lesions at the RPE level, had vitrectomy and chorioretinal biopsy performed at the same time. The vitreous specimen revealed reactive inflammatory cells (such as small lymphocytes, macrophages and histiocytes), but the chorioretinal biopsy showed that there were malignant cells infiltrating both the retina and choroid. This was consistent with a large cell lymphomatous process that, upon immunostaining, was shown to be the rare entity, T-cell intraocular lymphoma. Choroidal involvement is rare in PIOL, and it should be noted that this patient also had a bone marrow biopsy that was consistent with, but not diagnostic of bone marrow involvement. The patient also had systemic symptoms, such as anorexia, cachexia (he had lost 40 pounds), and lethargy, prior to his death from unknown causes.

However, despite occasions in which vitrectomy fails to disclose tumor cells, there have been reports in which it was the vitrectomy specimen that revealed atypical lymphocytes consistent with PIOL/PCNSL, while the CSF was free from any abnormalities.[32] It is not surprising to find PIOL cells only in the vitreous and not in the CSF, as PIOL may not have CNS involvement in the early stages.

While cytologic examination can reveal the malignant lymphocytes of PIOL, it cannot distinguish between B- or T-cell PIOL. While most PIOLs are of B-cell lineage, T-cell PIOL occurs in rare cases. However, in our experience, the lymphoma cells of T-cell PIOLs tend not to be as uniformly large as in B-cell PIOLs and range in size from small to intermediate to large. They can simulate a reactive inflammatory process. In addition, the nuclei of PIOL T-cells can have a bilobed or indented appearance as opposed to the numerous indentations in the nuclei of B-cell PIOL cells we commonly see. However, T-cell PIOLs can certainly have indented nuclei similar to B-cell PIOL. Immunohistochemistry, in which we are able to stain for CD3, CD4, CD8, and CD56 (in the case of NK/T cell lymphomas) antigens as well using PCR to detect *TCR* gene rearrangements (such as those in the *TCR-γ* gene) can help us identify the rare cases of T-cell PIOL.[43–45] In addition, IL-10 levels may be elevated and may be higher compared with IL-6 levels, but TGF-β levels may be greatly increased in T-cell PIOL. Increased TGF-β and IL-10 levels have been associated with cutaneous T-cell lymphomas (CTCL),[46,47] and reviews of the cases of T-cell intraocular lymphoma have noted frequent association with such disease (e.g., mycosis fungoides).[45] Nevertheless, T-cell PIOL can occur independently of CTCL. Coupland and colleagues noted that due to a lack of immunohistochemical markers for T-cell PIOL, making such a diagnosis is often more difficult than making a diagnosis of B-cell PIOL.[45]

Obtaining Vitreous: Fine Needle or the Vitrector? Char noted that in two of nine patients, more than one vitreous biopsy was necessary to establish the diagnosis of PIOL because malignant cells could not be identified in the first biopsy specimen.[48] This highlights the importance of repeating a vitrectomy in cases where there is a strong clinical suspicion (i.e., steroid-recalcitrant vitritis in an older patient with creamy sub-RPE infiltrates) and other important clues, such as high IL-10 to IL-6 ratio (discussed later in this chapter). Char also noted that cellular detail could be lost in samples obtained with vitrectomy instrumentation (which uses a rotor-motor large suction instrument) as compared with aspirates obtained from a 20-gauge needle.[48] Char presents a micrograph depicting a vitreous specimen from a 20-gauge needle; cellular details are intact (atypical lymphocytes are readily identified). However, a vitreous specimen from the same case obtained from the vitrector shows cells that are distorted, making it difficult to see the features of atypia and neoplasticity.

Despite the view in the past that a vitreous aspirate produces less distortion of cellular material,[48] vitreous aspirate often yields a smaller amount of cellular material than PPV. For this reason, we recommend performing a PPV, including core vitrectomy, when attempting to diagnose PIOL. Diagnostic yield of PPV is often superior to that of vitreous aspirate and can collect a large amount of the neoplastic cells.[49] Others noted that PPV would probably provide more sample as compared with aspirate.[50] PPV can also help improve vision by removing the vitreous cells responsible for the blurry vision many patients complain about.[30] If cytologic analysis finds cells consistent with neoplastic cells demonstrating PCNSL or PIOL, consultation of a neurooncologist and treatment may begin. If a patient succumbs to the disease, is histopathologic confirmation of PIOL or PCNSL (or both) of the eye or brain, respectively, required? Although some have performed this confirmatory process,[32] the discovery of lymphoma cells in the CSF or vitreous is diagnostic of PCNSL and PIOL, respectively. No further histologic confirmation is required to begin treatment or to confirm the diagnosis postmortem.

We recommend that an undiluted core vitrectomy specimen be immediately mixed with tissue culture medium and rapidly transported to a cytopathology laboratory. The sample or the diluted vitreous fluid should also be submitted to the cytopathology laboratory after a complete diagnostic vitrectomy. Cytologic analysis is the first step in making the diagnosis, and other tests, such as immunohistochemistry, flow cytometry cytokine measurement, and microdissection combined with the molecular method of PCR to detect monoclonality, may be performed if enough vitreous sample remains.[51] Part of the diluted vitreous sample should also be sent to the microbiology laboratory for culture of different microorganisms. Figure 9.1 is the typical protocol that we require ophthalmologists to follow when sending vitrectomy specimens for examination at the NEI.

For those eyes with solitary subretinal lesions without much vitreous cells, an aspiration of the subretinal lesion can be considered to obtain tumor cells for cytological diagnosis.

Vitrectomy with IL-10 to IL-6 Ratio Analysis. B-cell PIOLs are noted to secrete high amounts of IL-10, an immunosuppressive cytokine.[52] By contrast, in uveitis, which consists of an infiltrate of mainly macrophages and T-cells, there are higher levels of the pro-inflammatory cytokine IL-6 produced. For this reason, IL-10 to IL-6 ratios greater than 1.0 are highly suggestive of PIOL. In cases where no malignant cells are identified in a vitreous sample, but the IL-10/IL-6 ratio is greater than 1.0, a repeat vitrectomy should be performed. At the NEI, we pioneered the use of IL-10 to IL-6 ratios in vitrectomy specimens of suspected PIOL cases after others had suggested the utility of identifying IL-10 levels or both IL-10 and IL-6 levels in NHLs and PCNSLs.[53,54,92] In one of our studies, we found that the specimens with an IL-10 to IL-6 ratio greater than 1.0 had a sensitivity and specificity of 75% (the mean IL-10 to IL-6 ratio was 5.23 for 35 PIOL vitrectomy specimens and that of 64 uveitis vitrectomy specimens was 0.23).[56] Correctly classifying PIOL based on an IL-10/IL-6 greater than 1.0 was accomplished 74.7% of the time, and sensitivity and the specificity for the cutoff rule was 74.3% and 75.0%, respectively.[57] It is important to note that as PIOL and uveitis are complementary disease groups, a reversal in sensitivity and specificity were observed. Thus, uveitis had a sensitivity of 75.0% and a specificity of 74.3%.[57]

Cytocentrifugation. The Cytocentrifuge is an excellent way to obtain as many cells as possible with little distortion. As noted previously, this is important because as many well-preserved cells as possible are required to make a confident diagnosis of PIOL/PCNSL. The Cytocentrifuge is essentially

1.   Fresh vitreous specimen, 1-2 mL is immediately placed into a tube containing tissue   culture medium (RPMI) for a total volume of 2-5 mL and centrifuged at 1,000 rpm (200   g force) for 10 minutes at room temperature.

2.   Gently pipette off supernatants and place in a second tube for use in ELISA assay (cytokine analysis) and for PCR for virus detection. If such analyses are not available at your institution, freeze contents of tube and consider sending to institutions, such as the   NEI, that can perform these analyses. See below for mailing instructions (Step 7).

With Cytospin centrifuge	*Without Cytospin centrifuge*
3. Resuspend the sediment in 0.2-1 ml RPMI for cytocentrifuging. Each cytospin chamber contains 1-2 drops (0.1 ml) of fluid (mixture of vitreous cells and RPMI) depending on the degree of cloudiness so will yield 2-10 slides.	3. Resuspend the 1-2 ml of sediment in 3-4 ml RPMI (a total volume of 5 ml). Centrifuge again for 5 minutes at 1,000 rpm.
	4. Carefully pipette out the clear supernatant.
4. Spin in cytocentrifuge for 5 minutes at 500 rpm. Use coated slides (usually 5-10 slides).	5. Circle a coated slide with indelible marker pen. Place the bottom 1-2 mL of cellular mixture within the circled area on 5-10 slides. Pipette
5. Take the slides out of cytospin centrifuge chambers and air dry.	75-100 L on each slide. Air dry the slides.

6.   Stain for Wright-Giemsa, Diff Quick, and/or immunostaining (if needed). If you are sending un-stained slides to the NEI, put the slides in slide mailers and pack securely. See Step 7 below for mailing instructions.

7.   Mail the slides and collected supernatants on dry ice. Make sure to label all specimens and include a clinical history when you send the specimens. State clearly your request: cytology and/or molecular analysis.

NEI Protocol for the Preparation of Vitrectomy Specimens for
Examination[57,63,70,75–79,92,94,95]

Fig. 9.1 NEI vitrectomy preparation protocol.

a centrifugation system that employs the use of small chambers into which the fluid of interest, in the case of PIOL/PCNSL, CSF or vitreous, is placed. The chamber is connected to a silica membrane that traps water and other fluids, while allowing cellular material to pass through onto a glass slide. These cells may then be processed for staining using various techniques, such as the modified Papanicolaou technique, Giemsa, Diff Quick, or immunostaining. We recommend Giemsa and Diff Quick, then immunostaining for B- (including kappa and lambda) and T-cell markers. Hansen *et al.* noted that Cytocentrifugation appeared to result in a higher yield of cellular material from CSF samples analyzed for neoplastic cells compared with other techniques, such as the use of Nuclepore filtration.[41] In fact, Cytocentrifugation was able to yield cells diagnostic of lymphoma in three cases where Nuclepore filtration (which was noted to have problems with clogging and cellular loss) did not. It should be noted, however, that many centers do not currently have the Cytocentrifuge. Therefore, cytologic analysis still occurs using the technique of centrifugation in a conical tube, which as noted previously can distort cell shape, making it difficult at times to identify neoplastic cells. In addition, as the lymphoma cells are already fragile and if patients have been treated with corticosteroids for a supposed uveitis, the cells may be highly susceptible to traumatic forces, such as those experienced during centrifugation. Fortunately, the Cytocentrifuge is more affordable than before and this method may become increasingly utilized in different centers. This would enable ophthalmologists to more readily identify lymphoma cells and, therefore, begin treatment. See our recommendations for cytocentrifugation of the vitrectomy specimen in Fig. 9.1.

Flow Cytometry. Flow cytometry functions by using multiple aliquots of vitreous sample and adding a particular antibody against a cell surface antigen, such as an immunoglobulin (in the case of B-cells) or a T-cell receptor (in the case of T-cells). If cells bearing the antigen target are present, the antibody against the antigen will bind. Then, as cells pass single file through the cytometer, antibodies against the antigen-binding antibody already bound to the cell bind and fluoresce. This indicates the capture of a particular cell, and these cells are sent to an Eppendorf tube for collection. A problem encountered with flow cytometry is that, as with any machine, there is baseline background "noise" or error. Therefore, in cases where very few cells of interest may be present (as is often the case with PIOL), the background noise of the cytometer may obscure and hide the signal of the lymphoma cells that we attempt to identify.

However, some have noted that the preservation of cells from vitreous specimens can be poor, making cytologic analysis difficult. In such cases, flow cytometry can have utility. Davis, Viciana, and Ruiz reported on the analysis of 20 vitreous specimens using both cytologic analysis and flow cytometry; 10 cases were found to be intraocular lymphoma and 10 were found to be inflammatory conditions.[58] Four of the 10 intraocular lymphoma cases had been diagnosed previously with lymphoma; flow cytometry was diagnostic in two of these patients and non-diagnostic in the other two. It should be noted that in these four patients who previously had lymphomas, the prior disease was not necessarily intraocular. For example, one patient previously had mycosis fungoides, although this patient's intraocular lymphoma cells were found to be mainly CD8 positive rather than the typical CD4-positivity that is characteristic of mycosis fungoides tumor cells (as an aside, there have been rare reports of T-cell PCNSLs composed of CD8-positive lymphoma cells, for e.g. one involving a woman who had bilateral vitritis and choroidal infiltrates in the right eye; vitrectomy was non-diagnostic, but MRI showed a mass in the right frontoparietal region, and excision and immunophenotyping by flow cytometry disclosed a CD8-postive T-cell lymphoma[59]). Davis and colleagues found that flow cytometry was diagnostic of intraocular lymphoma in five of the six cases that had no prior history of lymphoma ("newly diagnosed" cases).[58] In these six cases it should be noted that CNS involvement (including intraocular) may not have been primary in all instances as one patient died of a diffuse lymphoma of the lungs. When this particular patient's X-rays were reviewed, subtle infiltrates not noted prior to the patient's death were found. The one case out of the six newly diagnosed cases in which flow cytometry was non-diagnostic, showed a vitreous cytologic analysis that suggested a lymphoproliferative process; ultimate confirmation of lymphomatous involvement of the CNS was made by brain biopsy. Davis and colleagues noted that, overall, in their study flow cytometry was able to make a diagnosis of ocular lymphoma in seven out of 10 cases and was non-diagnostic in three out of 10 cases.[58] Cytologic smears from a case of intraocular lymphoma and a case of ocular inflammation in association with systemic lupus erythematosis show some of the difficulties encountered with cytologic analysis. Smudge cells were revealed in the smears from the two different disease processes, and cytology was inadequate to make a diagnosis. The ocular lymphoma smear also contained small lymphocytes that could have been suggestive of a lymphoproliferative process, but were not diagnostic. Interestingly, flow cytometry of this particular vitreous sample showed a heterogeneous infiltrate. Brain biopsy confirmed that this patient had a CNS lymphoma. This case, as well as the cases in which flow cytometry was non-diagnostic in ocular lymphoma, illustrate the imperfections of flow cytometry. However, it is important to realize that flow cytometry can be a useful adjunct. One issue that flow cytometry cannot overcome and is noted by Davis *et al.*, is that not all B-cell lymphomas are able to produce surface immunoglobulins (kappa or lambda light chains are identified by flow cytometry as long as they are present on the cellular surface). In addition, T-cells may be found that can either suggest an inflammatory reaction or a rare T-cell intraocular lymphoma. Confirming that these T-cells are monoclonal would require the use of molecular analysis, such as PCR to identify rearrangements in the *TCR* gene as described by others.[45]

Later, Zaldivar *et al.* showed that in six cases of PIOL, cytologic analysis revealed lymphoma cells in all the cases.[60] These cases also had flow cytometry performed. One case had insufficient material for analysis by both cytology and flow cytometry of the first vitreous specimen, but a subsequent vitrectomy revealed lymphoma cells by both methods. Another case had positive cytology, but negative flow cytometry; subsequent vitrectomy revealed lymphoma cells by both techniques.

We recommend that cytologic analysis on vitrectomy specimens be first performed and the supernatant of the vitreous be evaluated for IL-10 and IL-6 levels. Then, adjunctive tests, such as, immunohistochemistry, molecular analysis, and flow cytometry, can be performed.

Immunohistochemistry of Cells. Taylor *et al.* were one of the first to describe the immunohistochemical profile of PCNSLs.[61] Their studies performed in the late 1970s showed that the majority of PCNSLs analyzed were of B cell lineage. While the immunophenotyping of PCNSL had been going on since the late 1970s, the immunohistochemical profiling of PIOL did not begin until the late 1980s and early 1990s.[62–64] Char and colleagues described nine patients who had vitrectomy performed.[48] Two methods were used to obtain vitreous samples: either vitreous aspirate via a 20-gauge needle for patients with minimal vitritis or core vitrectomy for cases with extensive vitritis. In all the cases, some of the vitreous sample was put through a filter and then stained using a modified Papanicolaou technique. The cells were examined for atypical features characteristic of PIOL (See Chapter 7 — Pathology of PIOL).[48,62,65,66] Some of the vitreous sample was put through a fluorescence activated cell sorter (FACS) machine and the subsequently distributed cells were immunostained. However, six cases did not stain and were categorized as being untypable. Char *et al.* noted that cytologic analysis was more accurate than lymphocyte subset analysis (at least with the reagents used in their study) in diagnosing PIOL.

The cells obtained from directly cytocentrifuged vitreous fluid are stained and their morphologies are better preserved and more easily visualized.[51,63,67–70] We have reported 14 cases of uveitis that had vitrectomy performed for analysis.[63] Four cases were infectious in origin, six cases were non-infectious uveitis, and three cases were PIOL. All the cases of PIOL were B-cell, and monoclonality was demonstrated in every case using monoclonal antibodies for the kappa (κ) or lambda (λ) light chain portions of the immunoglobulins. Wilson and colleagues also were successful in immunophenotyping cellular material obtained from vitreous specimens in five cases of intraocular lymphoma.[64] The obtained vitreous specimens were digested with hyaluronidase so that the cells could be suspended. The cells were then either analyzed using the immunoperoxidase method (two patients) or put through multicolor flow cytometric analysis (three patients). All the patients were found to have monoclonal B-cell lymphomas upon immunostaining.

Detecting Monoclonality as a Sign of Malignancy. As we noted in Chapter 3, malignant processes produce the clone of the tumor cell, which originally went awry. All the progeny produced from a malignant progenitor B (or rarely, T) lymphocyte will share the identical immunoglobulin gene configuration and will be monoclonal. In reactive processes, B lymphocytes, in response to antigenic peptides, will proliferate and produce immunoglobulins with different rearrangements in *VDJ* gene segments that make up an immunoglobulin. This rearrangement in the *VDJ* gene segments also precedes transformation in malignant processes. Similar processes occur in T-cell lymphomas, but rearrangements involve the *TCR* gene rather than the *IgH* gene as in B-cell lymphomas. Performing PCR to amplify the *IgH* or *TCR* gene products will show numerous bands on gel electrophoresis, indicating polyclonal products. However, in malignant B- and T-cell lymphomas only one band, indicating a monoclonal product will be seen. Thus, in monoclonal (malignant) processes, the tumor cells will all have the same gene rearrangements, and we can detect and confirm the same gene rearrangement (*e.g.,* in the *IgH* gene for B-cell PIOL and the *TCR* gene for T-cell PIOL) in PIOL tumor cells by using PCR.

Monoclonality in PIOL cells has been detected using PCR since 1999, when White and colleagues applied this technique to four patients with PIOL.[43] One patient had *bcl-2* gene translocation but no *IgH* gene rearrangement. Translocation of the *bcl-2* gene has been associated with follicular lymphoma.[71] Another case showed rearrangement of the *IgH* gene and no translocation of *bcl-2* or rearrangements of *TCR* genes. Interestingly, two cases were the rare T-cell lymphoma, as evidenced by the *TCR-γ* gene rearrangements detected by PCR. Two cases, one B-cell PIOL and one T-cell PIOL, had malignant lymphocytes that were readily detected upon cytologic analysis. Two other cases, one T-cell PIOL and the other a B-cell PIOL, had difficult cytologic analysis. The T-cell case had only few cells, with occasional large and atypical cells that were degenerated. The B-cell PIOL case had many necrotic cells and necrotic debris with rare malignant lymphocytes.

PCR can be a useful adjunctive test when the lineage of the lymphoma cells is in question. For example, while most PIOLs are B-cell in origin, there are occasional T-cell PIOLs that cannot be identified by cytologic inspection alone. Thus, the use of PCR to discover clonal rearrangements in the *TCR-γ* gene can be extremely useful as well as other tests, such as immunohistochemistry for T-cell antigens (CD3, CD4, CD8, or CD56 in the case of NK cells) and flow cytometry.

Microdissection. The core purpose of microdissection is the acquisition of a population of pure cells that may then be subjected to DNA, RNA, or protein analysis to characterize that particular population of cells. Microdissection using either a fine gauge (30-gauge) needle manually or laser capture has been an excellent technique for acquiring cells identified as being neoplastic and processing them for further analysis.[68,72–74] At the NEI we use both techniques. We have reported on the use of microdissection in numerous cases. Microdissection has enabled us to obtain enough lymphoma cells to characterize B-cell PIOL cells as being monoclonal by demonstrating the same rearrangement of the immunoglobulin heavy chain gene (*IgH*).[68,75–77]

Microdissection also enabled us to document a case of histologically and immunohistochemically confirmed B-cell PIOL in which there was heterogeneous rearrangement of the *IgH* gene.[76] We have performed microdissection with subsequent PCR analysis on 85 cases of PIOL diagnosed at the NEI, with 100% showing rearrangements of the *IgH* gene.[51,78] Microdissection can also be useful for uncovering rare cases of T-cell PIOL, by enabling us to attain a population of identified lymphoma cells and subjecting them to PCR for detection of monoclonal *TCR* gene rearrangements.[79]

Chorioretinal and Iris Biopsy. The biopsy of ocular tissues typically occurs when malignant cells have failed to be identified in the CSF and the vitreous of suspected PIOL cases. Failure to identify malignant cells in the vitreous can be due to degeneration of the cells obtained from the vitreous, paucity of cells in the vitreous, or lack of involvement of the vitreous with lymphomatous involvement confined to the retina or subretinal space below the RPE. We call the process in which cellular infiltrations in the retinochoroidal region involve the vitreous, "spill[ing] over."[80,81] In cases where there is no spillover of cells from the affected tissues, chorioretinal biopsy can obtain tissue from an area which upon ophthalmoscopic examination, appears to be involved by either a malignant or an inflammatory process. After successful experiments using animal models and the development of a device used to stabilize the globe and maintain its shape as well as decrease the amount of choroidal effusion (the Peyman eye basket) during the early-to-mid-1970s, Peyman's group developed an excellent way to perform a full-thickness resection or biopsy of the eye wall.[82–84] Peyman described how a chorioretinal biopsy might be accomplished in about nine simple steps.[85] The Peyman eye basket was sutured to the sclera and 2/3 of the scleral thickness was demarcated by a trephine. After dissection of the sclera with a Beaver blade, further demarcation of the sclera was achieved with a trephine. Diathermy was applied to the area, and the tissue for biopsy was excised using corneoscleral scissors. A vitrectomy was performed through the biopsy site, and the partial-thickness scleral flap was sutured back into place with injection of air into the eye so that intraocular pressure was reestablished. This technique helped to obtain a biopsy specimen that was morphologically intact and provided enough tissue for both histochemical and electron microscopic studies.[85] It was Peyman and colleagues who first described the use of chorioretinal biopsy in nine patients in whom diagnosis could not have been made otherwise (except for an enucleation), and, interestingly, one of the patients in their series had ocular reticulum cell sarcoma.[85] This patient was a 58-year-old Caucasian female who was noted to have vitreous haze and vitreous, retinal, and subretinal tumors in the right eye. Her vision was light perception. Diagnoses that were considered prior to the surgery included chorioretinitis or intraocular reticulum cell sarcoma, but no definite diagnosis had been made. After surgery using the technique of Peyman, histologic analysis revealed that it was ocular reticulum cell sarcoma that had destroyed the patient's vision.[85] This patient was the only one who did not retain preoperative visual acuity as compared with the other patients in the study who did not have the destructive malignancy. Later, Kirmani and colleagues described the use of choroidal biopsy in a patient whose right eye had a suspected malignancy, either primary or secondary.[86] Numerous tests performed to rule out infectious causes of uveitis (vitrectomy was not diagnostic and only revealed nonspecific chronic inflammatory cells) as well as tests to seek out a visceral malignancy (head CT, general physical and breast examinations, lumbar puncture, and bone marrow biopsy) were all negative. The only tests with positive findings were fluorescein angiography (early blockage of background choroidal vasculature and late staining of subretinal lesions) and ultrasonography (which showed that there were highly reflective echoes in the choroid and a serous elevation of the retina or RPE). These findings were not diagnostic per se, but they did prompt the authors to pursue a possible malignancy. Ultimately, an external choroidal biopsy was performed leading to the discovery of sub-RPE malignant lymphocytes, consistent with a diagnosis of primary intraocular RCS. Radio- and chemotherapies were then started.

At the NEI the use of external chorioretinal biopsies, similar to that described by Peyman, have proved useful in cases of uveitis where a diagnosis could not be established. The decision to perform chorioretinal biopsies is not approached cavalierly, but is often prompted when previous vitrectomies or CSF examinations are non-diagnostic. Chorioretinal biopsy is also initiated if a malignant or infectious etiology is likely or if the macula is threatened by lesions.[80] Our surgical technique for performing external chorioretinal biopsy is outlined here.[80,87] First, if the fundus can be visualized, we apply laser photocoagulation one to three days prior to surgery in a zone of the area to be biopsied. Otherwise, laser is placed after vitrectomy (discussed later). The conjunctiva is incised for 360°, and the rectus muscles are isolated and tied with silk suture. All the quadrants are inspected and we do not use the Peyman eye basket. Next, a 3-port PPV is performed and if laser was not placed due to haziness prior to the surgery, it is applied during vitrectomy. The vitreous specimen is sent for histopathologic and microbiologic analyses. Next, we mark out a site to be biopsied on the external sclera; typically, we mark out a 6 × 6 mm area that becomes a flap or "door" of the sclera through which the biopsy will take place. The scleral flap should be outlined beginning 5 to 6 mm posterior to the limbus. The infusion line is left in place, and a nearly full-thickness scleral flap with the above noted dimensions is made such that its hinge is posterior. When the flap of the sclera is retracted, the surgeon is able to visualize the choroid, which is practically bare; perhaps some fibers of overlying sclera remain. Next, a penetrating diathermy is placed through the choroid and retina along the outer margin of the inner choroidal bed. After turning off the infusion cannula, we make two incisions that are parallel to the limbus and are approximately 4 mm apart from each other by using a 75 blade. By inserting one blade of a 0.12 forceps through the incision, the full thickness of the choroid and retina may be grasped at one edge. Then, two more incisions, this time perpendicular to the limbus, are made using Vannas scissors yielding a block of chorioretinal tissue ranging in size from 2 × 3 to 4 × 4 mm. Care should be taken to grasp the full-thickness tissue only once using the forceps so that the architecture of the tissue is not destroyed. Prolapsed vitreous that occurs with removal of the chorioretinal block should be removed from the wound site using a vitreous cutter. Finally, the scleral flap is closed over the wound and sutured closed with interrupted 9-0 nylon. Fluid-gas exchange is performed using either 20% sulfuhexafluoride or 15% fluoropropane.

Chorioretinal biopsy has proved to be extremely valuable in cases where diagnosis was previously unestablished. In a series of seven patients in whom chorioretinal biopsy was performed at the NEI, the findings from the biopsy specimens enabled us to make a diagnosis in six of the patients and change therapy in five.[80] While none of these patients had PIOL, some of the lesions in these patients were very vaguely similar to those seen in ocular malignancy. For example, some patients presented with vitritis or uveitis unresponsive to corticosteroids. Other features of their diseases, however, were more suggestive of non-malignant etiologies. In each of these cases, it was the acquisition of chorioretinal tissue from biopsy that enabled proper diagnosis. It should be noted that prior to performing a chorioretinal biopsy, diagnoses that will be ruled in or out by performing this surgery and the proper tests to be performed on the biopsy tissue should be thought out. For example, in infectious cases of viral etiologies, electron microscopy may be helpful, revealing viral particles.[80] Planning should not only involve the retinal surgeons, but also the pathologist who can help in developing a plan, which when properly executed, will yield the most useful and pertinent results.

Johnston and colleagues also illustrated the importance of retinal and choroidal biopsies when all the other diagnostic tests have failed to yield diagnoses and when the empirical therapy did not result in abatement of the ocular lesions.[88] Diagnoses had not been attained in 14 patients who had uveitis and, as a last resort, retinal or choroidal biopsies were undertaken to establish either an infectious or a malignant cause. Four patients were discovered to have ocular tumors (three with PIOL and one with a metastasis) based on histologic analysis from the biopsy specimens. In addition, one other patient was ruled out for ocular lymphoma and was diagnosed as having a probable cytomegalovirus (CMV) retinitis. The surgical technique for choroidal biopsy that Johnston and colleagues used was similar to that described by us for retinochoroidal biopsy,[80] although it was only the choroid and not the retina that was perforated to obtain a choroidal biopsy.[88] For retinal, subretinal, or chorioretinal biopsies, an internal approach was utilized. A 3-port PPV was performed, and endodiathermy was applied to the area of the retina to be biopsied to cauterize retinal vessels around the margin of the biopsy site (usually at the junction of the involved and normal retina). The retinal tissue was then biopsied using vertical cutting scissors, leaving one corner of the tissue attached so that forceps could be used to grasp the tissue. Finally, the last corner was cut to remove the specimen. Endolaser was used to seal any retinal breaks, and the eye was filled with gas or silicone oil.

Later, Cassoux and colleagues described the surgical technique of endoretinal biopsy in three patients who were all suspect for ocular malignancy as a possible differential diagnosis.[89] All the patients underwent vitrectomy, with two patients also having concurrent endoretinal biopsies. The third patient underwent a second vitrectomy and endoretinal biopsy after cytologic analysis of the first vitreous sample failed to show any lymphoma cells, but did reveal a high IL-10 level. Biopsies in the first two patients revealed non-malignant processes and resulted in a change in treatment. Retinal biopsy in the third case with high vitreal IL-10 level revealed a diffuse large cell lymphoma infiltrating the retina and optic nerve head that was immunoperoxidase-positive for CD20 (B-cell antigen) and negative for CD3 (T-cell antigen). The histologic confirmation of a B-cell PIOL (lymphomatous disease was not found elsewhere in this patient) was important as it enabled the authors to begin chemotherapy[89] The surgical technique used by Cassoux and colleagues was similar to that described for internal retinochoroidal biopsy by Johnston and colleagues.[88] Cassoux *et al.* noted that the vitreous obtained from PPV was sent for cytology and IL-10 levels. Cassoux *et al.* also induced a localized retinal detachment (if one was not already present) by injecting sodium hyaluronate into the subretina. The bulging retina was then ready to be removed; it was cut around its perimeter with scissors and extricated with forceps. An application of endolaser photocoagulation was made about the biopsy site, with fluid-gas exchange finishing off the procedure.[89]

The biopsy tissue obtained is divided into three portions in the operating room (Fig. 9.2).[81] One-third of the tissue is placed into 4% glutaraldehyde for histopathologic studies including light and electron microscopic examinations. The second portion is snap frozen in optimal cutting temperature (OCT) embedding compound and is used for immunopathologic characterization. The third portion is sent for culture (our preference is for viral and other microorganisms cultures and/or tissue culture).[81]

While iris involvement is extremely rare in PIOL, it has been reported.[7,50,69,90,91] Iris involvement is more likely seen in systemic lymphoma

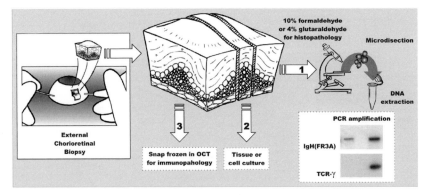

Fig. 9.2 Schematic diagram depicting external chorioretinal biopsy and processing. In this example, the specimen was submitted for routine histology, immunohistochemistry, tissue/cell/microbiology culture, and molecular analysis. The polymerase chain reaction (PCR) amplification illustrates a positive monoclonal immunoglobulin heavy chain (*IgH*) gene rearrangement (lane 1), negative control (lane 2), and positive control (lane 3).

that metastasizes to the eye. Findings on slit lamp examination that may lead one to suspect iris involvement in PIOL include engorged iridal vessels and iridal nodules. While iris biopsy is not typically an initial diagnostic procedure, it may be considered in cases where multiple vitrectomy specimens fail to reveal malignant cells and there is obvious iris involvement in the disease.

Again, chorioretinal and iris biopsies are typically performed as a last resort when other diagnostic tests that we have described in this chapter do not yield information leading to a diagnosis. Risks of biopsying, which include hypotony, hemorrhages, endophthalmitis, retinal detachment, and cataract formation, should be outweighed by the risk of allowing lesions that threaten the macula or are infectious or malignant in etiology, to progress. In addition, a plan should be designed so that proper testing of the biopsy tissue is carried out. This requires coordinating care amongst the surgeons, pathologist, microbiologist, and molecular biologist. The information obtained from the biopsy can often lead to a change in clinical treatment with benefits seen in the patient's vision and, in the case of PIOL, extension of the patient's life.

Figure 9.3 shows an algorithm that employs the diagnostic techniques we have covered in this chapter.

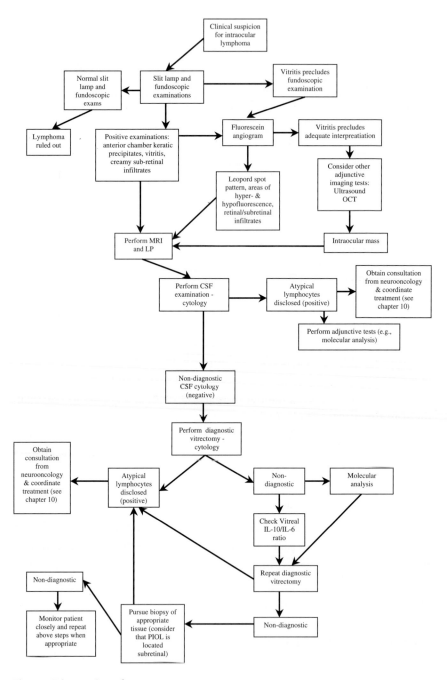

Fig. 9.3 Diagnostic pathway.

References

1. Dufour MH. (1904) Meningite sarcomateuse diffuse avec envahissement de la Moelle et de Racines. Cytologie positive et speciale du liquide cephalo-rachidien. *Rev Neurol* 12: 104–106.
2. Marks V, Marrack D. (1960) Tumour cells in the cerebrospinal fluid. *J Neurol Neurosurg Psychiatry* 23: 194–201.
3. Kline TS. (1962) Cytological examination of the cerebrospinal fluid. *Cancer* 15: 591–597.
4. Naylor B. (1964) The cytologic diagnosis of cerebrospinal fluid. *Acta Cytol* 8(2): 141–149.
5. Cooper EL, Ricker JL. (1951) Malignant lymphoma of the uveal tract. *Am J Ophthalmol* 34: 1153–1158.
6. Currey TA, Deutsch AR. (1965) Reticulum cell sarcoma of the uvea. *Southern Med J* 58: 919.
7. Vogel MH, Font RL, Zimmerman LE, Levine RA. (1968) Reticulum cell sarcoma of the retina and uvea. Report of six cases and review of the literature. *Am J Ophthalmol* 66(2): 205–215.
8. (1989) *The Oxford English Dictionary.* Oxford University Press, Oxford.
9. Seery CM, Davison PF. (1991) Collagens of the bovine vitreous. *Invest Ophthalmol Vis Sci* 32(5): 1540–1550.
10. Keene DR, Maddox BK, Kuo HJ, *et al.* (1991) Extraction of extendable beaded structures and their identification as fibrillin-containing extracellular matrix microfibrils. *J Histochem Cytochem* 39(4): 441–449.
11. Reardon AJ, Le Goff M, Briggs MD, *et al.* (2000) Identification in vitreous and molecular cloning of opticin, a novel member of the family of leucine-rich repeat proteins of the extracellular matrix. *J Biol Chem* 275(3): 2123–2129.
12. Brewton A, Mayne R. (1992) Mammalian vitreous humor contains networks of hyaluronan molecules: electron microscopic analysis using the hyaluronan-binding region (G1) of aggrecan and link protein. *Exp Cell Res* 198(2): 237–249.
13. Reardon AJ, Heinegard D, McLeod D, *et al.* (1998) The large chondroitin sulphate proteoglycan versican in mammalian vitreous. *Matrix Biol* 17(5): 325–333.
14. Hamburg A. (1959) Some investigations on the cells of the vitreous body. *Ophthalmologica* 138: 81–107.
15. Laicine EM, Haddad A. (1994) Transferrin, one of the major vitreous proteins, is produced within the eye. *Exp Eye Res* 59(4): 441–445.
16. Brown D, Hamdi H, Bahri S, Kenney MC. (1994) Characterization of an endogenous metalloproteinase in human vitreous. *Curr Eye Res* 13(9): 639–647.
17. Sebag J. (1987) Structure, function, and age-related changes of the human vitreous. *Bull Soc Belge Ophtalmol* 223 Pt 1: 37–57.

18. Nevins RC, Jr., Frey WW, Elliott JH. (1968) Primary, solitary, intraocular reticulum cell sarcoma (microgliomatosis). (A clinicopathologic case report). *Trans Am Acad Ophthalmol Otolaryngol* 72(6): 867–876.
19. Neault RW, Van Scoy RE, Okazaki H, MacCarty CS. (1972) Uveitis associated with isolated reticulum cell sarcoma of the brain. *Am J Ophthalmol* 73(3): 431–436.
20. Kennerdell JS, Johnson BL, Wisotzkey HM. (1975) Vitreous cellular reaction. Association with reticulum cell sarcoma of brain. *Arch Ophthalmol* 93(12): 1341–1345.
21. Minckler DS, Font RL, Zimmerman LE. (1975) Uveitis and reticulum cell sarcoma of brain with bilateral neoplastic seeding of vitreous without retinal or uveal involvement. *Am J Ophthalmol* 80(3 Pt 1): 433–439.
22. Barr CC, Green WR, Payne JW, *et al.* (1975) Intraocular reticulum-cell sarcoma: clinico-pathologic study of four cases and review of the literature. *Surv Ophthalmol* 19(4): 224–239.
23. Dean JM, Novak MA, Chan CC, Green WR. (1996) Tumor detachments of the retinal pigment epithelium in ocular/central nervous system lymphoma. *Retina,* 16(1): 47–56.
24. Machemer R. (1974) Advances in vitrectomy through the pars-plana (author's transl). *Klin Monatsbl Augenheilkd* 164(4): 572–579.
25. Machemer R. (1973) Subtotal vitrectomy through the pars plana. *Trans Am Acad Ophthalmol Otolaryngol* 77(2): OP198–OP201.
26. Machemer R, Buettner H, Norton EW, Parel JM. (1971) Vitrectomy: a pars plana approach. *Trans Am Acad Ophthalmol Otolaryngol* 75(4): 813–820.
27. Machemer R, Buettner H, Parel JM. (1972) Vitrectomy, a pars plana approach. Instrumentation. *Mod Probl Ophthalmol* 10: 172–177.
28. Machemer R, Norton EW. (1972) Vitrectomy, a pars plana approach. II. Clinical experience. *Mod Probl Ophthalmol* 10: 178–185.
29. Machemer R, Parel JM, Norton EW. (1972) Vitrectomy: a pars plana approach. Technical improvements and further results. *Trans Am Acad Ophthalmol Otolaryngol* 76(2): 462–466.
30. Michels RG, Knox DL, Erozan YS, Green WR. (1975) Intraocular reticulum cell sarcoma. Diagnosis by pars plana vitrectomy. *Arch Ophthalmol* 93(12): 1331–1335.
31. Klingele TG, Hogan MJ. (1975) Ocular reticulum cell sarcoma. *Am J Ophthalmol* 79(1): 39–47.
32. Parver LM, Font RL. (1979) Malignant lymphoma of the retina and brain. Initial diagnosis by cytologic examination of vitreous aspirate. *Arch Ophthalmol* 97(8): 1505–1507.
33. Penn I. (1983) Lymphomas complicating organ transplantation. *Transplant Proc* 15(4, Suppl. 1): 2790–2797.

34. Boubenider S, Hiesse C, Goupy C, *et al.* (1997) Incidence and consequences of post-transplantation lymphoproliferative disorders. *J Nephrol* **10**(3): 136–145.
35. Penn I. (1993) Incidence and treatment of neoplasia after transplantation. *J Heart Lung Transplant* **12**(6 Pt 2): S328–S336.
36. Penn I. (1996) Posttransplantation de novo tumors in liver allograft recipients. *Liver Transpl Surg* **2**(1): 52–59.
37. Ziemianski MC, Godfrey WA, Lee KY, Sabates FN. (1980) Lymphoma of the vitreous associated with renal transplantation and immunosuppressive therapy. *Ophthalmology* **87**(6): 596–601.
38. Del Vecchio PR, De Witt SH, Borelli JI, *et al.* (1959) Application of millipore filtration technique to cytologic material. *J Natl Cancer Inst* **22**(2): 427–431.
39. Bernhardt H, Young JM, Gourley RD. (1960) A simplified millipore filter technique for the isolation of cancer cells in body fluids. *Cancer* **13**: 631–633.
40. Wertlake PT, Markovits BA, Stellar S. (1972) Cytologic evaluation of cerebrospinal fluid with clinical and histologic correlation. *Acta Cytol* **16**(3): 224–239.
41. Hansen HH, Bender RA, Shelton BJ. (1974) The cyto-centrifuge and cerebrospinal fluid cytology. *Acta Cytol* **18**(3): 259–262.
42. Blumenkranz MS, Ward T, Murphy S, *et al.* (1992) Applications and limitations of vitreoretinal biopsy techniques in intraocular large cell lymphoma. *Retina* **12**(3): S64–70.
43. White VA, Gascoyne RD, Paton KE. (1999) Use of the polymerase chain reaction to detect B- and T-cell gene rearrangements in vitreous specimens from patients with intraocular lymphoma. *Arch Ophthalmol* **117**(6): 761–765.
44. Hoffman PM, McKelvie P, Hall AJ, *et al.* (2003) Intraocular lymphoma: a series of 14 patients with clinicopathological features and treatment outcomes. *Eye* **17**(4): 513–521.
45. Coupland SE, Anastassiou G, Bornfeld N, *et al.* (2005) Primary intraocular lymphoma of T-cell type: report of a case and review of the literature. *Graefes Arch Clin Exp Ophthalmol* **243**(3): 189–197.
46. Asadullah K, Docke WD, Haeussler A, *et al.* (1996) Progression of mycosis fungoides is associated with increasing cutaneous expression of interleukin-10 mRNA. *J Invest Dermatol* **107**(6): 833–837.
47. Bagot M, Nikolova M, Schirm-Chabanette F, *et al.* (2001) Crosstalk between tumor T lymphocytes and reactive T lymphocytes in cutaneous T cell lymphomas. *Ann N Y Acad Sci* **941**: 31–38.
48. Char DH, Ljung BM, Miller T, Phillips T. (1988) Primary intraocular lymphoma (ocular reticulum cell sarcoma) diagnosis and management. *Ophthalmology* **95**: 625–630.
49. Park SS, D'Amico DJ, Foster CS. (1994) The role of invasive diagnostic testing in inflammatory eye diseases. *Int Ophthalmol Clin* **34**(3): 229–238.

50. Siegel MJ, Dalton J, Friedman AH, *et al.* (1989) Ten-year experience with primary ocular 'reticulum cell sarcoma' (large cell non-Hodgkin's lymphoma). *Br J Ophthalmol* 73(5): 342–346.
51. Buggage RR, Chan CC, Nussenblatt RB. (2001) Ocular manifestations of central nervous system lymphoma. *Curr Opin Oncol* 13(3): 137–142.
52. Chan CC, Shen DF. (1999) Newer methodologies in immunohistochemistry and diagnosis. In BenEzra, D. (ed), *Uveitis Update*, pp. 1–13, Karger, Basel.
53. Blay JY, Burdin N, Rousset F, *et al.* (1993) Serum interleukin-10 in non-Hodgkin's lymphoma: a prognostic factor. *Blood* 82(7): 2169–2174.
54. Benjamin D, Knobloch TJ, Dayton MA. (1992) Human B-cell interleukin-10: B-cell lines derived from patients with acquired immunodeficiency syndrome and Burkitt's lymphoma constitutively secrete large quantities of interleukin-10. *Blood* 80(5): 1289–1298.
55. Salmaggi A, Eoli M, Corsini E, *et al.* (2000) Cerebrospinal fluid interleukin-10 levels in primary central nervous system lymphoma: a possible marker of response to treatment? *Ann Neurol* 47(1): 137–138.
56. Wolf LA, Reed GF, Buggage RR, *et al.* (2002) Levels of IL-10 and IL-6 in the vitreous are helpful for differential diagnosis of primary intraocular lymphoma and ocular inflammation. *ARVO Abstract*: #2221.
57. Wolf LA, Reed GF, Buggage RR, *et al.* (2003) Vitreous cytokine levels. *Ophthalmology* 110(8): 1671–1672.
58. Davis JL, Viciana AL, Ruiz P. (1997) Diagnosis of intraocular lymphoma by flow cytometry. *Am J Ophthalmol* 124(3): 362–372.
59. Novak JA, Katzin WE. (1995) Primary central nervous system T-cell lymphoma with a predominant CD8 immunophenotype. *Cancer* 75(8): 2180–2185.
60. Zaldivar RA, Martin DF, Holden JT, Grossniklaus HE. (2004) Primary intraocular lymphoma: clinical, cytologic, and flow cytometric analysis. *Ophthalmology* 111(9): 1762–1767.
61. Taylor CR, Russell R, Lukes RJ, Davis RL. (1978) An immunohistological study of immunoglobulin content of primary central nervous system lymphomas. *Cancer* 41(6): 2197–2205.
62. Char DH, Ljung BM, Deschenes J, Miller TR. (1988) Intraocular lymphoma: immunological and cytological analysis. *Br J Ophthalmol* 72(12): 905–911.
63. Davis JL, Solomon D, Nussenblatt RB, *et al.* (1992) Immunocytochemical staining of vitreous cells. Indications, techniques, and results. *Ophthalmology* 99(2): 250–256.
64. Wilson DJ, Braziel R, Rosenbaum JT. (1992) Intraocular lymphoma. Immunopathologic analysis of vitreous biopsy specimens. *Arch Ophthalmol* 110(10): 1455–1458.

65. Scroggs MW, Johnston WW, Klintworth GK. (1990) Intraocular tumors. A cytopathologic study. *Acta Cytol* **34**(3): 401–408.

66. Ridley ME, McDonald HR, Sternberg P, Jr., *et al.* (1992) Retinal manifestations of ocular lymphoma (reticulum cell sarcoma). *Ophthalmology* **99**(7): 1153–1160; discussion 1160–1151.

67. Akpek EK, Ahmed I, Hochberg FH, *et al.* (1999) Intraocular-central nervous system lymphoma: clinical features, diagnosis, and outcomes. *Ophthalmology* **106**(9): 1805–1810.

68. Shen DF, Zhuang Z, LeHoang P, *et al.* (1998) Utility of microdissection and polymerase chain reaction for the detection of immunoglobulin gene rearrangement and translocation in primary intraocular lymphoma. *Ophthalmology* **105**(9): 1664–1669.

69. Velez G, de Smet MD, Whitcup SM, *et al.* (2000) Iris involvement in primary intraocular lymphoma: report of two cases and review of the literature. *Surv Ophthalmol* **44**(6): 518–526.

70. Whitcup SM, de Smet MD, Rubin BI, *et al.* (1993) Intraocular lymphoma. Clinical and histopathologic diagnosis. *Ophthalmology* **100**: 1399–1406.

71. Tsujimoto Y, Croce CM. (1986) Analysis of the structure, transcripts, and protein products of bcl-2, the gene involved in human follicular lymphoma. *Proc Natl Acad Sci U S A* **83**(14): 5214–5218.

72. Emmert-Buck MR, Roth MJ, Zhuang Z, *et al.* (1994) Increased gelatinase A (MMP-2) and cathepsin B activity in invasive tumor regions of human colon cancer samples. *Am J Pathol* **145**(6): 1285–1290.

73. Emmert-Buck MR, Bonner RF, Smith PD, *et al.* (1996) Laser capture microdissection. *Science* **274**(5289): 998–1001.

74. Shen D, Zhuang Z, Matteson DM, *et al.* (1998) Detection of interleukin-10 and its gene expression in primary intraocular lymphoma by microdissection and reverse transcription PCR [ARVO Abstract]. *Invest Ophthalmol Vis Sci* **39**((4)): S290.

75. Shen DF, Herbort CP, Tuaillon N, *et al.* (2001) Detection of toxoplasma gondii DNA in primary intraocular b-cell lymphoma. *Mod Pathol* **14**(10): 995–999.

76. Buggage RR, Velez G, Myers-Powell B, *et al.* (1999) Primary intraocular lymphoma with a low interleukin 10 to interleukin 6 ratio and heterogeneous IgH gene rearrangement. *Arch Ophthalmol* **117**(9): 1239–1242.

77. Levy-Clarke GA, Byrnes GA, Buggage RR, *et al.* (2001) Primary intraouclar lymphoma diagnosed by fine needle aspiration biopsy of a subretinal lesion. *Retina* **21**(3): 281–284.

78. Chan CC. (2003) Molecular pathology of primary intraocular lymphoma. *Trans Am Ophthalmol Soc* **101**: 275–292.

79. Levy-Clarke GA, Chan CC, Nussenblatt RB. (2005) Diagnosis and management of primary intraocular lymphoma. *Hematol Oncol Clin North Am* **19**(4): 739–749.

80. Martin DF, Chan CC, de Smet MD, *et al.* (1993) The role of chorioretinal biopsy in the management of posterior uveitis. *Ophthalmology* 100(5): 705–714.
81. Nussenblatt RB, Whitcup SM. (2004) *Uveitis: Fundamental and Clinical Practice.* Mosby.
82. Peyman GA, Dodich NA. (1972) Full-thickness eye wall resection: an experimental approach for treatment of choroidal melanoma. I. Dacron-graft. *Invest Ophthalmol* 11(2): 115–121.
83. Peyman GA, Homer P, Kasbeer R, Vlchek J. (1975) Full-thickness eye wall biopsy. II. In primates. *Invest Ophthalmol* 14(7): 565–567.
84. Peyman GA, Meisels HI, Batko KA, Vlchek JK. (1975) Full-thickness eye wall biopsy. I. An experimental approach to the tissue diagnosis and study of choroidal and retinal lesions. *Invest Ophthalmol* 14(6): 484–487.
85. Peyman GA, Juarez CP, Raichand M. (1981) Full-thickness eye-wall biopsy: long-term results in 9 patients. *Br J Ophthalmol* 65(10): 723–726.
86. Kirmani MH, Thomas EL, Rao NA, Laborde RP. (1987) Intraocular reticulum cell sarcoma: diagnosis by choroidal biopsy. *Br J Ophthalmol* 71(10): 748–752.
87. Chan CC, Palestine AG, Davis JL, de Smet MD, *et al.* (1991) Role of chorioretinal biopsy in inflammatory eye disease. *Ophthalmology* 98(8): 1281–1286.
88. Johnston RL, Tufail A, Lightman S, *et al.* (2004) Retinal and choroidal biopsies are helpful in unclear uveitis of suspected infectious or malignant origin. *Ophthalmology* 111(3): 522–528.
89. Cassoux N, Charlotte F, Rao NA, *et al.* (2005) Endoretinal biopsy in establishing the diagnosis of uveitis: a clinicopathologic report of three cases. *Ocul Immunol Inflamm* 13(1): 79–83.
90. Raju VK, Green WR. (1982) Reticulum cell sarcoma of the uvea. *Ann Ophthalmol* 14(6): 555–560.
91. Corriveau C, Easterbrook M, Payne D. (1986) Lymphoma simulating uveitis (masquerade syndrome). *Can J Ophthalmol* 21(4): 144–149.
92. Chan CC, Whitcup SM, Solomon D, Nussenblatt RB. (1995) Interleukin-10 in the vitreous of primary intraocular lymphoma. *Am J Ophthalmol* 120(5): 671–673.
93. Whitcup SM, Stark-Vancs V, Wittes RE, *et al.* (1997) Association of interleukin-10 in the vitreous and cerebral spinal fluid and primary nervous system lymphoma. *Arch Ophthalmol* 115: 1157–1160.
94. Levinson RD, Hooks JJ, Wang J, *et al.* (1998) Triple viral retinitis diagnosed by polymerase chain reaction or the vitreous biopsy in a patient with Richter syndrome. *Am J Opthalmol* 126(5): 732–733.
95. Chan CC, Wallace DJ. (2004) Intraocular lymphoma: update on diagnosis and management. *Cancer Control* 11(5): 285–295.

Chapter 10

Management and Treatment of PIOL

Without treatment, PIOL is often rapidly fatal, especially when associated with PCNSL.[1] Patients with untreated PCNSL have a mean survival of just under three months.[2] Currently, the five-year survival rate ranges from less than 20% to 34% with our best therapies.[3,4] It is imperative, then, that a prompt diagnosis is made so that life-extending treatment may be initiated. In fact, in recent years, with increased awareness of PIOL, our diagnostic prowess has improved. However, there is still room for improvement in our therapeutic proficiency. What makes the treatment of PIOL difficult is that no truly definitive treatment exists. Large, multi-center clinical trials are difficult to perform because of the rarity of this malignancy. Despite this there have been shifts in treatments, and these have had some benefits in extending the lives of patients with PIOL.

Treating a patient with PIOL involves cooperative, well-orchestrated efforts among ophthalmologists, neuro-oncologists, and/or hemato-oncologists. In many ways, the treatment of PIOL patients is a new territory for both fields, and careful planning of treatment by these specialists will ensure that the patient receives the best chance for extending survival.

Historical Therapies

Surgery. When central nervous system (CNS) reticulum cell sarcoma (RCS), now known as primary CNS lymphoma (PCNSL), was recognized as a distinct primary malignancy affecting the brain, one method that was commonly employed in an attempt to combat the disease was surgical intervention. In fact, surgery was a typical intervention for many extranodal lymphomas during the period from the 1950s to the mid-1960s.[5]

Patients presenting with focal neurological deficits and symptoms suggested to surgeons that a probable intracranial mass was present. The precise nature of the mass (such as, glioma, astrocytoma, or RCS), however, could not be known for certain until at least a craniotomy with biopsy or resection was performed to obtain tissue for histopathologic examination.

While surgery was helpful, especially in cases of discrete, solitary masses, this therapy was noted to be an inadequate way to treat PCNSL. Henry and colleagues at the Armed Forces Institute of Pathology (AFIP) in Washington, D.C. examined 83 cases of primary malignant lymphoma of the CNS; 11 cases (13%) were of the RCS histologic type.[6] Of the 81 cases in which focality of CNS lesions were determined, 45 cases (56%) had unifocal lesions and 36 cases (44%) had lesions that were multifocal. Sixty-eight of these patients came to autopsy, and Henry *et al.* noted that because many patients had multifocal lesions, surgery was perhaps not the best mode of therapy.[6] Schaumburg, Plank, and Adams have reported on 25 patients with primary CNS RCS, histologically proven at autopsy or by biopsy.[7] Five patients underwent surgical excision of their cerebral lesions without subsequent X-ray therapy. Mean survival time was just 2.5 months for these patients. Three of these patients were noted at autopsy to have multifocal lesions. Others have also noted in their studies that the disease was multifocal in up to 25 % of their cases.[1] Considering the diffuse infiltrating growth pattern of PCNSL, performing extensive surgical resection, especially in the brain, is not only difficult, but does not provide any proven benefit with respect to morbidity and mortality.

Corticosteroids. One of the ways corticosteroids act on lymphoma cells is mediated through glucocorticoid and glucocorticoid-like receptors on the lymphoma cell plasma membrane and activating pathways leading to apoptosis.[8–10] Using glucocorticoid receptor-like-bearing murine lymphoma cells, Gametchu noted that exposure to dexamethasone induced cell membrane lysis.[9] Such actions helped explain the response of some tumors, such as non-Hodgkin's lymphomas (NHLs), to corticosteroids.[11,12] Indeed, in the cases of PCNSL and PIOL, we are well aware that corticosteroid use can lead to at least partial improvements in the tumor size. Unfortunately, this response is often short-lived. Some have shown that upregulation of the antiapoptotic protein, BCL-2, can confer resistance to glucocorticoid-mediated cytotoxicity.[13] We have seen some PCNSLs and

PIOLs that express the translocation t(14;18), involving the immunoglob-ulin (*Ig*) gene and *bcl-2*, which may lead to uncontrolled cell growth. At the National Eye Institute (NEI), we recently found that of 72 PIOL patients, 40 (55%) expressed the *bcl-2* t(14;18) translocation at the major break-point region (Mbr), while 15 of 68 (22%) expressed the translocation at the minor cluster region (mcr).[14] This may explain why some patients never exhibit a response to corticosteroid treatment (unresponsive) for PIOL that is initially mistaken for uveitis and may imply that expression of BCL-2 protein can circumvent glucocorticoid action in some cases of PIOL. At other times, PIOL that masquerades as uveitis and, consequently, is treated with corticosteroids, can experience a temporary improvement in symptoms of blurred vision and floaters. However, later, the "uveitis" becomes resistant to the corticosteroid used.[15] In other instances, "uveitis" recurs or worsens (rebounds) upon discontinuation of the corticosteroid treatment due to PIOL cells in the eye. As pathologists, we are all too aware of the effects that corticosteroids have on lymphoma cells that are already fragile. Often, prior corticosteroid use for a supposed uveitis or a mistaken cerebral inflammation or edema (when there is a PCNSL lesion[16,17]) can lead to even more fragile, more easily destroyed cells.[18] This produces diag-nostic difficulties because biopsy tissue obtained from brain or vitreous of corticosteroid-treated patients will often disclose necrotic, non-diagnostic cells.[18–20] It is advisable to defer biopsy in patients suspected of having PCNSL or PIOL if they have recently been treated with corticosteroids. In fact, if PCNSL or PIOL is suspected, use of corticosteroids should be put on hold until these malignant entities have been satisfactorily ruled out.[21]

Historical Radiation Therapy. X-rays, originally discovered by the German physicist, Wilhelm Conrad Roentgen, had been noted to cause the regression of a mole in 1897. For his contribution to the world of physics, Roentgen was awarded the Nobel Prize in Physics in 1901. Later, X-ray experiments involving the sterilization of rams were conducted without any external signs of damage. These observations suggested a therapeutic potential for X-rays.[22]

Cerebral RCS was noted to be sensitive to X-ray treatment and, in some cases, surgery was combined with radiotherapy.[7,23] Schaumburg and colleagues noted that in their group of 25 primary CNS RCS patients, 10 underwent surgery (including one patient who had a biopsy) and radiotherapy and the average survival time being 31.75 months.[7] Compare this with the 11-month mean survival time of the six patients who did not undergo treatment of any sort (excluding a patient who survived for eight years without treatment) in the study by Schaumburg *et al.* In addition, one patient had been alive for 2.5 years following surgery and radiotherapy, and another was alive after five months. The question is whether surgical resection of the tumor, in addition to radiotherapy, was beneficial. Considering that neuropathology was diffuse and multifocal in 14 cases (56%), surgical excision seems like an unnecessary procedure except in emergency cases where herniation and immediate death were to be averted by prompt excision or resection.

The study by Jellinger and colleagues from two centers, one in Vienna, Austria and the other in Budapest, Hungary, also showed the therapeutic advantage of radiation therapy.[1] At the Vienna site, 36 patients were identified with primary CNS malignant lymphoma. While the mean survival after surgery was 0.9 ± 0.3 months in surgery-only patients, those who underwent both surgery and irradiation survived for a mean of 17.2 ± 9.5 months.[1] Similarly, at the Budapest site (68 patients), those patients who underwent surgery survived a mean of one month, while those who had both surgery and irradiation survived 13 months.[1]

While PIOL and PCNSL cells are radiosensitive, the relapse rates associated with radiation therapy are disappointingly high (see Table 10.1).[1,24,25] Char and colleagues described 20 patients with PIOL (four patients, 20%) or PIOL/PCNSL (16 patients, 80%), with 18 patients (90%) having bilateral ocular disease (see Table 10.1).[26] Half of the patients in the study by Char *et al.* were alive at the time of report, and the other half had succumbed to their tumors. Of those alive, two received ocular radiation only (45 Gy) and eight received combined ocular and CNS irradiation (45 Gy) followed by chemotherapy (intrathecal methotrexate). It also appears that each of these 10 patients underwent unilateral enucleations. Of the 10 patients who succumbed to their tumors, four patients had both ocular and CNS irradiation (45 Gy), four had ocular and CNS irradiation (45 Gy) followed by intrathecal methotrexate, one had systemic chemotherapy only (cyclophosphamide, vinblastine, procarbazine, and prednisone), and one had enucleation only.[26,27] The variety of treatment regimens used in these patients underscores the uncertainty that existed at that time as to which treatment was the most efficacious.

Contemporary Treatment of PIOL

Radiation Therapy. The therapeutic use of radiation has a most serendipitous beginning. After leaving a canister of radium open in his vest pocket for an afternoon, Freund discovered two weeks later that he had developed erythema and ulceration of the skin underneath the area where the canister of radium had been.[22] The potential of radiation as a therapeutic agent had been identified.

Whole brain radiation therapy (WBRT) has been shown to lead to a dramatic initial response with decrease in size or regression of PCNSL lesions.[28] Despite such a response, recurrence is frequent and this is evidenced by a poor survival rate of only 4% after five years.[28,29]

In an important prospective phase II study of 41 patients with PCNSL by the Radiation Therapy Oncology Group (RTOG), radiation was administered as sole initial therapy, in which 40 Gy was delivered to the entire brain plus a 20 Gy boost to contrast enhancing lesions.[28] Of the 26 patients who had CT scans available for review four months after radiation therapy, 61.5% had a complete response (median survival of 19.8 months in these patients); 19.2% had a nearly complete response (median survival of 24.2 months); and 19.2% had a partial response (median survival of 9.9 months). Nelson *et al.* noted that as the nearly-complete responders could have progressed to complete response and their median survival was of 24.2 months, they were included with the group of complete responders. However, despite these encouraging response rates, the median overall survival was just 12.2 months (from the time of diagnosis; 11.6 months from starting radiation treatment) and the two-year survival rate was only 28%. Of the 41 patients, 28 patients (68.3%) had failures, with the commonest site of failure being the original site of disease (25 patients, 89.3%).[28] Could an increase in dosage of radiation from that used in the RTOG study, perhaps lead to better outcomes? An increase in dose to above 40 Gy (used in the RTOG study) is unlikely to improve outcomes, as noted by Corry and colleagues, who showed that there was no change in outcome measures on increasing the amount of radiation administered after 40 Gy.[30]

In 10 patients with PIOL/PCNSL, Akpek and colleagues noted that four patients received radiation therapy as treatment, and three of these patients were alive at the time of report with follow-up periods ranging from one to 14 months.[31] A combination of radiation and chemotherapy was performed in two patients (one was alive after 38 months of follow-up and another was dead after 16 months of follow-up). Another three patients had no treatment, and two of these patients were alive after one and two months of follow-up. The third patient without treatment was lost to follow-up.[31]

Chemotherapy. While WBRT has good initial response rates, the rate of recurrence with this mode of therapy has left much to be desired. Consequently, there has been a shift toward the use of chemotherapeutic agents as a primary agent for the treatment of PCNSL and PIOL.[32] In addition, some of the toxic effects of radiation therapy (discussed in *Adverse Effects* later in this chapter) can be avoided (although chemotherapeutic drugs confer their own adverse effects on patients) and chemotherapy can be delivered in two ways, either systemically or locally (intrathecally or intravitreally).

The use of high-dose cytosine arabinoside (ARA-C), a pyrimidine antagonist that terminates DNA chain elongation and disrupts the cell-cycle, has been described by Strauchen and colleagues for PIOL (see Table 10.1).[33] Six patients with intraocular lymphoma were described; four had undergone no previous treatment and two had received prior therapy. One patient had received systemic chemotherapy for a previous systemic lymphoma, and another patient was previously treated with radiation for PCNSL/PIOL and had eventually relapsed. Intravenous infusion of ARA-C ($2000–3000$ mg/m^2) occurred every 12 hours for three doses or every week for three doses. Four patients exhibited partial responses to ARA-C, which consisted of a reduction in vitreous cells and improvement in visual acuity. These patients then underwent radiation therapy, and although "good results" were obtained no further details in terms of the nature of the improvement, including whether or not there was recurrence of lesions or follow-up time periods, were noted. One patient exhibited no response to ARA-C and, due to post-vitrectomy complications, underwent enucleation. Finally, one patient who had previously undergone ocular radiation therapy for PIOL and had relapsed in the brain 1.5 years later, exhibited a complete ocular response (no vitreous cells were seen and a subretinal nodule had regressed) and response in the brain (whether complete or partial in not clear) to ARA-C. After completing the initial three doses of ARA-C, monthly administration of ARA-C for this patient was continued for six months. When the chemotherapeutic agent was discontinued, recurrent ocular involvement was noted. The patient was put back on monthly administration of ARA-C and again completely responded, at least with respect to the eye.

Methotrexate has now become the single most important chemotherapeutic agent in the treatment of PCNSL and PIOL.[4,34] Methotrexate is an antimetabolic drug that is analogous to folate. Therefore, it is able to inhibit the cellular enzyme, dihydrofolate reductase. Consequently, the *de novo* synthesis of purines, one of the important building blocks of nucleic acids, is inhibited. Methotrexate is capable of blocking cellular metabolism, specifically the synthesis (S) phase of the cell-cycle. It is an important therapeutic target for cells that are actively dividing, as in cancer. In addition, in a prodrug fashion, methotrexate becomes polyglutamated within the cell, allowing it to stay there and continue inhibiting dihydrofolate reductase, even after methotrexate levels have fallen.[35] Interestingly, methotrexate is not a first-line treatment for most non-Hodgkin's lymphomas. Some of the first applications of methotrexate occurred in patients with recurrent PCNSL following radiation treatment.[36,37] In the cases of PCNSL and PIOL, methotrexate must be delivered in high doses to overcome the blood-brain and blood-retina barriers, respectively. Methotrexate appears to enter the eye at lower concentrations than the brain. For example, methotrexate doses of 1 to 8 g/m^2 are usually infused for PCNSL, but there have been suggestions that higher doses may be required for PIOL. In a study examining intraocular concentrations of methotrexate after high-dose (8 g/m^2) systemic administration in a single patient with PCNSL, vitreal concentrations of methotrexate were 100–fold lower than serum.[38] Batchelor and colleagues found that in nine patients receiving 8 g/m^2 of intravenous methotrexate in an induction-consolidation-maintenance format, micromolar concentrations were reached in both the vitreous (ranging from 1.46 to 24.20 μM) and the aqueous (ranging from 3.08 to 19.47 μM) four hours after systemic methotrexate infusion, which can be therapeutic. However, no later time points were studied (see Table 10.1).[39] Others have noted that perhaps vitreous administration has utility in certain situations.[40–42]

The vitreous can be accessed relatively easily in the case of PIOL, and intravitreal injections of methotrexate have shown some benefits.

Generally, intravitreal injections of methotrexate have been used in patients who have refractory or recurrent PIOL. de Smet and colleagues described a 50-year-old woman with PCNSL and bilateral PIOL seen at the NEI.[40] Despite achieving clinical remission by negative CSF on systemic and intrathecal chemotherapy, the ocular disease did not remit, although it slightly improved with each systemic cycle of chemotherapy. After a single injection of methotrexate (0.4 mg) and thiotepa (2 mg) into the vitreous of this patient, greater than 1 μmol/L methotrexate was achieved for five days (a level deemed to be tumoricidal) and exhibited first-order kinetic rate of elimination (i.e., a constant fraction of drug was eliminated per unit time). The intraocular tumor remitted which was corroborated with nearly undetectable IL-10 levels. Smith and colleagues discussed the role of intravitreal methotrexate after other chemotherapy treatments had been administered via non-local routes (oral, ventricular via Ommaya reservoir, intravenous, and intraarterial with or without blood-brain barrier disruption) (although one patient did have prior ocular irradiation) in 16 patients with 26 involved eyes.[41] While the median number of intravitreal injections each patient received was 19, the median number of injections needed to clear the tumor from the eye was 8.5. In three patients, bilateral ocular recurrence was noted 12 to 24 months after remission had been achieved with intravitreal methotrexate. These ocular recurrences were associated with cerebral recurrences. However, reinstituting the intravitreal injections produced remission of the ocular tumors in all three cases.[41] Management of intracerebral disease is important as six patients in Smith's study died due to progression of lesions in the brain; none of these patients had intraocular tumors at autopsy.

Blood Brain Barrier Disruption and Intraarterial Chemotherapy. Different chemotherapeutics target specific aspects of cell function to prevent tumor growth. However, even some of the most effective therapeutics must be delivered appropriately to their desired site of action. Indeed, because the blood-brain barrier serves to block large (greater than 400 daltons) and water soluble (hydrophilic) compounds, many chemotherapeutic drugs that work well on systemic non-Hodgkin's lymphomas (NHLs) do not have a significant action on PCNSL or PIOL lesions that exist behind the blood-brain or blood-retina barriers, respectively. Rapoport *et al.* showed that the blood-brain barrier, which is made up of vascular endothelial cells and their tight junctions, could be "opened" by infusing cerebral-supplying arteries with hypertonic solutions.[43–48] Such abilities suggested a therapeutic potential for combining the opening of the barrier with chemotherapeutic agents that were typically excluded from the brain parenchyma, such as, cyclophophosphamide, doxorubicin, and vincristine. Rapoport *et al.* noted that the mechanism of action of blood-brain barrier disruption (BBBD) (which on first hearing may sound a bit aggressive; Rapoport and colleagues use the more gentle term "opening") is mediated by shrinkage of the endothelial cells that line the cerebral vasculature. This leads to a widening of the tight junctions between endothelial cells, responsible for the blood-brain barrier, such that larger and more hydrophilic molecules than usual may pass through.[44,45]

In the early 1990s, Neuwelt and colleagues described the efficacy of blood-brain barrier disruption in PCNSL by producing BBBD through infusing mannitol into an artery shown radiographically to supply the tumor.[32] Of the 30 patients with PCNSL, 13 were treated with radiation and 17 were treated with chemotherapy delivered to an osmotically disrupted blood-brain barrier. The BBBD with chemotherapy followed a specific protocol. First, the DNA alkylating agent, cyclophosphamide 15 mg/kg was intravenously (IV) infused so that it could be activated into its active phosphoramide mustard form by the liver's P-450 enzyme (this drug does cross the blood-brain barrier). Then, BBBD was produced by infusing mannitol into a tumor region-supplying artery (based on the location of tumor found on CT or MRI) as well as the two internal carotid arteries and one vertebrobasilar artery, such that entire chemotherapy of the brain could be accomplished. Following BBBD, methotrexate 2.5 g was infused intraarterialy. The benefit of infusing methotrexate intra-arterially is that it may be infused directly toward the brain rather than into the systemic circulation where systemic adverse effects may more likely occur. Finally, the DNA and RNA synthesis-inhibitor procarbazine (100 mg/day) and dexamethasone (24 mg/day) were administered orally over a period of two weeks after the blood-brain barrier disruption.[32] Radiation was administered to these patients only if there was progression of disease or a recurrence. Of the 11 assessable patients from the radiation-only group (group 1) and 16 assessable patients from the group receiving BBBD in combination with chemotherapy and radiation (group 2), the first group's median survival was 17.8 months, while the second group's median survival was 44.5 months.[32] Therefore, BBBD and chemotherapy proved to be a life-extending treatment modality.

While we can disrupt the blood-brain barrier through the infusion of hypertonic compounds, others have pointed out that the tumor itself has the potential to disrupt the barrier by its physical destruction of nearby vasculature. Therefore, BBBD may not be requisite prior to chemotherapeutic administration.[28] Indeed, PCNSL lesions are often located perivascularly. However, lesions that have diffuse spread beyond the cerebral vascular systems, deep into the parenchyma, may be more difficult to reach by chemotherapy and BBBD, whether produced by osmosis or by the tumor itself. In addition, the blood-brain barrier may still be intact despite tumor presence.[49]

Combining Modalities: Chemotherapy and Radiation Therapy. While there is no standard of care for PIOL, we are discovering insights into ways to optimize our treatment approach for this malignancy. Because some have shown that there is no significant difference between the survival rates of patients with PCNSL and those of patients with concurrent PCNSL and PIOL, and in light of the fact that up to 80 to 90%[26,27,50–52] of PIOL patients will eventuate to CNS disease, the presence of CNS disease is a prognostic factor. Therefore, it is recommended that both the brain and eyes be treated.[53]

We should remember that PIOL and PCNSL are most often of the diffuse large B-cell (DLBCL) histologic subtype of non-Hodgkin's lymphoma (NHL). Therefore, previous use of certain chemotherapeutics in systemic NHLs helped provide the impetus for using these agents in NHLs occurring within the CNS. For example, the combined treatment of chemotherapy and radiation therapy was also examined by O'Neill *et al.* in a study of 46 patients with PCNSL.[54] Preirradiation chemotherapy was administered in two cycles with an interval of four weeks and consisted of cyclophosphamide, doxorubicin (Adriamycin), vincristine (Oncovorin), and prednisone (CHOP therapy). Four weeks following the second cycle of chemotherapy, WBRT was instituted in a dose of 50.4 Gy. Four weeks following whole brain radiation therapy (WBRT), postirradiation chemotherapy was administered in the form of high dose arabinoside cytosine (also known as ARA-C or cytarabine) with each cycle spaced from the other by four weeks. The overall median survival for the patients studied was just 10.4 months, which was not any better than that noted in the Radiation Therapy Oncology Group (RTOG) study.[28] However, O'Neill pointed to an important prognostic indicator — age. Younger patients (60 years of age or less) had a better survival that very nearly approached statistical significance as compared with patients over the age of 60 years.[54]

Glass and colleagues described 25 PCNSL patients who received intravenous methotrexate prior to whole brain radiation therapy WBRT.[55] About half of the group had been reported previously and received two to four cycles of 3 g/m^2 of methorexate every three weeks.[56] They were included in Glass's report for long-term follow-up. The new group of patients followed a schedule of methotrexate (3 g/m^2) every 10 days for three to six cycles. Complete response to methotrexate was achieved in 14 patients (56%); 10 of these patients immediately had WBRT (ranging from 30.0–41.4 Gy) following methotrexate treatment with 100% maintaining complete response. Partial responses (greater than 50% decrease in tumor cross-sectional area, but less than a complete response) were achieved in eight patients (32%). All eight underwent WBRT (ranging from 30.0–30.6 Gy) with subsequent conversion to complete response in seven patients (87.5%). Three patients experienced progression of their disease and two went on to have WBRT. Of the 22 assessable patients who responded to the provided therapy, recurrence occurred in 13 (59.1%) in a median time of 32 months from the time of diagnosis. In those responding to the therapy, the median survival time from the time diagnosis was made was 42.5 months.[55] Recall that in the first RTOG study in which radiation was the sole therapy, although nearly 100% of the assessable patients responded to the radiation treatment, even the highest median survival time experienced by some of the responders was 18.3 months less than the responders in Glass and colleagues' study of pre-WBRT methotrexate administration.[28,55] Radiation dosages were lower in the chemotherapy-first study of Glass (only two patients had received WBRT doses of 44.0 and 41.4 Gy, respectively) as compared with the RTOG study's 40 Gy. Therefore, administration of methotrexate prior to irradiation increased long-term survival in PCNSL patients.

In a second study evaluating treatment modalities for PCNSL, the RTOG set out to determine the efficacy of pre-irradiation chemotherapy on PCNSL and compare the differences with their initial radiation-only study.[28,57] For patients who had a negative CSF cytology at the outset of the protocol, the treatment regimen included two cycles of CHOD chemotherapy (similar to CHOP therapy, but dexamethasone was used instead of prednisone). After the second cycle, a CT (or MRI) scan was obtained to determine the response to treatment. Those patients exhibiting responses went on to a third and final cycle of chemotherapy. However, if CT scan revealed that there was progression of the PCNSL lesion, the patients were given radiation therapy rather than moving on to the third cycle of chemotherapy. In addition, patients exhibiting positive CSF cytology received intrathecal methotrexate 12 mg/dose during the first and second cycles. If CSF cytology remained positive at the completion of intrathecal methotrexate administration, patients were considered as failing treatment and were taken off the protocol. Patients who had negative CSF cytology moved on to a third cycle of chemotherapy provided CT scan showed no progression, in which case the patients received radiation therapy. Patients who received a third cycle of chemotherapy also completed their treatment with radiation therapy. In the end, the median survival time for the entire group was a short 16.1 months, and when this median survival was compared with that of the RTOG's first study examining radiation treatment as sole therapy, no difference was found.[28] Interestingly, patients in the RTOG's second study of combined modalities having positive CSF cytology appeared to have longer two-year and median survivals (82% and 32 months, respectively) as compared with their CSF-negative counterparts (33% and 13 months, respectively), although these differences were not statistically significant.[57]

In an important study, 52 patients with PCNSL (10 of whom also had intraocular lymphoma) were committed to pre-irradiation chemotherapy (both systemic and intrathecal), radiation, and post-irradiation chemotherapy.[58] Pre-irradiation chemotherapy consisted of 3.5 g/m^2 of systemic methotrexate every other week for five cycles, with 12 mg of methotrexate infused via an Ommaya reservoir during the weeks when systemic methotrexate was not administered. Two other chemotherapeutic agents were also used during this pre-irradiation chemotherapy phase. One chemotherapeutic agent was vincristine, 1.4 mg/m^2, administered during systemic infusion of methotrexate. The other agent was procarbazine, administered at 100 mg/m^2/day for seven days during the first, third, and final cycles of systemic methotrexate infusion. The median overall survival for all patients was an impressive 60 months, the best to be seen in any large study of PCNSL/PIOL. Poor performance on the Karnofsky Performance Scale (KPS) with a value less than 80 was also associated with poor prognosis. Another poor prognostic factor was age greater than 60 years. Interestingly, older patients not undergoing radiation (22 patients) often succumbed to recurrent disease (45%), while older patients receiving radiation therapy frequently died due to complications associated with late neurotoxicity.[58]

Recently, the RTOG, in conjunction with the Southwest Oncology Group (SWOG), has provided us with another prospective study dealing with the treatment of PCNSL.[4] After reports of methotrexate's potential efficacy in treating PCNSL,[32,36,37,55] this newest RTOG set out to more definitively outline the benefits of using methotrexate. The treatment schema consisted of five cycles of chemotherapy administered over 10 weeks. Each cycle's chemotherapy regimen included methotrexate (2.5 g/m^2) and vincristine (1.4 mg/m^2, maximum of 2.8 mg). Procarbazine (100 mg/m^2/day for seven days) was given on the first, third, and final cycles of chemotherapy. Five cycles of intrathecal administration of methotrexate (12 mg, accomplished via an Ommaya reservoir) followed each week of intravenous infusion of methotrexate. In addition, dexamethasone was administered in a dose that was tapered weekly to discontinuation. WBRT was administered following completion of the chemotherapy portion of the protocol. This study was a large one by PCNSL standards, and data from 98 patients were presented; only one patient had ocular involvement. Relapse occurred in 33 patients (34%) with 28 (29%) relapsing in the CNS and five (5%) developing lymphoma outside the CNS. Median progression-free survival was 24 months, and the median overall survival was 36.9 months with a five-year survival rate of 32%. These findings helped to ensure methotrexate's leading role in our quest to most effectively treat PCNSL.

Ferreri and colleagues discussed 22 cases of PIOL, with 21 having concomitant PCNSL and one having purely intraocular disease (see Table 10.1).[53] Patients were treated with various regimens, and ocular remission (complete or partial response, or progressive disease) as well as ocular failure were examined. One patient received no treatment and succumbed to the lymphoma, and two patients died from toxicity associated with chemotherapy. The patient with exclusive ocular disease received only ocular irradiation and had complete remission with no relapse. Of eight patients receiving chemotherapy and radiation that had a field, including the eyes, one patient had ocular failure. Of eight patients receiving chemotherapy with or without radiation therapy that had a field excluding the eyes, three patients had ocular failure. The two patients receiving radiation therapy that included the eyes both exhibited ocular failure. The median time to ocular failure was significantly different statistically between these three groups, 20, 15, and 2.5 months, respectively. Thus, chemotherapy and ocular irradiation in combined PCNSL and PIOL disease significantly prolonged life as compared with radiation therapy alone.

Hormigo and colleagues presented two groups of patients, one group with exclusive PIOL (17 patients) and the other with concurrent PIOL and PCNSL (14 patients) (see Table 10.1).[16] Specific treatments for each patient varied, but generally chemotherapy (either single agents or multiple) alone or in combination with radiation (either ocular or WBRT) was instituted. Chemotherapeutic agents employed included methotrexate, ARA-C, procarbazine, vincristine, and thiotepa (the most common drug to be administered was methotrexate). In the group of patients with exclusive ocular disease; four underwent treatment with chemotherapeutics; eight received both chemotherapy and ocular irradiation; two were administered chemotherapy and ocular and whole-brain irradiation; and three received ocular irradiation only. In the group of patients having concurrent ocular and cerebral disease; four received chemotherapy, one received chemotherapy and WBRT; eight received chemotherapy and ocular and whole-brain irradiation, and two were administered ocular and whole-brain irradiation only. The median survival of patients with exclusive ocular disease was superior to patients with oculocerebral disease; median survival from the time of diagnosis in PIOL-only patients was 39 months, while in combined PIOL/PCNSL patients, survival was 24 months (P < 0.03). The median survival from the onset of visual symptoms was 60 months and 35 months for the group of patients with eye disease and the group of patients with oculocerebral disease, respectively. Clearly, PIOL in association with PCNSL shortens the length of time patients will survive and time until diagnosis is an important factor as earlier diagnoses mean that treatment may be started that much earlier.

Biologics Therapy. The CD20 molecule is a B-cell-specific differentiation antigen expressed on the plasma membrane and is involved in transitioning the B-cell from G_o to G_1 phase of the cell cycle.[59,60] It was found during the mid-1980s that two anti-CD20 murine IgG2a monoclonal antibodies, IF5 and B1, were potent inhibitors of B-cell differentiation to IgM and IgG secretory cells.[59,61] Interestingly and paradoxically, IF5 was shown to increase thymidine uptake, cell viability, RNA synthesis, and cell size, although there was no effect on mitotic activity.[59]

As CD20 is found practically exclusively to B-cells (some CD8-positive T-cells have been shown to express low levels of this B-cell antigen[62,63]) and is involved in B-cell growth and differentiation, the ability to inhibit CD20's action seemed like a logical target for B-cell diseases, namely B-cell lymphomas.

The drug, rituximab (Rituxan), was developed by IDEC Pharmaceuticals Corporation in the early 1990s as a human-murine chimeric monoclonal antibody specific to CD20 on both normal and malignant B-cells.[64,65] Rituximab, originally developed under the name IDEC-C2B8, works in two cytotoxic ways. One is that upon binding CD20, the monoclonal antibody drug is able to activate the complement system. This leads to the formation of the membrane attack complex (MAC) in the target cell's membrane, thereby destroying it. Such a mechanism of action in PCNSL was suggested in the case of a 19-year-old patient with PCNSL who was intraventricularly administered rituximab supplemented with autologous serum.[66] Additionally, rituximab's Fc portion is able to bind to Fc receptors found on cytotoxic cells, activating the formation of perforin molecules in the membranes of target B-cells and inducing apoptosis.

Rituximab has recently been used in some cases of PCNSL as a second-line therapy. Pels and colleagues described a 66-year-old male patient who had histologically confirmed PCNSL.[67] Despite treatment with a regimen of systemic and intraventricular polychemotherapy,[68] he suffered from a relapse that was treated with the same chemotherapy regimen as noted above. The patient relapsed a second time and procarbazine, CCNU, and vincristine chemotherapy were initiated. Nevertheless, a third relapse occurred and whole-brain radiation therapy was performed with partial remission. Unfortunately, the patient's mental faculties continued to decline and a gadolinium enhanced T1-weighted MRI revealed a hypointense and massive lesion occupying the left frontal lobe. Intravenous rituximab was initiated, but to no avail; no regression of the tumor was noted on repeat MRI. Therefore, intraventricular injections of rituximab were performed. Encouragingly, after one and four weeks, there were no lymphoma cells in the CSF and the patient exhibited slight improvement in clinical symptoms. However, there was no change in the size of the tumor and, in fact, two months after intraventricular injections there was enlargement of the tumor and a return of lymphoma cells within the CSF. The patient soon succumbed to the malignancy. This is the first case to be described in which rituximab was administered for refractory and relapsing PCNSL.

Because of its large molecular weight, rituximab has difficulty crossing the blood-brain barrier. This has been evidenced by SPECT scans tracking the lack of uptake of ^{123}I-rituximab into PCNSL lesions.[69] Others have tried intraventricular administration of rituximab and autologous serum as this combination proved to be tumoricidal *in vitro* as compared with rituximab alone or rituximab plus heat-inactivated autologous serum.[66] A patient had failed first-line treatments for PCNSL and received intraventricular rituximab injections (10 mg/9 mL, 40 mg/12 mL, and 50 mg/13 mL supplemented (diluted) with autologous serum. Although an improvement in the level of consciousness and abatement in the size of tumor and cerebral edema occurred eight weeks after intraventricular injections, no further administrations of rituximab were given and the patient succumbed to the lymphoma.[66]

May rituximab be used in PIOL? One of the problems with using rituximab in PIOL is its difficulty in penetrating the blood-retina barrier.[70] An approach to overcome this problem is to inject rituximab intravitreally. This has not yet been tried in humans with PIOL, but recently, at the NEI, we examined the pharmacokinetics of rituximab when introduced into the vitreous of rabbits.[71] Sixteen rabbits were injected intravitreally with 100 μl of rituximab. The injection was given to one eye of each rabbit. Because there are two distinct compartments within the eye, the vitreous and aqueous, and there are distinctive flow constants moving drug introduced into the vitreous to the aqueous and from the aqueous out of the eye, it was important to consider these unique aspects in shaping the pharmacokinetics of rituximab. Vitreal and aqueous concentrations were monitored on the second, seventh, eleventh, and seventeenth days. Considering that the amount of rituximab in the aqueous compartment was 3% of that of the vitreal compartment at any time, the half-life of rituximab was very nearly that of the amount in the vitreous alone. Therefore, half-life was found to be 4.7 days.

These findings hold intriguing possibilities for treating both compartments (aqueous and vitreous) of the eye. This is important because either compartment may be involved in PIOL. For example, vitritis is the commonest finding in PIOL (66%), while anterior chamber involvement in the form of cell and flare or keratic precipitates is the next commonest finding (43%).[72] The more challenging location to treat is perhaps the subretina, and subretinal infiltrates are the third commonest finding in PIOL patients.[72] Kim and colleagues noted that intravenous or subconjunctival injections of rituximab may prove to be better routes of administration for targeting subretinal infiltrates.[71]

In treating PIOL, one must take into consideration the fact that the neoplastic process occurs behind an intact blood-retina barrier. The lymphoma cells are nourished by the choroid and do not seem to induce neovascularization to support themselves. Thus, anti-neovascularization agents, such as, monoclonal antibodies against VEGF, may be unlikely to be effective.

Radioimmunoconjugates may be another mode of therapy for lymphomas, such as, PIOL.[73] Essentially, radioisotopes are attached to immunoglobulins specific for certain antigens on tumor cells. Upon reaching its target, the radioisotope emits particles in a certain size field based on the energy with which each particle is emitted. Two radioistopes (yttrium or iodine) have been used in systemic NHL with encouraging results,[74,75] and it remains to be seen whether these therapies will be employed in PIOL and PCNSL, although overcoming the blood-brain and blood-retina barriers remains an issue.[69]

Similarly, cell toxins might be attached to immunoglobulins, as in the case of BL22, a monoclonal antibody specific for CD22 found on B cell PIOL and PCNSL cells.[76]

Intensive Chemotherapy with Stem Cell Rescue. It has been shown in relapsing systemic NHL that transplantation of autologous stem cells following high-dose chemotherapy can lead to significantly better overall survival as compared with conventional treatment.[77]

In a study of three patients with exclusive PIOL and eight patients with combined PIOL and PCNSL who failed first-and second-line treatments (which included combination chemotherapy and WBRT), five patients (two with exclusive ocular disease and three with oculocerebral disease) underwent salvage treatment with high-dose chemotherapy (in the form of thiotepa, busulfan, and cyclophosphamide) and autologous bone marrow transplantation.[78] All five patients had a complete response, although two patients did experience ocular relapse at two or six months after bone marrow transplantation.

Later, Soussain and colleagues described 22 patients (three with exclusive ocular disease, eight with oculocerebral disease, and 11 with exlusive cerbral disease) undergoing high-dose chemotherapy and stem cell rescue due to relapse or refractory disease.[79] Of the 20 patients undergoing the intensive chemotherapy and stem cell rescue, 16 (80%) exhibited a complete response and the three-year probability of survival was 60%. Thus, in select cases refractory to treatment, stem cell rescue may be an option worth considering.

Targeting Chemokines and their Receptors. At the NEI, we have implicated interactions between chemokines and chemokine receptors in playing a role in homing PIOL cells to specific locations in the eye. PIOL cells in the retina and subretinal (sub-RPE) area were shown to express the B-cell chemokine receptors, CXCR4 and CXCR5, while infiltrating reactive lymphocytes located in the choroid did not by immunohistochemistry.[80] Retinal pigment epithelial (RPE) cells, on the other hand, showed mild positivity for CXCL13 (also known as BLC), the ligand for CXCR5. Interestingly, in another study, we showed that RPE cells that were not infiltrated by PIOL cells showed more abundant *CXCL13* and *CXCL12* (ligand for CXCR4) transcripts (mRNA) as compared with RPE cells, which had already been infiltrated by tumor.[81] This suggests that one way PIOL cells infiltrate various portions of the retina and subretina is by "following" a path of chemokine expression.

Could chemokine receptor antagonists play a role in treating PIOL? Work in the AIDS arena has brought to light an intriguing antagonist of CXCR4, known as AMD-3100.[82] CXCR4 (in addition to CD4) is used by the human immunodeficiency virus (HIV) to fuse to and thereby gain entry into the T-cell. By inhibiting CXCR4, AMD-3100 has been shown to inhibit *in vitro* replication of T-tropic strains of HIV-1 and HIV-2. CCR5 is expressed by both T-cells and macrophages, which is used by macrophage-tropic strains of HIV-1 to fuse to and gain entry into macrophages. This receptor has also been a target for antagonists to inhibit

HIV infection.[83] These antagonists may prove to be of use in NHLs, such as, PIOL, although experiments involving these drugs have not yet been performed.

Adverse Effects Associated with Therapy

While our therapeutic options can help extend the lives of patients with PIOL and PCNSL, they are not completely benign. Like any other pharmacologic agent, certain adverse effects are associated with treatment.

Complications of Radiation Therapy. Radiation therapy has many dire toxic effects. Many of these present themselves after some delay. One of the most devastating adverse effects of radiation therapy is the production of irreversible decline in cognitive function. High doses of radiation therapy, doses in excess of 60 Gy, can lead to brain parenchyma necrosis.[28] Abrey and colleagues noted that delayed neurotoxicity (characterized by gait ataxia, dementia, urinary incontinence, and decline in Karnofsky performance scale) affected 32% of PCNSL patients receiving combined therapy with methotrexate followed by WBRT and cytarabine.[84] A significant risk factor for developing neurotoxicity was age greater than 60 years.

In Hoffman's study, the most common complication was severe cataract in five (50%) patients; keratoconjunctivitis sicca in four (40%); punctate keratopathy in two (20%); radiation retinopathy in two (20%); optic atrophy in one (10%); glaucoma due to rubeosis iridis in one (10%); and carcinoma *in situ* of the limbus in one (10%).[85] We have experience of successful eradication of PIOL in two patients treated with radiation. Although no PIOL cells were found in the autopsied eyes, they revealed cataracts, loss of photoreceptor cells, and gliosis.

In addition, radiation therapy prior to instituting BBBD and chemotherapy can result in decreased amounts of chemotherapeutic passing through the BBB.[86] An animal model has shown that with irradiation, changes in the vasculature, such as endothelial hyperplasia, stromal fibrosis, and basement membrane changes, lead to decreased chemotherapeutic agent delivery to the brain whether delivered one month or one day prior to methotrexate administration.[87] Dahlborg and colleagues showed that patients receiving BBBD and chemotherapy had better mean survival times (41 months) as compared with patients receiving radiotherapy (16 months).[88]

Complications of Methotrexate Therapy. Some of the common toxicities associated with methotrexate include stomatitis, myelosuppresion, alopecia, and gastrointestinal upset. Toxicity generally occurs when there is delayed excretion of methotrexate or when persistently high levels of the drug exist due to methotrexate-induced renal damage. Although hemoperfusion[89] and hemodialysis[90] may be used in cases where there is life-threateningly high concentrations of methotrexate, many of the toxicities can be prevented or alleviated by administering leucovorin after methotrexate is delivered systemically or intrathecally.[91] Colestimide, an anion exchange resin (occasionally used in hypercholesterolemia), which binds to methotrexate has also been noted to expedite the clearance of high doses of methotrexate.[92]

Polymorphisms in DNA have been associated with disease, such as age-related macular degeneration.[93–99] Could polymorphisms also be associated with drug-related neurotoxicity? This intriguing possibility has been raised by Linnebank and colleagues who noted that in patients with PCNSL undergoing treatment (systemic chemotherapy with methotrexate, ifosfamide, cyclophosphamide, cytarabine, vincristine, vindesine, and dexamethasone and intraventricular chemotherapy with methotrexate, cytarabine, and prednisolone), the presence of at least one of three functional polymorphisms involved in methionine synthase activity conferred a relative risk of 4.7 for white matter changes associated with methotrexate.[100] Methionine synthase is involved in CNS myelination, and methotrexate's depletion of a key substrate required by methionine synthase is hypothesized to be involved in the white matter changes. However, others have shown that there was no influence of a single polymorphism in the gene encoding an enzyme involved in methionine metabolism on toxicity associated with treatment of pediatric systemic NHL with high-dose methotrexate in pediatric patients with systemic NHL.[101] No significant differences in toxicity associated with high-dose methotrexate exist between younger patients (less than 60 years of age) and older patients (over 60 years of age) with PCNSL and having normal renal function.[102]

Intravitreal methotrexate carries the risk of corneal epitheliopathy; this was observed in 15 of 26 eyes (58%) that were submitted to intravitreal injections.[41] We have also observed damage of limbal stem cells secondary to long-term intravitreal methotrexate. In addition, progression of cataracts is associated with intravitreal injections of methotrexate. In 19 of 26 treated eyes, cataracts were noted to progress.[41] However, in 12 of these

19 cataractous eyes, vitrectomies had been performed prior to intravitreal methotrexate injections and vitrectomies in and of themselves are known to cause progression of cataracts.[103,104] Other risks associated with injections into the vitreous include vitreous hemorrhage, endophthalmitis, retinal detachment, and increased intraocular pressure.

Complications of Blood-Brain Barrier Disruption and Intraarterial Chemotherapy Administration. Seizures have been noted to occur in up to 6% of patients receiving BBBD.[105] These occurrences may be averted by the administration of anticonvulsant prior to the initiation of BBBD. The most serious complication arising from the administration of chemotherapeutics intraarterially rather than intravenously is increased risk of thrombotic events.[105] Other complications arising out of BBBD and intraarterial chemotherapy administration include increased intracranial pressure and neuropsychotic toxicities.

Complications of Rituximab. Neurotoxic effects have not been described with the intrathecal administration of rituximab,[67,106] and as with other intravitreal injections, there is a risk of endophthalmitis, vitreous hemorrhage, or retinal detachment. Recently, intravenous infusion of ^{123}I-rituximab into four patients with PCNSL (unifocal lesions in two patients and multifocal in two others) and serial SPECT scans at 1, 24, and 48 hours post-infusion have been described.[69] The authors showed that only very faint accumulation of ^{123}I-rituximab in the region of edema about three of the patients' respective tumors was noted and a questionable accumulation of drug within the tumor was seen in one patient on the last scan. In fact, the activity in the tumor was lower than that of the background of the body, leaving the drug available to accumulate in the peripheral blood and bone marrow rather than the intended target located in the CNS.[69]

Recommended Therapeutic Approach. We have learned much over the years in treating PIOL and PCNSL. All PIOL patients must be evaluated by neurooncologists. For immunocompetent patients under 60 years of age, it would be wise to learn from the experience of the most recent RTOG study,[58] especially when PIOL occurs with concomitant PCNSL. Thus, a first-line therapy for PIOL patients should start with high-dose methotrexate (which can be combined with other chemotherapeutic agents) followed by WBRT of 36–40 Gy with an ocular-inclusive field (posterior two-thirds of both eyes, even if ocular disease is unilateral) dose of 30 Gy.[53] For patients with exclusive PIOL, similar treatments with high-dose methotrexate-based regimens should be instituted.[42] Because of the natural tendency of the disease in PIOL patients to eventually develop into cerebral disease and considering that relapses on therapy can occur in the brain, ocular and whole-brain irradiation may be considered in some patients with isolated ocular lymphoma. However, for immunocompetent patients over the age of 60 years (one of two identified poor prognostic factors), the combination of high-dose chemotherapy and WBRT can have severe neurologic sequelae. Deterioration in neurologic functioning could lead to a decrease in the Karnofsky Performance Status (KPS) scale (the second of two well-identified poor prognostic factors[28]) and bode poorly for the patient over 60 years of age. Consequently, chemotherapy without radiation therapy in this group of patients is recommended. In cases where ocular disease relapses or is refractory to high-dose methotrexate-based regimens, intravitreal methotrexate may be considered. Two other cases exist, however, where local chemotherapy may be administered: high tumor burden in the eye (adjunctive to systemic chemotherapy) and in cases where systemic administration of chemotherapeutics is contraindicated.[34]

Treatment for AIDS-related PCNSL/PIOL. While AIDS patients have a higher incidence of PCNSL than immunocompetent patients, the incidence rates for this particular group of immunocompromised patients have decreased since the introduction of highly-active anti-retroviral therapy (HAART).[107] Thus, the use of HAART plays an important role in maintaining optimal immune status. For example, without maintenance of an adequate T-cell population, latent EBV infection induces B-cell activation, thereby promoting the pathway towards the development of PCNSL in AIDS patients (for review see Cheung[108]). Radiation therapy has been recommended for use in AIDS PCNSL patients with reports of less than four-month median survival from the time of appearance of CNS symptoms in those receiving radiation as compared with a median survival of just 27 days in those not receiving whole-brain irradiation.[109] Interestingly, those not undergoing radiation most often died from tumor progression, while those receiving brain irradiation more commonly died from opportunistic infections. In fact, the occurrence of PCNSL in AIDS patients is heralded by very low CD4+ counts (less than 50 cells/mm^3), a point at which these patients

Table 10.1 Treatments and Outcomes in PCNSL & PIOL Studies

Patient Characteristics Treatment Regimen	N	Outcome	Author
4 PCNSL/PIOL pts			Char, *et. al.*[25]
5 PIOL pts			
OWBRT	4	2 pts died after 1 and 31 mos f/u	
+ Chemo[a]	3		
ORT (50 Gy)	1		
ORT (45 Gy) + Chemo[a]	1		
16 PCNSL/PIOL pts		Mean survival 41 months in 10 living patients	Char, *et. al.*[26]
4 PIOL pts			
OWBRT 45 Gy	4		
ORT 45 Gy	2		
OWBRT 45 Gy + IT-MTX	12		
S-MTX	1		
Enucleation	10[b]		
6 PIOL pts			Strauchen, *et. al.*[33]
ARA-C (2000–3000 mg/m²) X 3	2	1 eventuated to enucleation	
		1 maintained complete response on ARA-C	
+ WBRT	4	Partial response, "Good results" w/WBRT	

(*Continued*)

Table 10.1 (*Continued*)

Patient Characteristics Treatment Regimen	N	Outcome	Author
21 PIOL/PCNSL pts		2-year OS 39 +/− 11%	Ferreri, *et. al.*[53]
1 PIOL pt			
Chemo → OWBRT	8	OS of 47+ months	
Chemo → WBRT or no OWBRT	10	OS of 9.5+ months	
RT	3	OS of 10 months	
No Tx	1	—	
PIOL/PCNSL	7		Batchelor, *et. al.*[39]
PIOL	2		
Induction			
8 g/m² IV-MTX q14 days until complete response			
Consolidation			
8 g/m² IV-MTX q14 days X 2 doses		Micromolar concentrations of MTX present in both ocular chambers 4 h after completing infusion in 8/8	
Maintenance			
8 g/m² IV-MTX q28 days X 11 doses	7/9	Ocular response to treatment; 3/7 experienced recurrent ocular disease	
	2/9	Refractory ocular disease requiring ORT → complete response	
		7 pts with PIOL/PCNSL had complete response of CNS disease	

(*Continued*)

Table 10.1 (*Continued*)

Patient Characteristics Treatment Regimen	N	Outcome	Author
17 PIOL pts		OS of 39 months from diagnosis	Hormigo, *et. al.*[15]
		OS of 60 months from onset ocular sx	
Chemo	4		
Chemo + ORT	8		
Chemo + OWBRT	2		
ORT	3		
14 PIOL/PCNSL pts		OS of 24 months from diagnosis	
		OS of 35 months from onset ocular symptoms	
Chemo	4		
Chemo + OWBRT	8		
Chemo + WBRT	1		
OWBRT	2		

[a]Chemo was variable and included IT-MTX as well as unstated IT and systemic chemotherapeutics.

[b]These patients also received either ORT or OWBRT + IT-MTX.

PIOL/PCNSL = combined ocular and cerebral disease; PIOL = exclusive ocular disease; OWBRT = ocular and whole-brain radiation therapy; ORT = ocular radiation therapy; IT = intrathecal; S = systemic; MTX = methotrexate; ARA-C = cytarabine; IV = intravenous.

are at their most susceptible to a host of opportunistic organisms.[110] Clearly, AIDS PCNSL and PIOL patients present a challenge to treatment.

References

1. Jellinger K, Radaskiewicz TH, Slowik F. (1975) Primary malignant lymphomas of the central nervous system in man. *Acta Neuropathol Suppl (Berl)* **Suppl 6**: 95–102.
2. Fine HA, Mayer RJ. (1993) Primary central nervous system lymphoma. *Ann Intern Med* **119**(11): 1093–1104.
3. Panageas KS, Elkin EB, DeAngelis LM, *et al.* (2005) Trends in survival from primary central nervous system lymphoma, 1975–1999: a population-based analysis. *Cancer* **104**(11): 2466–2472.
4. DeAngelis LM, Seiferheld W, Schold SC, *et al.* (2002) Combination chemotherapy and radiotherapy for primary central nervous system lymphoma: Radiation Therapy Oncology Group Study 93–10. *J Clin Oncol* **20**(24): 4643–4648.
5. Freeman C, Berg JW, Cutler SJ. (1972) Occurrence and prognosis of extranodal lymphomas. *Cancer* **29**(1): 252–260.
6. Henry JM, Heffner RR, Jr., Dillard SH, *et al.* (1974) Primary malignant lymphomas of the central nervous system. *Cancer* **34**(4): 1293–1302.
7. Schaumburg HII, Plank CR, Adams RD. (1972) The reticulum cell sarcoma — microglioma group of brain tumours. A consideration of their clinical features and therapy. *Brain* **95**(2): 199–212.
8. Baxter JD, Harris AW. (1975) Mechanism of glucocorticoid action: general features, with reference to steroid-mediated immunosuppression. *Transplant Proc* **7**(1): 55–65.
9. Gametchu B. (1987) Glucocorticoid receptor-like antigen in lymphoma cell membranes: correlation to cell lysis. *Science* **236**(4800): 456–461.
10. Wyllie AH. (1980) Glucocorticoid-induced thymocyte apoptosis is associated with endogenous endonuclease activation. *Nature* **284**(5756): 555–556.
11. Goldin A, Sandberg JS, Henderson ES, *et al.* (1971) The chemotherapy of human and animal acute leukemia. *Cancer Chemother Rep* **55**(4): 309–505.
12. Claman HN. (1972) Corticosteroids and lymphoid cells. *N Engl J Med* **287**(8): 388–397.
13 Sentman CL, Shurter JR, Hockenberry D, *et al.* (1991) Bcl-2 inhibits multiple forms of apoptosis but not negative selection in thymocytes. *Cell* **67**: 879.
14. Wallace DJ, Shen DF, Reed GF, *et al.* (2006) Detection of the bcl-2 t(14;18) translocation and proto-oncogene expression in primary intraocular lymphoma. *Invest Ophthalmol Vis Sci* **47**(7): 2750–2756.

15. Hormigo A, Abrey L, Heinemann MH, DeAngelis LM. (2004) Ocular presentation of primary central nervous system lymphoma: diagnosis and treatment. *Br J Haematol* **126**(2): 202–208.
16. Herrlinger U, Schabet M, Bitzer M, *et al.* (1999) Primary central nervous system lymphoma: from clinical presentation to diagnosis. *J Neurooncol* **43**(3): 219–226.
17. Herrlinger U. (1999) Primary CNS lymphoma: findings outside the brain. *J Neurooncol* **43**(3): 227–230.
18. Basso U, Brandes AA. (2002) Diagnostic advances and new trends for the treatment of primary central nervous system lymphoma. *Eur J Cancer* **38**(10): 1298–1312.
19. Geppert M, Ostertag CB, Seitz G, Kiessling M. (1990) Glucocorticoid therapy obscures the diagnosis of cerebral lymphoma. *Acta Neuropathol (Berl)* **80**(6): 629–634.
20. Peterson K, Gordon KB, Heinemann MH, DeAngelis LM. (1993) The clinical spectrum of ocular lymphoma. *Cancer* **72**(3): 843–849.
21. Whitcup SM, Chan CC, Buggage RR, *et al.* (2000) Improving the diagnostic yield of vitrectomy for intraocular lymphoma [letter; comment]. *Arch Ophthalmol* **118**(3): 446.
22. Cox JD, Ang KK. (2003) *Radiation Oncology: Rationale, Technique, Results.* Mosby, St. Louis.
23. Adams RD. (1975) Certain notable clinical attributes of the histiocytic sarcomas of the central nervous system. *Acta Neuropathol Suppl (Berl)* **Suppl 6**: 177–180.
24. Freeman LN, Schachat AP, Knox DL, *et al.* (1987) Clinical features, laboratory investigations, and survival in ocular reticulum cell sarcoma. *Ophthalmology* **94**: 1631–1639.
25. Char DH, Ljung BM, Deschenes J, Miller TR. (1988) Intraocular lymphoma: immunological and cytological analysis. *Br J Ophthalmol* **72**(12): 905–911.
26. Char DH, Ljung BM, Miller T, Phillips T. (1988) Primary intraocular lymphoma (ocular reticulum cell sarcoma) diagnosis and management. *Ophthalmology* **95**: 625–630.
27. Char DH, Margolis L, Newman AB. (1981) Ocular reticulum cell sarcoma. *Am J Ophthalmol* **91**(4): 480–483.
28. Nelson DF, Martz KL, Bonner H, *et al.* (1992) Non-Hodgkin's lymphoma of the brain: can high dose, large volume radiation therapy improve survival? Report on a prospective trial by the Radiation Therapy Oncology Group (RTOG): RTOG 8315. *Int J Radiat Oncol Biol Phys* **23**(1): 9–17.
29. Deangelis LM, Yahalom J, Rosenblum M, Posner JB. (1987) Primary CNS lymphoma: managing patients with spontaneous and AIDS-related disease. *Oncology (Williston Park)* **1**(6): 52–62.

30. Corry J, Smith JG, Wirth A, *et al.* (1998) Primary central nervous system lymphoma: age and performance status are more important than treatment modality. *Int J Radiat Oncol Biol Phys* **41**(3): 615–620.

31. Akpek EK, Ahmed I, Hochberg FH, *et al.* (1999) Intraocular-central nervous system lymphoma: clinical features, diagnosis, and outcomes. *Ophthalmology* **106**(9): 1805–1810.

32. Neuwelt EA, Goldman DL, Dahlborg SA, *et al.* (1991) Primary CNS lymphoma treated with osmotic blood-brain barrier disruption: prolonged survival and preservation of cognitive function. *J Clin Oncol* **9**(9): 1580–1590.

33. Strauchen JA, Dalton J, Friedman AH. (1989) Chemotherapy in the management of intraocular lymphoma. *Cancer* **63**(10): 1918–1921.

34. Levy-Clarke GA, Chan CC, Nussenblatt RB. (2005) Diagnosis and management of primary intraocular lymphoma. *Hematol Oncol Clin North Am* **19**(4): 739–749.

35. Chabner BA, Allegra CJ, Curt GA, *et al.* (1985) Polyglutamation of methotrexate. Is methotrexate a prodrug? *J Clin Invest* **76**(3): 907–912.

36. Herbst KD, Corder MP, Justice GR. (1976) Successful therapy with methotrexate of a multicentric mixed lymphoma of the central nervous system. *Cancer* **38**(4): 1476–1478.

37. Ervin T, Canellos GP. (1980) Successful treatment of recurrent primary central nervous system lymphoma with high-dose methotrexate. *Cancer* **45**(7): 1556–1557.

38. Henson JW, Yang J, Batchelor T. (1999) Intraocular methotrexate level after high-dose intravenous infusion. *J Clin Oncol* **17**(4): 1329.

39. Batchelor TT, Kolak G, Ciordia R, *et al.* (2003) High-dose methotrexate for intraocular lymphoma. *Clin Cancer Res* **9**(2): 711–715.

40. de Smet M, Vancs VS, Kohler D, *et al.* (1999) Intravitreal chemotherapy for the treatment of recurrent intraocular lymphoma. *Br J Ophthalmol* **83**(4): 448–451.

41. Smith JR, Rosenbaum JT, Wilson DJ, *et al.* (2002) Role of intravitreal methotrexate in the management of primary central nervous system lymphoma with ocular involvement. *Ophthalmology* **109**(9): 1709–1716.

42. Chan CC, Wallace DJ. (2004) Intraocular lymphoma: update on diagnosis and management. *Cancer Control* **11**(5): 285–295.

43. Rapoport SI. (1970) Effect of concentrated solutions on blood-brain barrier. *Am J Physiol* **219**(1): 270–274.

44. Rapoport SI, Hori M, Klatzo I. (1972) Testing of a hypothesis for osmotic opening of the blood-brain barrier. *Am J Physiol* **223**(2): 323–331.

45. Rapoport SI. (2001) Advances in osmotic opening of the blood-brain barrier to enhance CNS chemotherapy. *Expert Opin Investig Drugs* **10**(10): 1809–1818.

46. Rapoport SI. (2000) Osmotic opening of the blood-brain barrier: principles, mechanism, and therapeutic applications. *Cell Mol Neurobiol* **20**(2): 217–230.

47. Rapoport SI, Hori M, Klatzo I. (1971) Reversible osmotic opening of the blood-brain barrier. *Science* **173**(4001): 1026–1028.

48. Rapoport SI, Matthews K, Thompson HK, Pettigrew KD. (1977) Osmotic opening of the blood-brain barrier in the rhesus monkey without measurable brain edema. *Brain Res* **136**(1): 23–29.

49. Neuwelt EA, Barnett PA, Bigner DD, Frenkel EP. (1982) Effects of adrenal cortical steroids and osmotic blood-brain barrier opening on methotrexate delivery to gliomas in the rodent: the factor of the blood-brain barrier. *Proc Natl Acad Sci USA* **79**(14): 4420–4423.

50. Baehring JM, Androudi S, Longtine JJ, *et al.* (2005) Analysis of clonal immunoglobulin heavy chain rearrangements in ocular lymphoma. *Cancer* **104**(3): 591–597.

51. Rockwood EJ, Zakov ZN, Bay JW. (1984) Combined malignant lymphoma of the eye and CNS (reticulum-cell sarcoma). *J Neurosurg* **61**: 369–374.

52. Chan CC, Buggage RR, Nussenblatt RB. (2002) Intraocular lymphoma. *Curr Opin Ophthalmol* **13**(6): 411–418.

53. Ferreri AJ, Blay JY, Reni M, *et al.* (2002) Relevance of intraocular involvement in the management of primary central nervous system lymphomas. *Ann Oncol* **13**(4): 531–538.

54. O'Neill BP, O'Fallon JR, Earle JD, *et al.* (1995) Primary central nervous system non-Hodgkin's lymphoma: survival advantages with combined initial therapy? *Int J Radiat Oncol Biol Phys* **33**(3): 663–673.

55. Glass J, Gruber ML, Cher L, Hochberg FH. (1994) Preirradiation methotrexate chemotherapy of primary central nervous system lymphoma: long-term outcome. *J Neurosurg* **81**(2): 188–195.

56. Gabbai AA, Hochberg FH, Linggood RM, *et al.* (1989) High-dose methotrexate for non-AIDS primary central nervous system lymphoma. Report of 13 cases. *J Neurosurg* **70**(2): 190–194.

57. Schultz C, Scott C, Sherman W, *et al.* (1996) Preirradiation chemotherapy with cyclophosphamide, doxorubicin, vincristine, and dexamethasone for primary CNS lymphomas: initial report of radiation therapy oncology group protocol 88–06. *J Clin Oncol* **14**(2): 556–564.

58. Abrey LE, Yahalom J, DeAngelis LM. (2000) Treatment for primary CNS lymphoma: the next step. *J Clin Oncol* **18**(17): 3144–3150.

59. Golay JT, Clark EA, Beverley PC. (1985) The CD20 (Bp35) antigen is involved in activation of B cells from the G0 to the G1 phase of the cell cycle. *J Immunol* **135**(6): 3795–3801.

60. Clark EA, Shu G. (1987) Activation of human B cell proliferation through surface Bp35 (CD20) polypeptides or immunoglobulin receptors. *J Immunol* 138(3): 720–725.
61. Golay JT. (1986) Functional B-lymphocyte surface antigens. *Immunology* 59(1): 1–5.
62. Hultin LE, Hausner MA, Hultin PM, Giorgi JV. (1993) CD20 (pan-B cell) antigen is expressed at a low level on a subpopulation of human T lymphocytes. *Cytometry* 14(2): 196–204.
63. Katopodis O, Liossis SN, Viglis V, *et al.* (2003) Expansion of CD8+ T cells that express low levels of the B cell-specific molecule CD20 in patients with multiple myeloma. *Br J Haematol* 120(3): 478–481.
64. (1994) Phase II results using a new antibody in the treatment of lymphoma. *Oncology (Williston Park)* 8(12): 84, 87.
65. Anderson DR, Grillo-Lopez A, Varns C, *et al.* (1997) Targeted anti-cancer therapy using rituximab, a chimaeric anti-CD20 antibody (IDEC-C2B8) in the treatment of non-Hodgkin's B-cell lymphoma. *Biochem Soc Trans* 25(2): 705–708.
66. Takami A, Hayashi T, Kita D, *et al.* (2006) Treatment of primary central nervous system lymphoma with induction of complement-dependent cytotoxicity by intraventricular administration of autologous-serum-supplemented rituximab. *Cancer Sci* 97(1): 80–83.
67. Pels H, Schulz H, Manzke O, *et al.* (2002) Intraventricular and intravenous treatment of a patient with refractory primary CNS lymphoma using rituximab. *J Neurooncol* 59(3): 213–216.
68. Pels H, Deckert-Schluter M, Glasmacher A, *et al.* (2000) Primary central nervous system lymphoma: a clinicopathological study of 28 cases. *Hematol Oncol* 18(1): 21–32.
69. Dietlein M, Pels H, Schulz H, *et al.* (2005) Imaging of central nervous system lymphomas with iodine-123 labeled rituximab. *Eur J Haematol* 74(4): 348–352.
70. Mordenti J, Thomsen K, Licko V, *et al.* (1999) Intraocular pharmacokinetics and safety of a humanized monoclonal antibody in rabbits after intravitreal administration of a solution or a PLGA microsphere formulation. *Toxicol Sci* 52(1): 101–106.
71. Kim H, Csaky KG, Chan CC, *et al.* (2006) The pharmacokinetics of rituximab following an intravitreal injection. *Exp Eye Res* 82(5): 760–766.
72. Velez G, de Smet MD, Whitcup SM, *et al.* (2000) Iris involvement in primary intraocular lymphoma: report of two cases and review of the literature. *Surv Ophthalmol* 44(6): 518–526.
73. Schaedel O, Reiter Y. (2006) Antibodies and their fragments as anti-cancer agents. *Curr Pharm Des* 12(3): 363–378.

74. Kaminski MS, Zelenetz AD, Press OW, *et al.* (2001) Pivotal study of iodine I 131 tositumomab for chemotherapy-refractory low-grade or transformed low-grade B-cell non-Hodgkin's lymphomas. *J Clin Oncol* **19**(19): 3918–3928.

75. Krasner C, Joyce RM. (2001) Zevalin: 90yttrium labeled anti-CD20 (ibritumomab tiuxetan), a new treatment for non-Hodgkin's lymphoma. *Curr Pharm Biotechnol* **2**(4): 341–349.

76. FitzGerald DJ, Kreitman R, Wilson W, *et al.* (2004) Recombinant immunotoxins for treating cancer. *Int J Med Microbiol* **293**(7–8): 577–582.

77. Philip T, Guglielmi C, Hagenbeek A, *et al.* (1995) Autologous bone marrow transplantation as compared with salvage chemotherapy in relapses of chemotherapy-sensitive non-Hodgkin's lymphoma. *N Engl J Med* **333**(23): 1540–1545.

78. Soussain C, Merle-Beral H, Reux I, *et al.* (1996) A single-center study of 11 patients with intraocular lymphoma treated with conventional chemotherapy followed by high-dose chemotherapy and autologous bone marrow transplantation in 5 cases. *Leuk Lymphoma* **23**(3–4): 339–345.

79. Soussain C, Suzan F, Hoang-Xuan K, *et al.* (2001) Results of intensive chemotherapy followed by hematopoietic stem-cell rescue in 22 patients with refractory or recurrent primary CNS lymphoma or intraocular lymphoma. *J Clin Oncol* **19**(3): 742–749.

80. Chan CC. (2003) Molecular pathology of primary intraocular lymphoma. *Trans Am Ophthalmol Soc* **101**: 275–292.

81. Chan CC, Shen D, Hackett JJ, *et al.* (2003) Expression of chemokine receptors, CXCR4 and CXCR5, and chemokines, BLC and SDF-1, in the eyes of patients with primary intraocular lymphoma. *Ophthalmology* **110**(2): 421–426.

82. Hendrix CW, Flexner C, MacFarland RT, *et al.* (2000) Pharmacokinetics and safety of AMD-3100, a novel antagonist of the CXCR-4 chemokine receptor, in human volunteers. *Antimicrob Agents Chemother* **44**(6): 1667–1673.

83. Wu L, LaRosa G, Kassam N, *et al.* (1997) Interaction of chemokine receptor CCR5 with its ligands: multiple domains for HIV-1 gp120 binding and a single domain for chemokine binding. *J Exp Med* **186**(8): 1373–1381.

84. Abrey LE, DeAngelis LM, Yahalom J. (1998) Long-term survival in primary CNS lymphoma. *J Clin Oncol* **16**(3): 859–863.

85. Hoffman PM, McKelvie P, Hall AJ, *et al.* (2003) Intraocular lymphoma: a series of 14 patients with clinicopathological features and treatment outcomes. *Eye* **17**(4): 513–521.

86. Kroll RA, Neuwelt EA. (1998) Outwitting the blood-brain barrier for therapeutic purposes: osmotic opening and other means. *Neurosurgery* **42**(5): 1083–1099; discussion 1099–1100.

87. Remsen LG, McCormick CI, Sexton G, *et al.* (1995) Decreased delivery and acute toxicity of cranial irradiation and chemotherapy given with osmotic blood-brain barrier disruption in a rodent model: the issue of sequence. *Clin Cancer Res* 1(7): 731–739.

88. Dahlborg SA, Henner WD, Crossen JR, *et al.* (1996) Non-AIDS primary CNS lymphoma: first example of a durable response in a primary brain tumor using enhanced chemotherapy delivery without cognitive loss and without radiotherapy. *Cancer J Sci Am* 2(3): 166.

89. Frappaz D, Bouffet E, Cochat P, *et al.* (1988) [Hemoperfusion on charcoal and hemodialysis in acute poisoning caused by methotrexate]. *Presse Med* 17(23): 1209–1213.

90. Thierry FX, Vernier I, Dueymes JM, *et al.* (1989) Acute renal failure after high-dose methotrexate therapy. Role of hemodialysis and plasma exchange in methotrexate removal. *Nephron* 51(3): 416–417.

91. Flombaum CD, Meyers PA. (1999) High-dose leucovorin as sole therapy for methotrexate toxicity. *J Clin Oncol* 17(5): 1589–1594.

92. Makino K, Kochi M, Nakamura H, *et al.* (2005) Effect of oral colestimide on the elimination of high-dose methotrexate in patients with primary central nervous system lymphoma — case report. *Neurol Med Chir (Tokyo)* 45(12): 650–652.

93. Tuo J, Smith BC, Bojanowski CM, *et al.* (2004) The involvement of sequence variation and expression of CX3CR1 in the pathogenesis of age-related macular degeneration. *Faseb J* 18(11): 1297–1299.

94. Klein RJ, Zeiss C, Chew EY, *et al.* (2005) Complement factor H polymorphism in age-related macular degeneration. *Science* 308(5720): 385–389.

95. Edwards AO, Ritter R, 3rd, Abel KJ, *et al.* (2005) Complement factor H polymorphism and age-related macular degeneration. *Science* 308(5720): 421–424.

96. Haines JL, Hauser MA, Schmidt S, *et al.* (2005) Complement factor H variant increases the risk of age-related macular degeneration. *Science* 308(5720): 419–421.

97. Hageman GS, Anderson DH, Johnson LV, *et al.* (2005) A common haplotype in the complement regulatory gene factor H (HF1/CFH) predisposes individuals to age-related macular degeneration. *Proc Natl Acad Sci USA* 102(20): 7227–7232.

98. Zareparsi S, Branham KE, Li M, *et al.* (2005) Strong association of the Y402H variant in complement factor H at 1q32 with susceptibility to age-related macular degeneration. *Am J Hum Genet* 77(1): 149–153.

99. Conley YP, Thalamuthu A, Jakobsdottir J, *et al.* (2005) Candidate gene analysis suggests a role for fatty acid biosynthesis and regulation of the complement

system in the etiology of age-related maculopathy. *Hum Mol Genet* **14**(14): 1991–2002.

100. Linnebank M, Pels H, Kleczar N, *et al.* (2005) MTX-induced white matter changes are associated with polymorphisms of methionine metabolism. *Neurology* **64**(5): 912–913.

101. Seidemann K, Book M, Zimmermann M, *et al.* (2006) MTHFR 677 (C → T) polymorphism is not relevant for prognosis or therapy-associated toxicity in pediatric NHL: results from 484 patients of multicenter trial NHL-BFM 95. *Ann Hematol*: 1–10.

102. Jahnke K, Korfel A, Martus P, *et al.* (2005) High-dose methotrexate toxicity in elderly patients with primary central nervous system lymphoma. *Ann Oncol* **16**(3): 445–449.

103. Melberg NS, Thomas MA. (1995) Nuclear sclerotic cataract after vitrectomy in patients younger than 50 years of age. *Ophthalmology* **102**(10): 1466–1471.

104. Holekamp NM, Shui YB, Beebe DC. (2005) Vitrectomy surgery increases oxygen exposure to the lens: a possible mechanism for nuclear cataract formation. *Am J Ophthalmol* **139**(2): 302–310.

105. Doolittle ND, Miner ME, Hall WA, *et al.* (2000) Safety and efficacy of a multicenter study using intraarterial chemotherapy in conjunction with osmotic opening of the blood-brain barrier for the treatment of patients with malignant brain tumors. *Cancer* **88**(3): 637–647.

106. Pels H, Schulz H, Schlegel U, Engert A. (2003) Treatment of CNS lymphoma with the anti-CD20 antibody rituximab: experience with two cases and review of the literature. *Onkologie* **26**(4): 351–354.

107. Wolf T, Brodt HR, Fichtlscherer S, *et al.* (2005) Changing incidence and prognostic factors of survival in AIDS-related non-Hodgkin's lymphoma in the era of highly active antiretroviral therapy (HAART). *Leuk Lymphoma* **46**(2): 207–215.

108. Cheung TW. (2004) AIDS-related cancer in the era of highly active antiretroviral therapy (HAART): a model of the interplay of the immune system, virus, and cancer. "On the offensive — the Trojan Horse is being destroyed" — Part B: Malignant lymphoma. *Cancer Invest* **22**(5): 787–798.

109. Baumgartner JE, Rachlin JR, Beckstead JH, *et al.* (1990) Primary central nervous system lymphomas: natural history and response to radiation therapy in 55 patients with acquired immunodeficiency syndrome. *J Neurosurg* **73**(2): 206–211.

110. Levine AM. (1992) Acquired immunodeficiency syndrome-related lymphoma. *Blood* **80**(1): 8–20.

Chapter 11

Prognosis in PIOL

The word "prognosis" comes from Greek and literally means *foreseeing* or *fore-knowing*. In medicine, prognosis is an ever-present projection. A good prognosis is like a good weather forecast as doctors and patients expect a certain amount of recovery and return to normalcy. A good prognosis is supplanted perhaps only by cure of the disease.

Diagnoses of PCNSL and PIOL have historically been associated with a poor prognosis. Although we have made great strides in understanding the fascinating pathological, cytological, immunological, and molecular characteristics of these unique lymphomas and our treatment tactics have improved survival over the years, PCNSL and PIOL often recur. This frequently bodes poorly for the patient's life. Currently, the five-year survival rate ranges from less than 20 to 34% with our best therapies.[1,2] Apart from the lesions of PIOL and PCNSL themselves, the characteristics of the patient, such as age and performance status, have been recognized as prognostic indicators. Yet, the ability to foresee a patient's future does not necessarily dictate fate, at least, not for physicians. Instead, prognosis serves to guide a physician's treatment with the intent to change that prognosis for the better and add meaningful time to a patient's life.

Historical Attempts at Prognostication

Some have noted that PCNSL (known as central nervous system (CNS) reticulum cell sarcoma (RCS) until the late 1980s) has different cytological patterns based upon the lymphoma classification schema of the Working Formulation, Lukes & Collins, and Kiel classification systems.[3–7] For example, in Jellinger and Paulus' review of 590 PCNSL histologic variants from the literature, which included 20 of their own cases, the most common histologic type (using the New Working Formulation) to be noted was diffuse large-cell (43.4%).[8] Other histologic subtypes included diffuse large-cell immunoblastic (19.7%), diffuse small cleaved cell (9.5%), small non-cleaved cell (8.8%), atypical and unclassifiable (7.1%), diffuse mixed-cell (7.1%), lymphoblastic non-convoluted (2.9%), and small lymphocytic (1.5%).[8] Earlier, Jellinger *et al.* had suggested that the development of a staging system for CNS RCS could be defined, and this would have some prognostic utility.[9] They noted that the lymphoblastic lymphoma cytologic subtype, which was characterized by densely packed, uniform cells with cleaved nuclei, numerous mitoses, and prominent nucleoli, had a poorer prognosis after surgical and radiation therapy as compared with immunoblastoma and immunocytoma cytologic subtypes of primary CNS malignant lymphoma.[9] While the mean survival time for patients receiving surgery and irradiation for immunoblastic lymphoma (40 cases) and immunocytoma (19 cases) were 25 and 15 months, respectively, the mean survival time for patients with lymphoblastic lymphoma (9 cases) receiving the same therapy was just six months at a center in Budapest, Hungary.[9] Similarly, at a center in Vienna, Austria, the mean survival time for patients receiving surgery and irradiation for immunoblastic lymphoma (15 cases) and immunocytoma (16 cases) were 10 and 13 months, respectively, while the mean survival time for patients with lymphoblastic lymphoma (5 cases) was only 4.5 months.[9] Regardless of the cytologic subtypes, however, most PCNSLs were noted to be intermediate- or high-grade lymphomas.[8]

Age and the ability to perform daily tasks have been recognized as important prognostic factors. Pollack and colleagues reviewed the cases of 27 PCNSL patients seen at their facility from the mid-1970s to the mid-1980s.[10] Patients below 60 years of age had significantly better one, two, and five year survival rates than patients who were over the age of 60. Pollack also found that of 24 patients responding to treatment (which varied among the patients and included surgery, chemotherapy, and radiotherapy), 15 (62.5%) had recurrences of their lymphomas. Those receiving treatment for recurrent disease (10 patients) had significantly better survivals as compared with patients not receiving treatment for recurrent disease (5 patients).[10] In addition, Pollack and colleagues looked at three physical features of the tumor itself to determine significance on prognosis: tumor multiplicity, tumor size, and tumor location/cerebral structure involvement. Only tumor location, with respect to affectation of deep structures (specifically, periventricular areas) significantly boded poorly for patients compared with those with lesions affecting the cerebrum or cerebellum.[10]

A patient's ability to perform tasks associated with normal life can help guide a physician towards different treatment or palliative care pursuits. Patients able to care for themselves and exhibiting no-to-minor signs and symptoms of disease, may be able to handle more robust forms of treatment geared at increasing survival. Patients displaying obvious signs and symptoms of disease as well as an inability for self-care may not be good candidates for aggressive therapies; palliative care may be more beneficial for these patients. The Karnofsky Performance Status (KPS) was developed by Karnofsky and colleagues in the late 1940s as a means to measure primary lung carcinoma patients' abilities entering palliative treatment with nitrogen mustard to perform basic daily activities.[11] The scale had three broad definitions: ability to proceed with normal, daily activities by oneself without special care; ability to live at home and care for oneself for the most part, but with the requirement of some assistance and an inability to work; and inability to care for oneself with the requirement of institutionalized or hospital care, and potentially the presence of a rapidly progressing disease. Within these three broad definitions were specific criteria, ranging from completely "normal" to "dead" that were attained by the ascription of a certain percentage of completely normal (i.e. normal was assigned 100% and dead assigned 0%). Percentages were measured in tens, and those with a percentage score greater that 70% would be, for the most part, fairly able to perform all activities of daily living. Perhaps the high scoring patients in this group would show only minimal signs or symptoms of disease.[11] The KPS, then, was an attempt to quantify some basic self-care functions.

In addition to PCNSL patients below 60 years of age, those having a KPS $\geq$ 70 also had significantly better one, two, and five year survival rates than patients with a KPS $\leq$ 70.[10]

A scale later developed by the Eastern Cooperative Oncology Group (ECOG) also assessed a patient's performance status.[12] This performance status scale had six grades ranging from zero (defined as a patient who is fully active and has no restrictions) to five (defined as a patient who is dead). The ECOG scale can be converted into percentages as used by the

KPS. Thus, ECOG grades of 0, 1, 2, 3, 4, and 5 are similar to KPS percentages of 90–100, 70–80, 50–60, 30–40, 10–20, and 0, respectively.[12] The ECOG score, like the KPS, has also been used to assess patients' abilities to perform daily activities, as a means to make prognosis in PCNSL.[13]

Others made note of certain other findings associated with PCNSLs, such as, elevated protein content in the CSF and tumor location. However, no attempts were made at correlating these features with survival.[9,14] For example, Henry *et al.* noted that of 41 cases of PCNSL (at the time still known as reticulum cell sarcoma), 35 cases (85.4%) had elevated protein levels of over 60 mg/100 mL CSF.[14] This was similar to Jellinger and colleagues' CSF protein findings in their 68 PCNSL patients; 85% had elevated CSF protein.[9] Later, these features were studied and recognized as prognostic factors by some.

Modern Prognosis

Age. Age, along with performance status, has been a consistent prognostic indicator in studies of PCNSL.[2,15–17] Age less than 60 years is associated with better survival than age greater than 60. However, 37 to 65% of patients with PCNSL or PIOL are over the age of 60.[18–20] Those over the age of 60 also experience significant neurotoxicity associated with radiation therapy. This results in a decline in cortical functioning. Abrey and colleagues showed that age greater than 60 was associated with neurotoxic effects involving dementia, decline in Karnofsky performance score, ataxia, and urinary incontinence that appeared in a median of just over a year.[21] Later, Abrey and colleagues again showed that age was an important determinant in prognosis as patients older than 60 years fared worse than younger patients.[17] They used a high-dose methotrexate-based regimen and compared patients older than 60 years who had radiation therapy following chemotherapy with patients older than 60 years who had chemotherapy only.[17] Regardless of having received radiation therapy or not, older age was a poor prognostic factor. It is interesting, however, to note the difference in the cause of death between those who had received radiation therapy and those who had not. Patients who had received chemotherapy frequently died due to relapse of lymphoma, while those who had received radiation therapy following chemotherapy often died from delayed neurotoxic effects.[17]

Importantly, it has been shown that patients over the age of 60 can tolerate high-dose methotrexate, currently the most effective treatment for PCNSL and PIOL. Provided renal function is normal, older patients should receive as aggressive methotrexate doses as their younger counterparts, especially in the light of the fact that older patients have a worse prognosis.[22]

Occasionally, some have suggested that age can dictate what type of therapy a patient should receive or the dosage,[23] although Reni and colleagues have shown that age and performance status are *independent* prognostic factors.[18] Indeed, as noted previously, dosage using first-line methotrexate treatment should not differ between patients younger or older than 60 years provided renal function is adequate.[22]

Performance Status. There are several ways of imparting quantitative value to the qualitative assessment of a patient's ability to carry out daily activities such as the ECOG, World Health Organization (WHO) and KPS. Performance status has consistently been shown to be an important prognostic indicator in PCNSL. For example, Corry showed that a WHO status score of less than or equal to one was associated with a significantly better median survival time than scores greater than one.[24] Hematologists and oncologists, key players involved in the treatment of patients with PCNSL and PIOL, have been noted to preferentially use the ECOG system.[13]

Relapse. Prognosis at relapse is poor. In Abrey *et al.*'s study, of 27 patients who achieved a clinical response to treatment using high-dose systemic methotrexate as well as intrathecal methotrexate followed by radiation therapy and cytarabine, 15 (55.6%) relapsed (median disease-free survival was 41.3 months).[21] As we noted earlier, Abrey *et al.* showed that in patients over the age of 60, relapse was associated with the lack of radiation therapy.[17] While those older than 60 years who did receive radiation after chemotherapy did not succumb to relapse as often as their counterparts not receiving radiation, this group succumbed to delayed neurotoxic effects that included dementia, ataxia, and fatigue.[17]

Gender. Corry and colleagues showed that in 62 patients with PCNSL, male patients had a significantly better median survival of 27.5 months compared with female patients' median survival of 11.5 months.[24]

However, more recently, Ferreri and colleagues have shown that gender does not seem to be significantly involved in the prognosis of PCNSL.[25]

Histologic Subtype. Based on the current WHO-REAL classification system, most PCNSLs are immunohistologically classified as diffuse large B-cell lymphomas (DLBCLs).[26] While cytologic examination is the gold standard for discovering malignant lymphocytes associated with PCNSL and PIOL, the histologic appearance of the tumor has not been associated with any type of prognostic significance.[25] In Ferreri and colleagues' review of 378 patients with PCNSL, and using the Working Formulation classification schema for identifying histologic subtypes (low grade, intermediate grade, and high grade subtypes[3]), no significant association was found between the histology of the tumor and the overall survival of PCNSL patients.[25]

Molecular Profiling. While histologic classification may not be significantly involved with our ability to make prognoses in PCNSL and PIOL, the recent advances made in molecular biology now enable us to characterize lymphomas and other cancers by the specific genes they express. Thus, the particular genetic signature for a tumor may be involved with prognosis. As we have mentioned in Chapter 3, three subtypes of DLBCL have been identified by gene expression profiling.[27] Germinal center B-cell (GCB) DLBCLs have a gene expression profile that is similar to normal B-cell counterparts found in the germinal centers of lymphoid organs. One important characteristic of the GCB genetic signature is the expression of the *bcl-6* transcription repressor protein,[27] which is a marker unique to B cells of germinal center derivation.[28–30] Activated B-cell (ABC) DLBCLs have an expression profile more like that of peripheral B-cells, which have been mitogenically stimulated. A third type of DLBCL, known as primary mediastinal (or type 3), has a gene expression profile unlike GCB and ABC DLBCLs. In adults, GCB DLBCLs make up approximately 50% of systemic NHL DLBCLs, while the ABC subtype makes up approximately 30%.[27] GCB subtypes are associated with a better outcome than are ABC subtypes. For example, patients with DLBCLs of the GCB subtype have been shown to have a better survival following chemotherapy compared with their ABC subtype counterparts.[31] Primary mediastinal DLBCL is also considered a clinically favorable subtype.[32] DLBCLs expressing the pro-apoptotic protein BAX have been shown to have better overall and disease-free survivals than those DLBCLs in which there is a relative lack of expression of this protein.[33] ·

While there is mounting evidence that gene expression profiling has prognostic utility in the systemic NHL realm, can these findings be applied to the much rarer PCNSL and PIOL? We already know that most PCNSLs and PIOLs are of the DLBCL histologic subtype; recent evidence has further characterized these unique lymphomas as exhibiting, most often, a GCB genetic signature.[34]

Molecular analyses have revealed that PCNSL and PIOL cells, which are most commonly derived from malignant B lymphocytes, exhibit rearrangements in the immunoglobulin heavy chain (*IgH*) gene.[35–37] *IgH* gene rearrangement, as discussed in Chapter 3, precedes malignant transformation in B lymphocytes. Recently, genotypic anomalies and changes in the expression of related proteins suggest a molecular prognosis may one day be achievable. Pels and colleagues recently analyzed the variable region genes of 18 PCNSLs via polymerase chain reaction (PCR) on the *IgH* gene.[38] The patients had all undergone treatment with either methotrexate-based chemotherapy (16 patients) or radiation and chemotherapy (two patients). Half of the patients exhibited complete response to treatment and the other half showed progressive disease. Although no statistical significance was reached, patients with complete response to treatment showed a trend towards higher mutation frequencies of the *IgH* gene as compared with patients who had progressive disease despite therapy. In addition, there was a trend towards preferential usage of the *VH4* gene segment in the *IgH* gene in PCNSL patients with progressive disease (seven patients) as compared with patients responding completely to treatment (five patients).[38] Coupland and colleagues also analyzed the *IgH* gene using PCR in eight of 16 patients, but in this instance, the patients had PIOL (six of 14 patients had concurrent cerebral disease).[37] Four patients showed usage of the *VH4* gene segment and four showed usage of the *VH3* gene segment, suggesting a relationship between PIOL and PCNSL. Furthermore, in both studies the ratio of replacement mutations and silent mutations within the framework region (FR) of the *V* gene segment was less than 1.5. These values indicated a tumor cell was antigen-selected.[37,38] Coupland's group also revealed that in three patients with oculocerebral disease, lymphoma cells obtained from the eye and brain lesions in each patient and undergoing *IgH*-PCR had the same monoclonal PCR product. This further supported a close relationship between PIOL and PCNSL.[37,39]

The translocation involving the oncogene, *bcl-2* and the *IgH* gene leads to increased expression of the oncoprotein and is a well-known mechanism in the genesis of B-cell lymphoma.[40–42] The *bcl-2* t(14;18) translocation brings the *bcl-2* gene under the control of the *IgH* enhancer, resulting in deregulated BCL-2 protein expression. The BCL-2 protein is capable of preventing apoptosis, and *in vitro* evidence suggests a role in drug resistance.[43,44] The precise role that the t(14;18) translocation plays in B-cell lymphoma, including PCNSL and PIOL, has yet to be determined.[33,45] The *bcl-2* translocation has been detected in PIOL,[46,47] and recent analysis performed at the National Eye Institute (NEI) on the clinical outcomes in 23 PIOL patients revealed no significant association between the translocation and survival or relapse.[42] Interesting, though, was the finding that patients with *bcl-2* translocation were significantly younger than patients without this translocation,[42] and youth, a fact we have already mentioned, is a significant prognostic factor involved in PCNSL. In addition, Larocca and colleagues have shown that most PCNSLs exhibit expression of the BCL-6 protein, indicating a germinal center derivation in keeping with most DLBCLs.[48] Of four PIOL cases tested at the NEI for expression of *bcl-6* mRNA, all were found to exhibit overexpression.[42] While no correlations have been drawn between the expression of *bcl-6* and survival in PCNSLs (or PIOLs) as has been performed for systemic DLBCLs, future studies may reveal a similar pattern that can hold prognostic significance.

Sites of Tumor Involvement. Blay and colleagues had shown in a review of 226 PCNSL patients that involvement of the corpus callosum or subcortical grey structures was significantly correlated with poor survival.[16] More recently, the involvement of deep brain structures has been noted to be an independent prognostic factor.[25] In a retrospective review of 370 PCNSL patients, the affectation of deep brain structures by PCNSL, including paraventricular structures, the brainstem, the basal ganglia, and the cerebellum was associated with significantly worse overall survival rates as compared with a lack of involvement of these structures.[25]

CSF Protein Levels. High cerebrospinal fluid (CSF) protein levels have been shown to be independently correlated with survival.[16,25] Blay and colleagues in their retrospective series of 226 patients with PCNSL showed that those with CSF protein level higher than 0.6 g/L had poor survival.[16] Likewise, Ferreri *et al.* showed that elevated CSF protein level was independently associated with poor survival.[25]

LDH Levels. Increased levels of lactate dehydrogenase (LDH), the enzyme involved in the intercatalysis of lactate and pyruvate, are associated with increased tissue destruction. In cancer, this may signify that there are malignant lymphocytes which are rapidly dividing and may be associated with more aggressive disease. As in systemic NHL, elevated levels of LDH have been associated with poor prognosis in PCNSL.[25,49]

Methotrexate Therapy. The use of high-dose methotrexate chemotherapy has improved survival in patients with PCNSL and PIOL. In fact, in PCNSL patients, the use of methotrexate imparts a better prognosis compared with other forms of therapy. However, recently it has been noted that the methylation of CpG islands of the reduced folate carrier gene (*RFC-1*) may confer a certain amount of resistance in PCNSL patients undergoing methotrexate chemotherapy. It was found that PCNSL patients exhibiting methylation of the promoter of *RFC-1* had a lower expression of the RFC protein compared with PCNSL patients who had an unmethylated promoter and control patients with systemic DLBCLs.[50] The RFC protein is important for the transport of not only folates across the membranes of cells, but also methotrexate (a folate analogue).[51] Therefore, a lower expression of RFC protein can result in tumors being less responsive to methotrexate-based therapies, as in PCNSL and PIOL. At the NEI, we recently came across a case of PIOL that was initially responsive, but later became resistant to intravitreal methotrexate (Sen *et al.*, unpublished data). Immunohistochemistry on the PIOL cells revealed that most of the cells had decreased expression of RFC and folate binding protein (FBP, proteins involved in binding folic acid[52,53]). Some cells showed expression of the multi-drug resistance protein (MRP, a protein that mediates efflux of methotrexate and has been shown to be associated with methotrexate resistance *in vitro*[54]), while normal lymphocytes showed expression in none of these patients. The PIOL cells obtained from a patient who had responded to treatment showed the reverse expression of proteins as compared with cells from the non-responding patient (i.e., there was increased expression of RFC and FBP, but decreased expression of MRP). Ocular radiation treatment was resorted to in the patient unresponsive to methotrexate, and complete response was noted after over three years of follow-up. Further studies may typify subsets of PIOL that are more responsive to therapies other than methotrexate.

Time to Make Diagnosis. Most cases of PIOL that are initially discovered to be restricted to the eye will eventuate to involve the brain.[55] Thus, another factor in the prognosis of PIOL is the time to make diagnosis from symptom onset. As a masquerade syndrome, PIOL has a long and notorious history of being diagnosed as a uveitis and treated as such until resistance to uveitis therapy prompted further explanation. Today, most cases of PIOL are diagnosed within the first year.[56] Thus, earlier diagnoses of PIOL may catch the disease at an early stage and prior to development of cerebral disease. For example, Hormigo and colleagues noted that early systemic treatment of PIOL patients prior to cerebral involvement resulted not only in better disease control, but improved overall survival in patients with ocular disease only as compared with those having oculocerbral disease.[57]

Putting it all Together. Ferreri and colleagues have developed the International Extranodal Lymphoma Study Group (IELSG) scoring system, a prognostic scoring system for PCNSLs.[25] This prognostic scoring system incorporates age, performance status, LDH and CSF protein levels, and deep brain structure involvement. Scores range from 0 to 5; those with scores of 0–1 are considered to be at "low risk," 2–3 are at "intermediate risk," and 4–5 are at "high risk." Age greater than 60 years, ECOG score greater than 1, elevated CSF protein, elevated LDH, and involvement of deep brain structures each yield 1 point on the IELSG scoring system (see Tables 11.1 and 11.2). Molecular factors may prove to be an additional prognostic factor. In the end, the power of a prognostic scoring system lies in its ability to serve as a tool to stratify patients into different groups in which specifically tailored treatments may be administered to maximize response and extend life. However, the utility of a prognostic scoring system or even individual prognostic factors have yet to be applied to PIOL specifically. Although PIOL is rarer than PCNSL, future studies may reveal important features of PIOL relevant to prognostication. Alternatively, it may be found that many or all of the prognostic features involved in PCNSL can be applied to PIOL.

Table 11.1 Prognostic Variables and their Scores — The International Extranodal Lymphoma Study Group (IELSG) Prognostic Scoring System[25]

Variable	Value (favorability)	PCNSL[1] PS[2]
Age	≤ 60 years (favorable)	0
	> 60 years (unfavorable)	1
ECOG[3] Performance Status	0–1 (favorable)	0
	2–4 (unfavorable)	1
LDH[4] Serum Level	Normal (favorable)	0
	Elevated (unfavorable)	1
Protein CSF[5] Concentration	Normal (favorable)	0
	Elevated (unfavorable)	1
Involvement of Deep Brain Structures (periventricular regions, basal ganglia, brainstem, cerebellum)	No (favorable)	0
	Yes (unfavorable)	1

[1]PCNSL = primary central nervous system lymphoma; [2]PS = prognostic score; [3]ECOG = Eastern Cooperative Oncology Group; [4]LDH = lactate dehydrogenase; [5]CSF = cerebrospinal fluid.

Table 11.2 Total IELSG Prognostic Score[25]

Total PCNSL[1] PS[2]	2 Year OS[3] Rate
0–1	80%
2–3	48%
4–5	15%

[1]PCNSL = primary central nervous system lymphoma; [2]PS = prognostic score; [3]OS = overall survival.

Prognosis in PIOL. Although there is currently no defined prognostic scoring system for PIOL, it is helpful to summarize features of this special lymphoma that may likely be involved in the prognosis of the disease. Age, a consistently valuable prognostic factor in PCNSL, is important in PIOL as well. As in PCNSL, PIOL patients tend to be in their fifth to sixth decades of life.[58] We may be able to also derive prognostic information based upon the location of the PIOL lesion. For example, lesions confined to the sub-RPE space may indicate an early stage of the disease or perhaps disease that is less aggressive than lesions that have infiltrated the retina by breaking through the usual RPE barrier or show infiltration of the vitreous and optic nerve. Correlating patient outcomes with fundus and fluorescein angiographic changes may help elucidate these possibilities. Molecular pathology is becoming an increasingly important way to subcategorize systemic DLBCLs, which appear to have different prognoses; recent findings in PIOL suggest similarities to PCNSL in terms of germinal center derivation and *VH* gene segment usage. Drug sensitivity will likely play an important role serving as a prognostic index; this has not only been suggested in PCNSL, but in PIOL as well. For example, resistance to methotrexate may indicate subsets of PIOL that are better treated with other forms of therapy. Drug sensitivity plays a role in the response a tumor has to instituted treatment and may account for lesions in some patients progressing (i.e., progressive disease), and lesions in other patients showing a complete response. Regression and response may be followed by performing ophthalmoscopic examination, fluorescein angiography, and MRI and measuring the vitreal IL-10/IL-6 ratio. The precise role that CNS involvement has in PIOL remains to be defined, but the recent description of cases of oculocerebral disease in which eye and brain lesions have the same molecular pathology[37,39] reveal that prognostic factors involved in PCNSL may be transferred to PIOL, either in part or in whole. On the other hand, it may become evident that PIOL may impart its own unique features to combined oculocerebral disease. Finally, it remains a mystery as to why some PIOLs do not progress to cerebral disease. Recall that up to 80% or more of PIOLs eventuate to involve the brain, while 25% of PCNSLs later show ocular involvement.[59,60] Are there characteristics that prevent some PIOLs from progressing to involve the brain? May these characteristics serve as prognostic indices? Answers to these questions and the development of a useful prognostic scoring system for PIOL are goals we are intent on achieving.

References

1. Panageas KS, Elkin EB, DeAngelis LM, *et al.* (2005) Trends in survival from primary central nervous system lymphoma, 1975–1999: a population-based analysis. *Cancer* **104**(11): 2466–2472.
2. DeAngelis LM, Seiferheld W, Schold SC, *et al.* (2002) Combination chemotherapy and radiotherapy for primary central nervous system lymphoma: Radiation Therapy Oncology Group Study 93–10. *J Clin Oncol* **20**(24): 4643–4648.

3. (1982) National Cancer Institute sponsored study of classifications of non-Hodgkin's lymphomas: summary and description of a working formulation for clinical usage. The Non-Hodgkin's Lymphoma Pathologic Classification Project. *Cancer* **49**(10): 2112–2135.
4. Lennert K. (1975) Morphology and classification of malignant lymphomas and so-called reticuloses. *Acta Neuropathol Suppl (Berl)* **Suppl 6**: 1–16.
5. Lukes RJ, Collins RD. (1974) A functional approach to the classification of malignant lymphoma. *Recent Results in Cancer Research* **46**: 18–30.
6. Lukes RJ, Collins RD. (1974) Immunologic characterization of human malignant lymphomas. *Cancer* **34**(4 Suppl): suppl:1488–1503.
7. Lukes RJ, Collins RD. (1975) New approaches to the classification of the lymphomata. *Br J Cancer* **31 Suppl 2**: 1–28.
8. Jellinger K, Paulus W. (1992) Primary central nervous system lymphomas — an update. *J Cancer Res Clin Oncol* **119**(1): 7–27.
9. Jellinger K, Radaskiewicz TH, Slowik F. (1975) Primary malignant lymphomas of the central nervous system in man. *Acta Neuropathol Suppl (Berl)* **Suppl 6**: 95–102.
10. Pollack IF, Lunsford LD, Flickinger JC, Dameshek HL. (1989) Prognostic factors in the diagnosis and treatment of primary central nervous system lymphoma. *Cancer* **63**(5): 939–947.
11. Karnofsky DA, Abelmann WH, Craver LF, Burchenal JH. (1948) The use of nitrogen mustards in the palliative treatment of carcinoma. *Cancer* **1**: 634–656.
12. Oken MM, Creech RH, Tormey DC, *et al.* (1982) Toxicity and response criteria of the Eastern Cooperative Oncology Group. *Am J Clin Oncol* **5**(6): 649–655.
13. Ferreri AJ, Reni M. (2005) Prognostic factors in primary central nervous system lymphomas. *Hematol Oncol Clin North Am* **19**(4): 629–649, vi.
14. Henry JM, Heffner RR, Jr., Dillard SH, *et al.* (1974) Primary malignant lymphomas of the central nervous system. *Cancer* **34**(4): 1293–1302.
15. Bessell EM, Graus F, Punt JA, *et al.* (1996) Primary non-Hodgkin's lymphoma of the CNS treated with BVAM or CHOD/BVAM chemotherapy before radiotherapy. *J Clin Oncol* **14**(3): 945–954.
16. Blay JY, Conroy T, Chevreau C, *et al.* (1998) High-dose methotrexate for the treatment of primary cerebral lymphomas: analysis of survival and late neurologic toxicity in a retrospective series. *J Clin Oncol* **16**(3): 864–871.
17. Abrey LE, Yahalom J, DeAngelis LM. (2000) Treatment for primary CNS lymphoma: the next step. *J Clin Oncol* **18**(17): 3144–3150.
18. Reni M, Ferreri AJ, Garancini MP, Villa E. (1997) Therapeutic management of primary central nervous system lymphoma in immunocompetent patients: results of a critical review of the literature. *Ann Oncol* **8**(3): 227–234.

19. Shibamoto Y, Tsuchida E, Seki K, *et al.* (2004) Primary central nervous system lymphoma in Japan 1995–1999: changes from the preceding 10 years. *J Cancer Res Clin Oncol* **130**(6): 351–356.

20. Jahnke K, Korfel A, Komm J, *et al.* (2005) Intraocular lymphoma 2000–2005: results of a retrospective multicentre trial. *Graefes Arch Clin Exp Ophthalmol*: 1–7.

21. Abrey LE, DeAngelis LM, Yahalom J. (1998) Long-term survival in primary CNS lymphoma. *J Clin Oncol* **16**(3): 859–863.

22. Jahnke K, Korfel A, Martus P, *et al.* (2005) High-dose methotrexate toxicity in elderly patients with primary central nervous system lymphoma. *Ann Oncol* **16**(3): 445–449.

23. Yamanaka R, Morii K, Shinbo Y, *et al.* (2005) Modified ProMACE-MOPP hybrid regimen with moderate-dose methotrexate for patients with primary CNS lymphoma. *Ann Hematol* **84**(7): 447–455.

24. Corry J, Smith JG, Wirth A, *et al.* (1998) Primary central nervous system lymphoma: age and performance status are more important than treatment modality. *Int J Radiat Oncol Biol Phys* **41**(3): 615–620.

25. Ferreri AJ, Blay JY, Reni M, *et al.* (2003) Prognostic scoring system for primary CNS lymphomas: the International Extranodal Lymphoma Study Group experience. *J Clin Oncol* **21**(2): 266–272.

26. Harris NL, Jaffe ES, Diebold J, *et al.* (1999) The World Health Organization classification of neoplastic diseases of the hematopoietic and lymphoid tissues. Report of the Clinical Advisory Committee meeting, Airlie House, Virginia, November, 1997. *Ann Oncol* **10**(12): 1419–1432.

27. Alizadeh AA, Eisen MB, Davis RE, *et al.* (2000) Distinct types of diffuse large B-cell lymphoma identified by gene expression profiling. *Nature* **403**(6769): 503–511.

28. Onizuka T, Moriyama M, Yamochi T, *et al.* (1995) BCL-6 gene product, a 92- to 98-kD nuclear phosphoprotein, is highly expressed in germinal center B cells and their neoplastic counterparts. *Blood* **86**(1): 28–37.

29. Cattoretti G, Chang CC, Cechova K, *et al.* (1995) BCL-6 protein is expressed in germinal-center B cells. *Blood* **86**(1): 45–53.

30. Flenghi L, Ye BH, Fizzotti M, *et al.* (1995) A specific monoclonal antibody (PG-B6) detects expression of the BCL-6 protein in germinal center B cells. *Am J Pathol* **147**(2): 405–411.

31. Rosenwald A, Wright G, Chan WC, *et al.* (2002) The use of molecular profiling to predict survival after chemotherapy for diffuse large-B-cell lymphoma. *N Engl J Med* **346**(25): 1937–1947.

32. Rosenwald A, Wright G, Leroy K, *et al.* (2003) Molecular diagnosis of primary mediastinal B cell lymphoma identifies a clinically favorable subgroup

of diffuse large B cell lymphoma related to Hodgkin lymphoma. *J Exp Med* **198**(6): 851–862.

33. Sohn SK, Jung JT, Kim DH, *et al.* (2003) Prognostic significance of bcl-2, bax, and p53 expression in diffuse large B-cell lymphoma. *Am J Hematol* **73**(2): 101–107.

34. Montesinos-Rongen M, Kuppers R, Schluter D, *et al.* (1999) Primary central nervous system lymphomas are derived from germinal- center B cells and show a preferential usage of the V4–34 gene segment. *Am J Pathol* **155**(6): 2077–2086.

35. Endo S, Zhang SJ, Saito T, *et al.* (2002) Primary malignant lymphoma of the brain: mutation pattern of rearranged immunoglobulin heavy chain gene. *Jpn J Cancer Res* **93**(12): 1308–1316.

36. Chan CC. (2003) Molecular pathology of primary intraocular lymphoma. *Trans Am Ophthalmol Soc* **101**: 275–292.

37. Coupland SE, Hummel M, Muller HH, Stein H. (2005) Molecular analysis of immunoglobulin genes in primary intraocular lymphoma. *Invest Ophthalmol Vis Sci* **46**(10): 3507–3514.

38. Pels H, Montesinos-Rongen M, Schaller C, *et al.* (2005) VH gene analysis of primary CNS lymphomas. *J Neurol Sci* **228**(2): 143–147.

39. Coupland SE, Hummel M, Stein H, *et al.* (2005) Demonstration of identical clonal derivation in a case of "oculocerebral" lymphoma. *Br J Ophthalmol* **89**(2): 238–239.

40. Monni O, Joensuu H, Franssila K, *et al.* (1997) BCL2 overexpression associated with chromosomal amplification in diffuse large B-cell lymphoma. *Blood* **90**(3): 1168–1174.

41. Pezzella F, Jones M, Ralfkiaer E, *et al.* (1992) Evaluation of bcl-2 protein expression and 14;18 translocation as prognostic markers in follicular lymphoma. *Br J Cancer* **65**(1): 87–89.

42. Wallace DJ, Shen DF, Reed GF, *et al.* (2006) Detection of the bcl-2 t(14;18) translocation and proto-oncogene expression in primary intraocular lymphoma. *Invest Ophthalmol Vis Sci* **47**(7): 2750–2756.

43. Hermine O, Haioun C, Lepage E, *et al.* (1996) Prognostic significance of bcl-2 protein expression in aggressive non-Hodgkin's lymphoma. Groupe d'Etude des Lymphomes de l'Adulte (GELA). *Blood* **87**(1): 265–272.

44. Hill ME, MacLennan KA, Cunningham DC, *et al.* (1996) Prognostic significance of BCL-2 expression and bcl-2 major breakpoint region rearrangement in diffuse large cell non-Hodgkin's lymphoma: a British National Lymphoma Investigation Study. *Blood* **88**(3): 1046–1051.

45. Iqbal J, Sanger WG, Horsman DE, *et al.* (2004) BCL2 translocation defines a unique tumor subset within the germinal center B-cell-like diffuse large B-cell lymphoma. *Am J Pathol* **165**(1): 159–166.

46. Buggage RR, Velez G, Myers-Powell B, *et al.* (1999) Primary intraocular lymphoma with a low interleukin 10 to interleukin 6 ratio and heterogeneous IgH gene rearrangement. *Arch Ophthalmol* **117**(9): 1239–1242.
47. Shen DF, Zhuang Z, LeHoang P, *et al.* (1998) Utility of microdissection and polymerase chain reaction for the detection of immunoglobulin gene rearrangement and translocation in primary intraocular lymphoma [In Process Citation]. *Ophthalmology* **105**(9): 1664–1669.
48. Larocca LM, Capello D, Rinelli A, *et al.* (1998) The molecular and phenotypic profile of primary central nervous system lymphoma identifies distinct categories of the disease and is consistent with histogenetic derivation from germinal center-related B cells. *Blood* **92**(3): 1011–1019.
49. (1993) A predictive model for aggressive non-Hodgkin's lymphoma. The International Non-Hodgkin's Lymphoma Prognostic Factors Project. *N Engl J Med* **329**(14): 987–994.
50. Ferreri AJ, Dell'Oro S, Capello D, *et al.* (2004) Aberrant methylation in the promoter region of the reduced folate carrier gene is a potential mechanism of resistance to methotrexate in primary central nervous system lymphomas. *Br J Haematol* **126**(5): 657–664.
51. Sirotnak FM, Tolner B. (1999) Carrier-mediated membrane transport of folates in mammalian cells. *Annu Rev Nutr* **19**: 91–122.
52. Davis RE, Nicol DJ. (1988) Folic acid. *Int J Biochem* **20**(2): 133–139.
53. Henderson GB. (1990) Folate-binding proteins. *Annu Rev Nutr* **10**: 319–335.
54. Hooijberg JH, Broxterman HJ, Kool M, *et al.* (1999) Antifolate resistance mediated by the multidrug resistance proteins MRP1 and MRP2. *Cancer Res* **59**(11): 2532–2535.
55. Corriveau C, Easterbrook M, Payne D. (1986) Lymphoma simulating uveitis (masquerade syndrome). *Can J Ophthalmol* **21**(4): 144–149.
56. Akpek EK, Ahmed I, Hochberg FH, *et al.* (1999) Intraocular-central nervous system lymphoma: clinical features, diagnosis, and outcomes. *Ophthalmology* **106**(9): 1805–1810.
57. Hormigo A, Abrey L, Heinemann MH, DeAngelis LM. (2004) Ocular presentation of primary central nervous system lymphoma: diagnosis and treatment. *Br J Haematol* **126**(2): 202–208.
58. Chan CC, Buggage RR, Nussenblatt RB. (2002) Intraocular lymphoma. *Curr Opin Ophthalmol* **13**(6): 411–418.
59. Hochberg FH, Miller DC. (1988) Primary central nervous system lymphoma. *J Neurosurg* **68**(6): 835–853.
60. Peterson K, Gordon KB, Heinemann MH, DeAngelis LM. (1993) The clinical spectrum of ocular lymphoma. *Cancer* **72**(3): 843–849.

Chapter 12

Hypotheses on the Origin of PIOL

"No human being is constituted to know the truth, the whole truth, and nothing but the truth; and even the best of men must be content with fragments, with partial glimpses, never the full fruition."

— *Physician, Sir William Osler, 1849–1919*

The pathogenesis of lymphoma in the brain and eye remains, at best, obscure. Indeed, as immunologic sanctuaries, the development of lymphoma in the eye and brain still remains an elusive enigma. However, advances in science have provided new fragments of information that enable us to obtain better glimpses and develop a better understanding of both PIOL and PCNSL. Several theories have been proposed as to how this malignancy might develop within the eye and brain.[1]

One theory is that neoplastic transformation occurs in one of the lymphocyte subpopulations from the lymphoid organ that may traffic through or inhabit the CNS and/or eye; for example, in the choroid plexus or arachnoid membrane of the brain[2] and/or sub-RPE space of the eye,[3] although these specific sites themselves are not necessarily the most frequent locations of PCNSL. Usually, there is no B lymphocyte trafficking through the CNS and eye. Conversely, neoplastic transformation might occur in a population of systemic normal lymphocytes possessing receptors with a tropism for CNS (both cerebral and ocular) ligands and that cause them to "home" in to the cerebral or ocular tissues. A third hypothesis notes that as immunologically privileged sites, the brain and eye have an inherent susceptibility to allowing cellular aberrancy to occur as compared with systemic sites with relatively more immune surveillance.[4] It has also been hypothesized that polyclonal inflammatory proliferations, perhaps in the face of an infection in the CNS or the eye, might then select for an aberrant monoclonal malignant cell population.[5–8] In addition, genetic susceptibility plays a role in the development of some cancers (e.g., prostate cancer[9]) and may play a part in PCNSL and PIOL. However, no studies have identified susceptibility markers. In this chapter, we will pursue these hypotheses and the attempts made at explaining how PIOL and PCNSL might arise.

Homing of Lymphoma Cells to the CNS and the Eye

In Chapter 7, we noted some of the characteristic pathology in PCNSL. The perivascular arrangement that PCNSL cells exhibit and from which they infiltrate the parenchyma is at first puzzling considering that the brain does not have any resident lymphocytes. In the case of PIOL in the eye (also normally devoid of lymphocytes), we do not notice such a perivascular arrangement, but rather, a distinctive localization to the area between the retinal pigment epithelium (RPE) and Bruch's membrane. How, then, do we attempt to explain the entry of malignant lymphoma cells into the CNS and RPE area?

The idea of "homing," a process in which lymphocytes are attracted to or called to certain sites by the interaction between cell-surface molecules, was pioneered by Gowans and colleagues in the late 1950s and 1960s.[10,11] Initially, controversy existed with respect to the replacement and fate of lymphocytes that flowed from the thoracic duct noted in various animals. Gowans and Knight collected lymphocytes from donor rats and labeled them *in vitro* with tritiated adenosine and tritiated thymidine (which would enable their path to be followed at various time points using radiographic imaging). They transfused these labeled lymphocytes into the blood of recipient rats.[10] The labeled lymphocytes were shown to home into lymph nodes and, then, later reappear in the thoracic duct lymph. Today, we know that the recirculation of lymphocytes and their ability to home in to the afferent high endothelial venules (HEVs) of lymph nodes is by virtue of the expression of surface receptors (e.g., L-selectins, in the family of adhesion molecules). These interact with ligands present on the endothelial cells. In uveitis, lymphocyte function-associated antigen (CD11a) is expressed on infiltrating inflammatory cells and its ligand (or receptor), intracellular adhesion molecule-1 (ICAM-1, CD54), is expressed on ocular blood endothelial and RPE cells. Thus, inflammatory cells are recruited inside the eye.[12] With the homing of normal lymphocytes in mind, the elucidation of mechanisms implicating the homing process in malignant lymphocytes and how this may relate to localization and metastasis has become a recent pursuit.

Cytokines and chemokines play important roles in immunologic processes. Cytokines are important cell-signaling molecules that are involved in the recruitment of immune cells to various tissues. For example, we see an increase in the constitutive expression of the glucocorticoid-induced tumor necrosis factor-related receptor ligand (GITRL) by retinal tissues when proinflammatory cytokines are present and the ligand, which can engage its receptor, GITR, expressed on subsets of CD4-positive T-cells, and then play a role in some immune processes in the eye.[13] Chemokines are a special family of cytokines that are involved specifically in leukocyte chemotaxis. In fact, the word "chemokine" is a portmanteau of **chemo**tactic cyto**kines**. All chemokines share homology in both their gene and amino acid sequences. The chemokine nomenclature is derived from the first two conserved cysteines (C) in their amino acid sequence. Thus, the group of chemokines in which the first two cysteines are adjacent to each other is known as the CC chemokine group. The group of chemokines in which the cysteines are separated by an amino acid (X) is known as the CXC chemokine group. CC and CXC chemokines bind to their own types of receptors (R), CCR and CXCR, respectively. Two other chemokine groups are known, the C chemokine group (having only one conserved cysteine) and the CX3C chemokine group (with one member, fractakine/neurotactin, and in which three amino acids separate the two cysteines). Chemokine receptors are integral membrane proteins that span the membrane seven times and are coupled to G proteins.[14] CXC chemokines have a specific amino acid sequence of glutamic acid-leucine-arginine that precedes the first cysteine residue. However, there are CXC chemokines that do not have this particular amino acid motif, and at least some of these are involved in lymphocyte chemoattraction. We might think of chemokines as attracting sensitive lymphocytes and monocytes/macrophages to specific sites in a specific direction by the chemokine concentration expressed by certain tissues. Thus, increasing concentrations of chemokines could serve to allow lymphocytes to migrate upon a path of ever-increasing chemokine concentrations to locations where the lymphocytes are needed. The interaction of chemokines with their receptors on lymphocytes, then, is involved in both immune cell surveillance and accumulation. Obviously, chemokine and chemokine receptor interactions are important for proper immune function, but can such interactions be involved in malignant conditions?

Studies looking at a variety of cancers, including breast carcinoma,[15] colorectal cancer,[16] and epithelial ovarian cancer[17] have implicated chemokines as partaking in a process that allows for tumor growth, localization, and metastasis in specific sites. In the eye, previous studies have shown that the RPE produces chemokines, such as, CCL2 (also known as monocyte chemoattractant protein, MCP),[18] CXCL8 (also known as interleukin 8, IL-8),[19] and CCL5 (also known as regulated on activation, normally T cell expressed and secreted, RANTES).[20] An improper expression of chemokines or their receptors may play a role in disease. Recently, our laboratory at the National Eye Institute (NEI) has shown that polymorphisms in the *CX3CR1* gene may produce a receptor expressed by macrophages with decreased affinity for the ligand CX3CL1. This may ultimately play a role in enhancing the risk for developing age-related macular degeneration (AMD).[21] A chemokine-chemokine receptor system that is somehow dysfunctional, then, has the potential to play a role in the development of disease processes, including cancer.

Recent evidence suggests that chemokines may be involved in PCNSL and PIOL. We noted previously that the homing of lymphocytes occurs in a specific direction based upon a chemokine gradient path. This may explain the characteristic locations in which we find PIOL cells. That is, we typically find PIOL cells located subretinally between the retinal pigment epithelium (RPE) and Bruch's membrane.[3,6] In other cases, we note that from subretinal foci, infiltrating protrusions of PIOL cells break through sections of the RPE and invade the retina. From the retina the PIOL cells may then be able to invade the vitreous and the optic nerve. Could the expression of chemokines in a gradient fashion lead to a characteristic mode of infiltration by PIOL cells? At the NEI we pursued this possibility by examining the chemokine expression by retinal tissues that included two enucleated eyes, a normal autopsy eye, and a chorioretinal biopsy from three PIOL patients.[22] Microdissection of PIOL cells (see Chapter 9), RPE cells with lymphomatous infiltration, and RPE cells without lymphomatous infiltration was performed, and DNA was extracted using a proteinase K-enriched solution. Reverse transcriptase polymerase chain reaction (RT-PCR) was done to quantify the expression of the chemokines *CXCL12* and *CXCL13* by RPE cells and their respective receptors, *CXCR4* and *CXCR5*, on PIOL cells. Interestingly, we found that RPE cells infiltrated by PIOL cells had a lower expression of *CXCL12* and *CXCL13* compared with their counterparts not yet invaded by PIOL. The RPE cells from the normal control eye did not express these chemokines either by immunohistochemistry or RT-PCR. Both CXCR5 and CXCR4 were expressed by PIOL cells.[22] Thus, in the development of PIOL, RPE cells, for as yet unknown reasons, may express the chemokines CXCL12 and CXCL13, which may, in part, serve to guide malignant PIOL cells from the initial sites of infiltration to involve more areas. The expression of similar chemokines may promote the infiltration of the retina and vitreous. An interesting divergence from this idea of a chemokine pathway that originates in the subretina are cases in the literature where there are no subretinal lesions, but only PIOL cells in the vitreous.[23] Additionally, adhesion molecules may also be involved in the homing of lymphoma cells to bring PCNSL and PIOL to fruition. In an immunocompromised murine model (severe combined immunodeficiency or SCID) mice were used by Bashir and colleagues to study the involvement of LFA-1 (CD11a, a receptor expressed on B and T lymphocytes) and ICAM-1 (CD54) might have in homing human-derived EBV-immortalized B cells heterotransplanted into the right frontal lobe of the mice.[24] Immunohistochemistry revealed staining of lymphoma for LFA-α and LFA-β, the two chains that make up LFA-1, as well as ICAM-1 and staining of ICAM-1 in the brain tumor blood vessels; cerebral tissues from control mice did not exhibit staining for ICAM-1. In addition to this murine model, Bashir, *et al.* performed immunohistochemistry on 12 PCNSL tissue samples (one case was from an AIDS patient). Staining for LFA-1α, LFA-1β, and ICAM-1 was noted in 11, 9, and 9 patients, respectively. Tumor blood vessels, which stained positive for ICAM-1, were noted in six out of seven tumors that exhibited definite tumor vasculature. However, in brain tissue from these patients without lymphomatous infiltration, staining for adhesion molecules did not occur. Thus, in both human PCNSL and the murine model, LFA-1 and ICAM-1 interactions potentially play a role in the homing of malignant lymphocytes to certain regions of the brain parenchyma,[24] although no specific anatomical location was noted in the human samples.

Derivation of Lymphoma Cells

We have discussed the involvement of chemokines and their receptors in homing malignant lymphoma cells into the eye and CNS. However, from which normal counterpart are these malignant cells derived? Are there molecular clues that may hint at the etiology involved in malignant transformation?

Chromosomal alterations and the expression of certain genes can provide us clues as to the stages of differentiation particular cells (both benign and malignant) may be in and seem to offer the potential of serving as a novel way to subtype some lymphomas.[25,26] Larocca and colleagues have demonstrated that most PCNSLs seem to be derived from the germinal center (GC) as evidenced by the frequent expression of BCL-6 in non-AIDS PCNSL (100% of such cases) and AIDS PCNSL (56% of such cases).[27] BCL-6 is a zinc finger/POZ transcriptional repressor protein involved in B-cell differentiation.[28] Germinal center B-cells express BCL-6, but not pre-GC B-cells nor the more differentiated plasma cells.[29-31] Interestingly, Larocca *et al.* showed that the expression of BCL-6 seemed to be mutually exclusive of expression of the Epstein-Barr virus (EBV) protein, LMP-1, and the anti-apoptotic protein, BCL-2. Two expression patterns were exhibited by the PCNSLs: BCL-6+/LMP-1−/BCL-2−, which had a histologic pattern of large noncleaved cells and BCL-6−/LMP-1+/BCL-2+, which histologically appeared as immunoblastic morphology. Considering that most of the PCNSLs expressed BCL-6, the histogenesis and pathogenesis of many PCNSLs may relate to the normal counterpart cell being the GC B-cell. Another point of interest in their work was that while mutations involving the 5' noncoding region of the *bcl-6* gene were noted (42.3% of AIDS PCNSLs and 59.1% of non-AIDS PCNSLs), there were no rearrangements involving this gene in the PCNSLs. Thus, the expression of BCL-6 seems to be evidence of a B-cell's derivation from the GC and is distinct from other B-cell lymphomas, such as, mantle cell and marginal zone lymphomas.[31]

Coupland's group also showed that in 50 patients with PIOL/PCNSL, most had immunohistochemical evidence of a GC derivation. Immunoglobulin transcription factors, including expression of Ig protein and BCL-6, were exhibited by 43 (86%) and 46 (92%) of the patients, respectively.[32] In addition, other immunoglobulin transcription factors, including the proteins BSAP/PAX5, MUM1/IRF4, Oct. 2, and its co-activator BOB.1/ OBF.1 were shown to be expressed by most of the PIOL/PCNSL cells (98 to 100% of cases). Interestingly, while 46 of 50 PIOL/PCNSL cases expressed immunoglobulin, only 27 of 50 cases of peripheral DLBCL expressed this protein. Another difference between PIOL/PCNSL cases and peripheral DLBCL cases was the expression of the transcription factor PU.1. Ten percent of PIOL/PCNSL cases exhibited expression of this protein, while 46% of peripheral DLBCL cases showed expression. The differences in expression of the PU.1 transcription factor and immunoglobulin are interesting considering that PIOL and PCNSLs are subsets of DLBCLs and denote some of the basic molecular differences between peripheral DLBCL and PIOL/PCNSLs.

In our recent study of 72 PIOL cases, 40 of 72 (55%) patients expressed *bcl-2* translocation, six of 26 (23%) expressed *bcl-10* gene, and four of four tested patients expressed *bcl-6* gene.[33] Again, PIOL exhibits a unique pattern when compared with systemic lymphomas, such as, follicular lymphoma, DLBCL, or PCNSL. Overall, the gene expression in PIOL seems more closely related to GC derived-DLBCL.

Multicentricity of PCNSL/PIOL

In any one patient with concurrent cerebral and ocular disease, are the lesions in each site due to multiple sites of malignant transformation or are the lesions more representative of separate sites of the same neoplastic process? It seems that a multicentric origin for PCNSL and PIOL is suggested.[6,34,35] Indeed, Coupland and colleagues have described three cases of combined PIOL and PCNSL in which lymphoma cells obtained from ocular and cerebral lesions underwent the polymerase chain reaction (PCR) of the *IgH* gene.[34,36] Each case showed that lymphoma cells obtained from ocular and cerebral lesions had the same PCR product, indicating separate foci of the same neoplastic condition. Whether lymphoma cells move between ocular and cerebral compartments via the optic nerve or cerebrospinal fluid (CSF) has not been determined, although in one animal model, lymphoma cells were noted to spread via the optic nerve.[37] This model will be discussed in detail in Chapter 13.

Coupland's group has shown that the PIOL cells are closely related to the PCNSL cells. Using PCR, it was shown that 4 of 8 cases of PIOL (one of these four cases having concurrent cerebral involvement) used the *VH* gene segment, VH4-34.[36] Previously, preferential usage of the VH4-34 segment of the *IgH* gene was shown in 5 of 10 cases of PCNSL.[38] Both studies suggested that PIOL and PCNSL were closely related to each other. They also suggested a germinal center derivation for both PIOL and PCNSL by virtue of the fact that somatic mutations in the V region of the *IgH* gene had occurred, perhaps implicating a selection for the expression of a functional antibody by the malignant lymphoma cells.[36]

Origin of PCNSL/PIOL in Immunocompromised Patients

Although not completely understood, the development of PCNSL and PIOL in immunocompromised patients is a little easier to explain. While in immunocompetent patients predisposing factors are yet to be identified, it is known that the development of PCNSL and PIOL in immunocompromised patients (including those with congenital immunodeficiency syndromes, those receiving iatrogenic immunosuppression after allograft organ transplantation, and HIV-infected patients) is associated with the reactivation of the latent Epstein Barr virus (EBV) infection in an immunodeficient milieu.[39–41] EBV preferentially infects B-cells and leads to the proliferation of B lymphocytes; these processes induced by EBV are implicated as playing a causative role in malignant lymphoproliferations, such as, Burkitt's lymphoma, Hodgkin's disease, and nasopharyngeal carcinoma.[42] Human herpes virus 8 (HHV-8) DNA in the PIOL cells has been detected by us in an AIDS patient and both EBV and HHV-8 DNAs in the PIOL cells of another AIDS patient.[43]

Infectious etiologies may also play a role in some PIOLs and PCNSLs found in immunocompetent patients. In our laboratory at the NEI, we described two HIV-negative patients who had retinochoroidal lesions reminiscent of ocular toxoplasmosis found to have PIOL by cytology and molecular analyses of diagnostic vitrectomy specimens.[8] Interestingly, these two patients exhibited *T. gondii* DNA, but not HHV-8 or EBV DNAs, in PIOL cells; normal cells did not contain infectious microorganism DNA or molecular evidence of monoclonality. *T. gondii* may play a role in other lymphoproliferative disorders.[43,44] HHV-8 has also been demonstrated in some cases of PIOL.[42] In 6 of 32 randomly selected cases at the NEI (two patients had AIDS), we found HHV-8 DNA using PCR amplification in

PIOL cells, but not ocular or inflammatory cells. Additionally, in two of 21 randomly selected cases (one patient had AIDS and the other was immunocompetent), EBV DNA was detected in the PIOL cells.[42] In all the AIDS-associated PIOLs, infectious molecular signatures have been always identified. In contrast, many PIOLs in immunocompetent patients have not been successfully isolated or found to contain microorganisms or infectious genes. In general, infectious etiologies may play a role in its pathogenesis.

Annotation

Certainly, we have better glimpses into the unique features of PIOL and perhaps one day we will have more than just fractured glimpses; a clearer, more distinct picture of this fascinating malignancy can be expected. We have seen that PIOL is very similar to PCNSL and these two lymphomatous processes, although a subset of DLBCL, exhibit molecular features that are unique as compared with the systemic counterpart of this immunohistologic group. In addition, localization of PIOL cells may be due to homing and interactions between chemokines and their receptors as well as adhesion molecules. It is still unknown, however, under what situations and with what stimulations lymphoma-homing chemokines and adhesion molecules are expressed. Furthermore, in most cases of PIOL in which no infectious etiology is found and in the immunocompetent patient, what factors are permissive to the development of an intraocular lymphoma? Theoretical physicist Stephen Hawking said, "to confine our attention to terrestrial matters would be to limit the human spirit." Indeed, as physicians and scientists we were never content with the early histologic descriptions of PIOL and PCNSL. Immunologic characterization and the recent exploration into the molecular realm of PIOL have brought us closer to the truth about lymphomatous development and treatment.

References

1. Fine HA, Mayer RJ. (1993) Primary central nervous system lymphoma. *Ann Intern Med* 119(11): 1093–1104.
2. Shibata S. (1989) Sites of origin of primary intracerebral malignant lymphoma. *Neurosurgery* 25(1): 14–19.

3. Chan CC, Buggage RR, Nussenblatt RB. (2002) Intraocular lymphoma. *Curr Opin Ophthalmol* **13**(6):411–418.

4. Paulus W. (1999) Classification, pathogenesis and molecular pathology of primary CNS lymphomas. *J Neurooncol* **43**(3): 203–208.

5. Hochberg FH, Miller DC. (1988) Primary central nervous system lymphoma. *J Neurosurg* **68**(6): 835–853.

6. Buggage RR, Chan CC, Nussenblatt RB. (2001) Ocular manifestations of central nervous system lymphoma. *Curr Opin Oncol* **13**(3): 137–142.

7. Chan CC, Shen DF, Whitcup SM, *et al.* (1999) Detection of human herpesvirus-8 and Epstein-Barr virus DNA in primary intraocular lymphoma. *Blood* **93**(8): 2749–2751.

8. Shen DF, Herbort CP, Tuaillon N, *et al.* (2001) Detection of toxoplasma gondii DNA in primary intraocular b-cell lymphoma. *Mod Pathol* **14**(10): 995–999.

9. Casey G, Neville PJ, Plummer SJ, *et al.* (2002) RNASEL Arg462Gln variant is implicated in up to 13% of prostate cancer cases. *Nat Genet* **32**(4): 581–583.

10. Gowans JL, Knight EJ. (1964) The route of re-circulation of lymphocytes in the rat. *Proc R Soc Lond B Biol Sci* **159**: 257–282.

11. Marchesi VT, Gowans JL. (1964) The migration of lymphocytes through the endothelium of venules in lymph nodes: an electron microscope study. *Proc R Soc Lond B Biol Sci* **159**: 283–290.

12. Whitcup SM, Chan CC, Li Q, Nussenblatt RB. (1992) Expression of cell adhesion molecules in posterior uveitis. *Arch Ophthalmol* **110**(5): 662–666.

13. Kim BJ, Li Z, Fariss RN, *et al.* (2004) Constitutive and cytokine-induced GITR ligand expression on human retinal pigment epithelium and photoreceptors. *Invest Ophthalmol Vis Sci* **45**(9): 3170–3176.

14. Rossi D, Zlotnik A. (2000) The biology of chemokines and their receptors. *Annu Rev Immunol* **18**: 217–242.

15. Muller A, Homey B, Soto H, *et al.* (2001) Involvement of chemokine receptors in breast cancer metastasis. *Nature* **410**(6824): 50–56.

16. Wang D, Wang H, Brown J, *et al.* (2006) CXCL1 induced by prostaglandin E2 promotes angiogenesis in colorectal cancer. *J Exp Med.*

17. Wang Y, Yang J, Gao Y, *et al.* (2005) Regulatory effect of e2, IL-6 and IL-8 on the growth of epithelial ovarian cancer cells. *Cell Mol Immunol* **2**(5): 365–372.

18. Elner SG, Strieter RM, Elner VM, *et al.* (1991) Monocyte chemotactic protein gene expression by cytokine-treated human retinal pigment epithelial cells. *Lab Invest* **64**(6): 819–825.

19. Elner VM, Strieter RM, Elner SG, *et al.* (1990) Neutrophil chemotactic factor (IL-8) gene expression by cytokine-treated retinal pigment epithelial cells. *Am J Pathol* **136**(4): 745–750.

20. Crane IJ, Kuppner MC, McKillop-Smith S, *et al.* (1998) Cytokine regulation of RANTES production by human retinal pigment epithelial cells. *Cell Immunol* 184(1): 37–44.

21. Tuo J, Smith BC, Bojanowski CM, *et al.* (2004) The involvement of sequence variation and expression of CX3CR1 in the pathogenesis of age-related macular degeneration. *Faseb J* 18(11): 1297–1299.

22. Chan CC, Shen D, Hackett JJ, *et al.* (2003) Expression of chemokine receptors, CXCR4 and CXCR5, and chemokines, BLC and SDF-1, in the eyes of patients with primary intraocular lymphoma. *Ophthalmology* 110(2): 421–426.

23. Zhou M, Chen Q, Wang W, *et al.* (2003) Two cases of primary intraocular lymphoma. *Zhonghua Yan Ke Za Zhi* 39(7): 442–444.

24. Bashir R, Coakham H, Hochberg F. (1992) Expression of LFA-1/ICAM-1 in CNS lymphomas: possible mechanism for lymphoma homing into the brain. *J Neurooncol* 12(2): 103–110.

25. Alizadeh AA, Eisen MB, Davis RE, *et al.* (2000) Distinct types of diffuse large B-cell lymphoma identified by gene expression profiling. *Nature* 403(6769): 503–511.

26. Bea S, Zettl A, Wright G, *et al.* (2005) Diffuse large B-cell lymphoma subgroups have distinct genetic profiles that influence tumor biology and improve gene expression-based survival prediction. *Blood.*

27. Larocca LM, Capello D, Rinelli A, *et al.* (1998) The molecular and phenotypic profile of primary central nervous system lymphoma identifies distinct categories of the disease and is consistent with histogenetic derivation from germinal center-related B cells. *Blood* 92(3): 1011–1019.

28. Chang CC, Ye BH, Chaganti RS, Dalla-Favera R. (1996) BCL-6, a POZ/zinc-finger protein, is a sequence-specific transcriptional repressor. *Proc Natl Acad Sci U S A* 93(14): 6947–6952.

29. Onizuka T, Moriyama M, Yamochi T, *et al.* (1995) BCL-6 gene product, a 92- to 98-kD nuclear phosphoprotein, is highly expressed in germinal center B cells and their neoplastic counterparts. *Blood* 86(1): 28–37.

30. Cattoretti G, Chang CC, Cechova K, *et al.* (1995) BCL-6 protein is expressed in germinal-center B cells. *Blood* 86(1): 45–53.

31. Flenghi L, Ye BH, Fizzotti M, *et al.* (1995) A specific monoclonal antibody (PG-B6) detects expression of the BCL-6 protein in germinal center B cells. *Am J Pathol* 147(2): 405–411.

32. Coupland SE, Loddenkemper C, Smith JR, *et al.* (2005) Expression of immunoglobulin transcription factors in primary intraocular lymphoma and primary central nervous system lymphoma. *Invest Ophthalmol Vis Sci* 46(11): 3957–3964.

33. Wallace DJ, Shen DF, Reed GF, *et al.* (2006) Detection of the bcl-2 t(14;18) translocation and proto-oncogene expression in primary intraocular lymphoma. *Invest Ophthalmol Vis Sci* 47(7):2750–2756.

34. Coupland SE, Hummel M, Stein H, *et al.* (2005) Demonstration of identical clonal derivation in a case of "oculocerebral" lymphoma. *Br J Ophthalmol* 89(2): 238–239.

35. Hormigo A, Abrey L, Heinemann MH, DeAngelis LM. (2004) Ocular presentation of primary central nervous system lymphoma: diagnosis and treatment. *Br J Haematol* 126(2): 202–208.

36. Coupland SE, Hummel M, Muller HH, Stein H. (2005) Molecular analysis of immunoglobulin genes in primary intraocular lymphoma. *Invest Ophthalmol Vis Sci* 46(10): 3507–3514.

37. Hochman J, Assaf N, Deckert-Schluter M, *et al.* (2001) Entry routes of malignant lymphoma into the brain and eyes in a mouse model. *Cancer Res* 61(13): 5242–5247.

38. Montesinos-Rongen M, Kuppers R, Schluter D, *et al.* (1999) Primary central nervous system lymphomas are derived from germinal-center B cells and show a preferential usage of the V4–34 gene segment. *Am J Pathol* 155(6): 2077–2086.

39. Levine AM. (1994) Lymphoma complicating immunodeficiency disorders. *Ann Oncol* 5 **Suppl** 2: 29–35.

40. Boubenider S, Hiesse C, Goupy C, *et al.* (1997) Incidence and consequences of post-transplantation lymphoproliferative disorders. *J Nephrol* 10(3): 136–145.

41. Gentil MA, Gonzalez-Roncero F, Cantarell C, *et al.* (2005) Effect of new immunosuppressive regimens on cost of renal transplant maintenance immunosuppression. *Transplant Proc* 37(3): 1441–1442.

42. Young TL, Murray PG. (2003) Epstein-Barr virus and oncogenesis: from latent genes to tumours. *Oncogene* 22(33): 5108–5121.

43. Chan CC. (2003) Molecular pathology of primary intraocular lymphoma. *Trans Am Ophthalmol Soc* 101: 275–292.

44. Denkers EY, Caspar P, Hieny S, Sher A. (1996) Toxoplasma gondii infection induces specific nonresponsiveness in lymphocytes bearing the V beta 5 chain of the mouse T cell receptor. *J Immunol* 156(3): 1089–1094.

45. Stein K, Hummel M, Korbjuhn P, *et al.* (1999) Monocytoid B cells are distinct from splenic marginal zone cells and commonly derive from unmutated naive B cells and less frequently from postgerminal center B cells by polyclonal transformation. *Blood* 94(8): 2800–2808.

Chapter 13

Experimental Models of PIOL

The development of a suitable animal model is critical in identifying the risk factors for disease development, elucidating fundamental molecular mechanisms in disease progression, and providing guidance as to whether or not a particular treatment is a potentially safe and efftective option for humans. Indeed, animal models continue to be highly valuable, perhaps now more so than ever. While we continue to make great strides in understanding the molecular basis and origins of PIOL, recent developments in the use of animal models have the potential to further our understanding of this special lymphomatous process.

One of the first considerations while creating an animal model of a human disease is the particular attribute or attributes of the human disease that will be mimicked in the animal. For example, as we are concerned with PIOL and PCNSL, do we use lymphoma cells obtained from an animal or a human? This is an important question because the immunologic status, whether immunocompromised or immunocompetent, of the animal may play a role in the disease process. If we attempt to use human lymphoma cells in an animal model, will there be an immunologic response to this xenograft? If so, perhaps the use of an animal that lacks an intact immune system may be used in the setting of human lymphoma, or pharmacologic immunosuppression of the host animal may be needed. On the other hand, if we decide to use an animal-derived lymphoma in the same animal model, does this lymphoma have features and characteristics that are similar to human lymphoma? That is, is there an animal analogue of a particular human lymphoma? Another important question is whether or not primary lymphomas of the brain or eye exist in animals commonly used as models.

Historical Experimental PCNSL Models in Animals

Spontaneously developed PCNSLs have been described in cats and dogs, but are rare occurrences.[1,2] To date, there has been a report of a potential PCNSL (the histologic diagnosis was malignant reticulosis) in two adult rats. This report emerged from a larger study that examined the development of various cerebral tumors in the setting of ethylene oxide exposure.[3] However, to our knowledge, there have not been any reports of spontaneous development of PCNSL or PIOL in the rat or mouse.

The establishment of a murine model of PCNSL dates back to the late 1970s when Epstein and colleagues performed xenograft transplantation of human lymphoma cells intracerebrally in nude, athymic (immuno-compromised) mice.[4] The lymphoma lines were all human-derived and histologically classified based on the Rappaport classification system. Histologic types included diffuse undifferentiated, diffuse histiocytic, nodular mixed histiocytic and lymphocytic, diffuse mixed histiocytic and lymphocytic, malignant histiocytosis, and nodular sclerosing type of Hodgkin's disease. It was noted that with inocula of $1-5 \times 10^5$ cells of the lymphoma lines into the cerebrum of the adult immunocompromised mice led to the development of clinical manifestations of CNS infiltration (e.g., cachexia, arched back, and slight megacephaly) as well as pathologic evidence of extensive cerebral infiltration, except for inoculation with Hodgkin's disease. In the case of inoculation with Hodgkin's lymphoma cells or normal thymocytes, there was no development of cerebral edema and, importantly, no development of intracranial malignant lesions. In the mice that did develop extensive intracranial tumors, the cytology of the malignant cells was similar to that of the humans from which they were derived. Interestingly, secondary cell culture of the xenografted intracranial tumors revealed infection of the tumor cells with the murine NIH/Swiss type-C xenotropic virus. This raised the possibility that the heterotrans-planted human lymphomas derived a certain degree of enhanced growth properties from the infection.[4]

Others noted that human-derived diffuse histiocytic lymphoma cells (Rappaport Classification) xenografted into nude, athymic mice were pro-tected from antibody directed against the tumor by the blood-brain bar-rier,[5] portending an obstacle to monoclonal antibody-directed therapy (such as with Rituximab[6]). While large molecules like antibodies had difficulty traversing the blood-brain barrier, perhaps this barrier also prevented extracerebral metastasis.

Romani and colleagues developed a murine model of intracerebral lymphoma using an immunogenic lymphoma line in mice immunosuppressed with cyclophosphamide.[7] Cytotoxic T-lymphocytes were sensitized to the lymphoma line and infused into the immunosuppressed mice. Immunosuppressed mice infused with sensitized cytotoxic T-lymphocytes of at least 10^6 cells exhibited regression of tumor as compared with immunosuppressed mice not receiving the adoptive immunotherapy. Later, it was suggested that perhaps the amount of protection a lymphomatous proliferation in the brain might experience from the host animal's immune system might be contingent upon the lack of expression of anti-graft cell surface markers.[8]

In an attempt to determine the spread of lymphoma in the CNS and its relation to the blood-brain barrier, Aho and colleagues performed extracerebral (intraperitoneal, intraarterial, intravenous, or intrathecal) or intracerebral (i.e. intraparenchymal) injections of rat leukemized T-cell lymphoma.[9] With intraperitoneal and intraarterial injections, the blood-brain barrier was disrupted by using a technique called cold injury. This technique involved the application of a mixture of dry ice and isopentane to the surgically exposed skull bone over the frontal lobe. In rats that were injected with lymphoid cells extracerebrally, the lymphoma spread into the dura and the subarachnoid space. Parenchymal disease developed at the terminal stages of the disease (17 days after inoculation) and was very similar to leukemic spread of disease in humans. This pattern of involvement was in contrast to intracerebral administration of the lymphoid cells in which the pattern of spread was more similar to PCNSL in humans with perivascular arrangement of the malignant cells in the cortex and infiltration into the white matter. In the face of blood-brain barrier disruption with cold injury, tumors were noted to infiltrate the CNS at disrupted sites. This suggested that a deficient barrier could open a portal to lymphomatous infiltration of the parenchyma.

Recent Murine Models of PIOL/PCNSL

Murine T-cell Models of PIOL. Assaf and colleagues described a murine model in which murine T-lymphoma cells were injected into the peritoneum of neonatal and young mice.[10] These tumorigenic revertant lymphoma cells, termed Rev-2-T-6 cells, had originally been derived from a substrate-adherent, non-tumorigenic S49 mouse T-cell lymphoma variant developed in Balb/c mice. In culture media, these lymphoma cells grow in suspension and when injected intraperitoneally into mice, they produce solid abdominal tumors. The histology of these tumors is high-grade malignant lymphoma of the small, non-cleaved cell type with a starry-sky appearance. In Assaf and colleagues' study, the lymphoma cells were injected intraperitoneally into syngeneic Balb/c mice (6 to 60 days postnatal). In all ages of mice, intraperitoneal injection of the Rev-2-T-6 cells produced solid abdominal tumors as expected. However, in the neonatal mice (6 to 11 days postnatal), up to 58% developed clinical signs of eye and CNS involvement, while none of the mice older than 13 days developed such signs. Clinical ocular findings appeared 24 to 30 days post-inoculation, were unilateral or bilateral, and included orbit and eyelid involvement and pseudohypopyon. In 22 young mice exhibiting clinical ocular signs of lymphoma infiltration and that were submitted to histopathologic examination, the orbit and optic nerve were most frequently involved (86% each, though, interestingly, optic nerve parenchymal involvement was not noted). The bulbar conjunctiva, eyelids, sclera, and cornea were involved in 57%, 49%, 31%, and 0% of the examined eyes, respectively. The uveal tract was involved in 37% of the eyes. As for intraocular structures, 29% and 17% of the examined eyes showed involvement of the anterior and posterior chambers, respectively. The vitreous and retina were involved in 14% and 3% of the eyes, respectively. Despite their lack of clinical signs of retinal and CNS involvement, older mice did show some involvement of these structures on histopathologic examination (up to 20% of inoculated older mice). The pattern of lymphoma cell infiltration in the young mice suggested that involvement of the brain was requisite for optic nerve involvement. The subarachnoid space was most frequently found to be involved upon histologic examination of the brain (up to 95% of mice), suggesting that this could be the primary site of tumor infiltration. However, the choroid plexus, cranial nerves, and cranial nerve ganglia were also frequently involved. Ocular involvement could occur in the setting of optic nerve involvement (suggesting extension along the optic nerve to the eye), but could also occur independently of infiltration of the optic nerve (suggesting another mode of involvement for the eye, perhaps hematogenous). The expression of cell adhesion molecules that are involved in CNS immune reactions[11] was also determined. Flow cytometry revealed that 60% of the Rev-2-T-6 cells expressed surface CD18, CD11a/LFA-1, CD54/ICAM-2, CD4 and 20% of the lymphoma cells expressed CD2. This was an intriguing model that described ocular infiltration of lymphoma from an intraperitoneal site. Choroidal and uveal involvement was more common than subretinal, retinal, and vitreal involvement and the fact that lymphoma cells were injected intraperitoneally producing abdominal tumors, made this model similar to intraocular lymphoma in a human secondary to a systemic lymphoma. Some aspects of this model were reminiscent of human PIOL, especially with the involvement of the subretina, retina, and vitreous. However, such an involvement was quite infrequent. Although the lymphoma cells were of T-cell origin, many of the cell surface adhesion molecules (e.g., CD11a/LFA-1, CD54/ICAM-2, and CD2) found to be expressed by flow cytometry on the Rev-2-T-6 cells were also expressed by lymphoma cells of B-cell origin.[12]

Later, Hochman's group used the Rev-2-T-6 cells and performed intraperitoneal injections into mice seven days postnatal.[13] Mice were examined for manifestations of clinical ocular and CNS involvement and sacrificed from seven to 31 days post-inoculation at which time eyes and brains were removed for histological analysis. Up to 58% and 10% of mice developed clinical ocular (e.g., anterior chamber and orbital involvement) and CNS (growth retardation) signs of lymphoma infiltration, respectively. Mice that developed clinical ocular signs of lymphoma (22 of 38, 58%) had a significantly shorter survival than mice without these signs. Various patterns of brain, optic nerve, intraocular, and orbital involvement with tumor were observed, ultimately with 17 patterns being described.[13] The different patterns of involvement suggested that intraocular involvement seemed to follow from cerebral involvement with extension along the optic nerve into the eye. Orbital involvement, on the other hand, did not seem to be dependent upon intraocular involvement, but other mechanisms of metastasis as this site could be involved even if no intraocular involvement was found by histopathology. As the uvea and anterior chamber involvement was always associated with the involvement of the optic nerve and brain and because there was also no case in which the optic nerve was involved without brain involvement, there seemed to be no retrograde extension from the eye to the brain. Hochman and colleagues also performed extensive histopathological examinations of the brain and cranial nerves at different time points, post-lymphoma inoculation, to determine which sites might be first infiltrated. From these analyses, it was found that the choroid plexus, cranial nerves, cranial nerve ganglia, and ventricular system were infiltrated before the subarachnoid space (recall that earlier, Hochman's group had found that the subarachnoid space was most frequently involved[10]). A potential pathway toward lymphomatous infiltration has been described based on this model. Similar to the earlier study by Assaf and colleagues,[10] this study was similar to a systemic lymphoma metastasizing to the brain and eye in neonatal mice.

Recently, our laboratory at the National Eye Institute (NEI), has developed a murine model of T-cell PIOL using the murine Rev-2-T-6 lymphoma line.[14] Sixteen adult (six-to-eight-week-old compared to seven days postnatal in a study by Hochman *et al.*[13]) immunocompetent Balb/c mice were injected with either 50,000 or 100,000 Rev-2-T-6 cells through the pars plana and into the vitreous of the left eye. The right eye was used as control and injected only with phosphate buffered saline (PBS). Nearly all mice from both inoculated groups developed ocular manifestations of a masquerade syndrome consisting of vitreous opacities, some becoming severe enough to preclude view of the posterior pole. Some mice also developed anterior chamber involvement as evidenced by pseudohypopyon as well as retinal lesions in the inoculated eye. Upon histologic examination, the lymphoma cells were found to localize to the vitreous and between the neurosensory retina and retinal pigment epithelium (RPE); this was confirmed using immunoperoxidase staining with an antibody directed against the p14 surface antigen of the Rev-2-T-6 lymphoma cells (no other ocular and inflammatory cells stained with this antibody). This finding further supports that the RPE cells play an important barrier role. Microdissection was then performed to isolate the Rev-2-T-6 cells. Reverse transcriptase polymerase chain reaction (RT-PCR) was done to examine the fold-change (compared to control) in mRNA expression of classical Th1 cytokines (*IL-2* and *IFN-γ*) and classical Th2 cytokines (*IL-4* and *IL-10*) as well as the pro-inflammatory cytokine, *IL-6*, and a T-cell chemokine receptor, *CCR1*, by both the microdissected and cultured Rev-2-T-6 cells. Products from RT-PCR showed that *IL-4* was weakly expressed by ocular, but not cultured, Rev-2-T-6 cells. *IL-10*, *IFN-γ*, and

CCR1 transcripts were expressed by both cultured and ocular lymphoma cells. This indicated that there were no impairments in the expression of these cytokines or the chemokine receptor when Rev-2-T-6 cells were introduced into the ocular milieu. *IL-2* and *IL-6* mRNA were expressed by neither cultured nor ocular lymphoma cells. Because IL-10/IL-6 ratios greater than 1.0 can be an important adjunctive test in making the diagnosis of B-cell PIOL in humans,[15,16] the vitreal IL-10/IL-6 ratio was measured in our Rev-2-T-6 inoculated model. Interestingly, for this murine T-cell model,[14] the vitreal IL-10 and IL-6 levels were 691 pg/mL and 481 pg/mL, respectively, yielding an IL-10/IL-6 ratio of 1.44. The vitreous from control eyes, which were injected only with phosphate buffer solution, had IL-10 and IL-6 levels that were below detection.

Classically, in humans, PIOL cells are overwhelmingly of B-cell lineage and, specifically, they are diffuse large B-cell lymphomas (DLBCL). In the case of our experiment, we used a murine T-cell lymphoma, and subretinal localization of tumor in our murine model mimicked that in humans. However, while human PIOL cells classically localize to the area between the RPE and Bruch's membrane,[17-20] in our murine model, the lymphoma cells localized to the area between the neuroretina and the RPE.[14] Nevertheless, this study was a landmark in its own right because it was a new experimental model for intraocular lymphoma. Previously, the only other intraocular lymphoma model available was that developed by Hochman's group as noted above. With our model (in which Hochman was involved), intraocular injection produced clinical and histopathological disease similar to the human disease. Importantly, and similar to the human analogue, the lymphoma cells in our model localized to the subretinal space and vitreous and did not induce neovascularization. We also used adult mice in our study, which more closely resembles human PIOL. The fact that the lymphoma cells in our model expressed the chemokine receptor CCR1 also raised the possibility that chemokine homing was a factor in tumor localization. Finally, the vitreal IL-10/IL-6 ratio greater than 1.0 in our murine model was similar to that seen in human PIOL during adjunctive testing.

Murine B-cell Models of PIOL. Our laboratory's development of a murine PIOL model via intravitreal injection of lymphoma cells proved to be a promising new way to study this malignancy.[14] As the Rev-2-T-6 intraocular murine model proved to be feasible, we decided to pursue a B-cell PIOL murine model that would more closely resemble the immunologic lineage found in human PIOL.

Recently, at the NEI, a human B-cell lymphoma, specifically Epstein Barr virus (EBV)-negative Burkitt's lymphoma, was inoculated into the eyes of mice.[21] The use of a human lymphoma line required that we use an immunodeficient mouse that would not mount a rejection response to the xenografted tissue. We inoculated cultured human Burkitt's lymphoma cells (that are available for purchase from a biological technology company) into the eyes of severe combined immunodeficiency (SCID) mice and found that in just over a week tumor developed in the eye that preferentially localized to the subretinal space. In fact, the localization was akin to that found in our previous intravitreal T-cell PIOL model[14] as the tumor localized to the area above the RPE and below the retina. The brain meningeals showed infiltration in some mice as well, indicating metastasis from the original ocular site. Importantly, we noted by flow cytometry that the Burkitt's lymphoma cells expressed CD22 and B-cell chemokine receptors CXCR4 and CXCR5 (with *in vivo* CXCR5 surface expression greater than CXCR4 expression by immunohistochemistry), whether cultured or obtained from the eye after inoculation and growth. In addition, IL-10 was noted to be constitutively expressed; a 60-fold increase in IL-10 mRNA by the lymphoma cells compared with the background level of IL-10 production. As we noted in Chapter 8, IL-10 is an important B-cell growth factor and is also involved in lymphomagenesis.[22,23] The generation of a B-cell model of PIOL was an important success for us because we had developed a model involving a lymphoma cell of B-cell lineage, similar to that of human PIOL. To determine if we could treat the PIOL, we developed and employed immunotoxin therapy. HA22 is a hybrid protein (one part monoclonal antibody binding domain and the other part an immunotoxin (covalently linked to the antibody protein), *Pseudomonas* exotoxin A (PE A)) that interacts with the CD22 molecule that is expressed on the surface of the inoculated lymphoma cells. This interaction of HA22 with CD22 leads to internalization of PE A and eventual cell death.[24] Upon intravitreal injection of HA22 into eyes that had been inoculated with tumor earlier, there was tumor-specific eradication of ocular disease. No metastases were noted. The ability to eradicate disease in our model of PIOL and potential for use in the human disease is certainly intriguing.

To further characterize our model of B-cell PIOL, we performed bilateral injections of the human Burkitt's lymphoma cells through the pars plana and into the vitreous of adult SCID mice. Control SCID mice were bilaterally injected with PBS.[25] After one week, we noted during funduscopic examination that some mice showed vitreous haze or cells, or tumor in the posterior pole. These findings were reminiscent of human PIOL masquerading as an idiopathic uveitis. After two weeks, funduscopy revealed that all the mice exhibited subretinal infiltrates. Control mice injected with PBS, on the other hand, did not show these lesions. We then performed histological analysis on the brains and eyes of the mice. We observed that the lymphoma cells localized to the vitreous and subretinal space above the RPE, a finding identical to that observed in our previous T-cell PIOL model and similar to our initial establishment of our B-cell PIOL model.[14,21] In severe cases, tumor was noted to invade the choroid, sclera, and even the orbit. When we compared the histology of our B-cell model of PIOL with that in our previous Rev-2-T-6 model,[14] we noted that there seemed to be more choroidal invasion by the lymphoma cells in the immunocompromised SCID mice (injected with human Burkitt's lymphoma) than in the immunocompetent Balb/c mice (injected with murine Rev-2-T-6 lymphoma). Perhaps the immunodeficient state in combination with a B-cell lymphoma played a part in the more substantial choroidal invasion in SCID mice. We also examined chemokine and chemokine receptor expression involved in our B-cell model and our previous T-cell model.[14] Specifically, we evaluated expression of the chemokines CXCL12 (a chemokine involved in the guidance of B-cell chemotaxis[26]) and CCL3 (involved in T-cell attraction) by the microdissected retina of both eyes inoculated with tumor and eyes injected only with PBS. We also examined the expression of the chemokine receptors CXCR4 (expressed by malignant B-cells[26]) and CCR1 (expressed by T-cells) by human Burkitt's and Rev-2-T-6 lymphoma cells, respectively, by evaluating mRNA expression after performing RT-PCR. We observed that retinas from Burkitt's lymphoma-inoculated SCID mice had a slight increase in *CXCL12* expression compared to control retinas (i.e., inoculated with PBS only). Microdissected retinas from the Rev-2-T-6-inoculated BALB/c mice had a nearly two-fold change in *CCL3* expression compared to PBS control eyes. In addition, we examined the expression of the chemokine receptors CCR1 (expressed on T-lymphocytes) and CXCR4 (expressed by B-lymphocytes) by lymphoma cells. Microdissected Burkitt's lymphoma cells had just over a three-fold change in *CXCR4* compared to human cDNA (control DNA). Microdissected Rev-2-T-6 cells had a slight increase in *CCR1* expression compared to mouse control DNA. These findings suggest that B-cell chemokines such as CXCL12 and T-cell chemokines like CCL3 in the retina might be involved in the homing of lymphoma cells (bearing the appropriate chemokine receptors, such as, CXCR4 and CCR1, respectively) to subretinal locations. Compared to controls, retina from BALB/c Rev-2-T-6 and SCID Burkitt's-inoculated mice had over a 10- and nearly a three-fold change in *IL-6* expression and over 5- and 4-fold changes in *TNF-α* expression, respectively. On the other hand, there was a decrease in the expression of *IL-10* by retinal cells from both groups of mice. A lack of an inflammatory response in SCID mice is suggested by a relatively lower fold-change in *IL-6* expression, which reflects that the SCID mice are immunocompromised. This B-cell model of PIOL, then, proved to be a useful way to study the human condition. Further definition of the role that chemokines and their receptors might play in homing PIOL cells to the subretina may possibly involve the use of molecules that interfere with chemokine-chemokine receptor interactions.

Where Do We Go From Here? The development of a B-cell model of PIOL that mimics the human condition is important. Indeed, this gives us the opportunity to analyze further other chemokines and cytokines that are involved in producing an intraocular milieu that is conducive to the establishment of PIOL. However, in our recent B-cell lymphoma model of PIOL, one important difference between human PIOL and our recent models developed at the NEI exists. Recall that human PIOL in the setting of an immunocompetent patient is most frequently a DLBCL. Our use of SCID mice has established a model of PIOL in an immunocompromised organism. Thus, in this respect, our model specifically mimics PIOL in immunocompromised humans, such as AIDS and transplant patients. In addition, the lymphoma line we used in our B-cell murine model was a human Burkitt's lymphoma line and not a DLBCL. We wondered if there were lymphoma lines, specifically murine, which mimicked the human DLBCL immunohistologic subtype. Currently, we are developing and investigating a DLBCL model in immunocompetant mice.

It is an exciting time for us at the NEI. We have developed promising models of PIOL in the mouse that mimic important features of human PIOL. Furthermore, we are working on a new model of PIOL using a murine DLBCL in an immunocompetent mouse, bringing us closer to a model more analogous to an immune-intact human PIOL. As the esteemed US news reporter Walter Cronkite noted, "In seeking truth, you have to get both sides of a story." Soon we will be able to tell a more complete story of PIOL — a story worth telling.

References

1. Callanan JJ, Jones BA, Irvine J, *et al.* (1996) Histologic classification and immunophenotype of lymphosarcomas in cats with naturally and experimentally acquired feline immunodeficiency virus infections. *Vet Pathol* 33(3): 264–272.
2. Zaki FA, Hurvitz AI. (1976) Spontaneous neoplasms of the central nervous system of the cat. *J Small Anim Pract* 17(12): 773–782.
3. Garman RH, Snellings WM, Maronpot RR. (1985) Brain tumors in F344 rats associated with chronic inhalation exposure to ethylene oxide. *Neurotoxicology* 6(1): 117–137.
4. Epstein AL, Herman MM, Kim H, *et al.* (1976) Biology of the human malignant lymphomas. III. Intracranial heterotransplantation in the nude, athymic mouse. *Cancer* 37(5): 2158–2176.
5. Adelman DC, Miller RA, Kaplan HS. (1980) Humoral immune responses to human lymphoma cell heterotransplants in the central nervous system of athymic, nude mice. *Int J Cancer* 25(4): 467–473.
6. Dietlein M, Pels H, Schulz H, *et al.* (2005) Imaging of central nervous system lymphomas with iodine-123 labeled rituximab. *Eur J Haematol* 74(4): 348–352.
7. Romani L, Bianchi R, Puccetti P, Fioretti MC. (1983) Systemic adoptive immunotherapy of a highly immunogenic murine lymphoma growing in the brain. *Int J Cancer* 31(4): 477–482.
8. Puccetti P, Giampietri A, Campanile F, *et al.* (1983) Antilymphoma graft responses in the mouse brain: a study of T-dependent functions. *Int J Cancer* 31(6): 769–774.
9. Aho R, Vaittinen S, Jahnukainen K, Kalimo H. (1994) Spread of malignant lymphoid cells into rat central nervous system with intact and disrupted blood-brain barrier. *Neuropathol Appl Neurobiol* 20(6): 551–561.

10. Assaf N, Hasson T, Hoch-Marchaim H, *et al.* (1997) An experimental model for infiltration of malignant lymphoma to the eye and brain. *Virchows Arch* **431**(6): 459–467.

11. Fabry Z, Raine CS, Hart MN. (1994) Nervous tissue as an immune compartment: the dialect of the immune response in the CNS. *Immunol Today* **15**(5): 218–224.

12. Pinto A, Carbone A, Gloghini A, *et al.* (1993) Differential expression of cell adhesion molecules in B-zone small lymphocytic lymphoma and other well-differentiated lymphocytic disorders. *Cancer* **72**(3): 894–904.

13. Hochman J, Assaf N, Deckert-Schluter M, *et al.* (2001) Entry routes of malignant lymphoma into the brain and eyes in a mouse model. *Cancer Res* **61**(13): 5242–5247.

14. Chan CC, Fischette M, Shen D, *et al.* (2005) Murine model of primary intraocular lymphoma. *Invest Ophthalmol Vis Sci* **46**(2): 415–419.

15. Wolf LA, Reed GF, Buggage RR, *et al.* (2002) Levels of IL-10 and IL-6 in the vitreous are helpful for differential diagnosis of primary intraocular lymphoma and ocular inflammation. *ARVO Abstract:* #2221.

16. Wolf LA, Reed GF, Buggage RR, *et al.* (2003) Vitreous cytokine levels. *Ophthalmology* **110**(8): 1671–1672.

17. Buggage RR, Chan CC, Nussenblatt RB. (2001) Ocular manifestations of central nervous system lymphoma. *Curr Opin Oncol* **13**(3): 137–142.

18. Tuaillon N, Chan CC. (2001) Molecular analysis of primary central nervous system and primary intraocular lymphoma. *Curr Mol Med* **1**(2): 259–272.

19. Chan CC, Wallace DJ. (2004) Intraocular lymphoma: update on diagnosis and management. *Cancer Control* **11**(5): 285–295.

20. Chan CC. (2003) Molecular pathology of primary intraocular lymphoma. *Trans Am Ophthalmol Soc* **101**: 275–292.

21. Li Z, Mahesh SP, Shen D, *et al.* (2006) Eradication of tumor colonization and invasion by a B cell specific immunotoxin in a murine model for human primary intraocular lymphom (PIOL). *Cancer Res* **66**: 10586–10593.

22. Blay JY, Burdin N, Rousset F, *et al.* (1993) Serum interleukin-10 in non-Hodgkin's lymphoma: a prognostic factor. *Blood* **82**(7): 2169–2174.

23. Bost KL, Bieligk SC, Jaffe BM. (1995) Lymphokine mRNA expression by transplantable murine B lymphocytic malignancies. Tumor-derived IL-10 as a possible mechanism for modulating the anti-tumor response. *J Immunol* **154**(2): 718–729.

24. Bang S, Nagata S, Onda M, *et al.* (2005) HA22 (R490A) is a recombinant immunotoxin with increased antitumor activity without an increase in animal toxicity. *Clin Cancer Res* **11**(4): 1545–1550.

25. Gonzales JA, Shen D, Zhou M, *et al.* (2006) Chemokine and chemokine receptor expression in two models of primary intraocular lymphoma. *ARVO Abstr.*: #2831.
26. Burger JA, Burger M, Kipps TJ. (1999) Chronic lymphocytic leukemia B cells express functional CXCR4 chemokine receptors that mediate spontaneous migration beneath bone marrow stromal cells. *Blood* **94**(11): 3658–3667.
27. Morse HC, III, Anver MR, Fredrickson TN, *et al.* (2002) Bethesda proposals for classification of lymphoid neoplasms in mice. *Blood* **100**(1): 246–258.

Chapter 14

Summary and Algorithm

Primary intraocular lymphoma remains an enigma, but certainly less so today than when it was first described in the late 1950s and 60s. The developments in the fields of immunology, molecular biology, and genetics have helped uncover some of the mysteries surrounding PIOL, albeit partially. However, there remain many unanswered questions involving this disease. Despite this, we are now well versed with the pathologic features of this lymphoma. Furthermore, we have become quite adept at being able to identify whether the patients we see in our clinics might have PIOL or another disease based upon the clinical features of this disease and the features of the patient (such as age and immune status). We are able to piece together an increasing likelihood of PIOL by using our clinical examination findings together with the results from imaging tests, such as fluorescein angiography.[1] However, we must identify the atypical lymphoma cells to make a definitive diagnosis that would enable us to begin treatment.[2,3] We are, then, competent at describing the features of PIOL: how it may appear clinically and histologically, what cells and tissues it affects, and what people (age) are more likely to develop this disease. What remain as mysteries are *why* and *how* this disease occurs and, specifically, *why* and *how* inside the eye. While these questions have existed for a long time we have, until very recently, lacked the proper tools that would enable us to answer them. With the progress made in molecular biology and genetics, we are better able to understand the fundamental characteristics of cancer. This enables us to not only seek answers to questions we have had all along, but to ask new and better questions about how and why a malignancy occurs.

PIOL affects two broad groups of people, those who are immunocompetent and those who are immunocompromised. Patients who are immunocompetent typically develop PIOL in their 50s and 60s. As their immune system is intact and involvements of microorganisms are not routinely found, it is still not known what factors lead to the development of PIOL in such patients.[4-10] Immunocompromised patients, on the other hand, tend to be younger and the development of disease in most of them is due to deficiency (whether congenital, acquired, or iatrogenic) of the immune system and reactivation of the latent Epstein Barr virus infection.[11-14]

Cytologic examination of the cerebrospinal fluid (CSF) or the vitreous reveals atypical, large lymphoid cells with a large, round nucleus (that may have numerous infoldings) and scant basophilic cytoplasm.[3,5,15-19] Within the granular nucleus are prominent irregular and frequently multiple nucleoli. Immunohistochemistry has revealed that the overwhelming majority of PIOL cells are of B-cell lineage and monoclonal (bearing B-cell markers, such as, CD19, CD20, CD22, and CD23 as well as kappa or lambda immunoglobulin light chains).[15,17,20] The rare cases of primary intraocular T-cell lymphomas bear CD3 and/or CD4 markers.[9,21] Monoclonal immunoglobulin H (*IgH*) or T-cell receptor (*TCR*) gene rearrangements, identified by the polymerase chain reaction (PCR), reveal the clonal derivation of PIOL cells from a malignant progenitor.[21-23]

Neoplastic PIOL B-cells secrete high amounts of IL-10, a cytokine that is both an immunosuppressive agent (which might be one way that the lymphoma cells escape tumor surveillance) and a B-cell growth factor (that may aid in proliferation of the tumor).[24,25] Our laboratory pioneered the use of measuring vitreal IL-10 and IL-6 levels, and this has been confirmed by other investigators.[26-29] IL-6, a proinflammatory cytokine is secreted in high amounts by the inflammatory cells of uveitis-macrophages and T-cells. IL-10 to IL-6 ratio (IL-10/IL-6) greater than 1.0, then, is an important adjunctive test that is suggestive of PIOL.[30] Special leukocyte-homing cytokines, known as chemokines, likely play a role in targeting the PIOL cells to the subretinal space between Bruch's membrane and the RPE. Indeed, we have seen the expression of chemokines and their receptors by RPE and PIOL cells, respectively, both in human PIOL and murine models of the disease.[31-33]

The recent developments made in DNA microarray technology have enabled us to uncover three pathogenetically distinct entities within the diffuse large B-cell (DLBCL) non-Hodgkin's lymphoma histologic sub-group.[34,35] The germinal center B-cell (GCB) subtype is characterized by mutations within the rearranged immunoglobulin gene and expression of BCL-6 protein. These properties occur specifically in B-cells undergoing interactions in the germinal center microenvironment or in B-cells that have passaged through the germinal center.[36] Two recurrent oncogenic events are noted to occur in GCB lymphomas, t(14;18) and *c-rel* expression on chromosome 2p.[37] Activated B-cell (ABC) subgroup lymphomas resemble a peripheral B-cell that has been mitogenically stimulated. These lymphomas exhibit constitutive expression of NF-κB and *bcl-2* overexpression.[37] A third subtype of DLBCL, known as primary mediastinal, has a genetic profile unlike the GCB and ABC subtypes. Most likely, we will find that PIOLs (which are extranodal DLBCLs), will belong to either the GCB or ABC subtype.

The expression of certain genes in PIOL will likely prove to play a role in prognosis. Genes for proteins involved in mediating influx or efflux of methotrexate, which is considered by most to be a first-line therapy for the treatment of PIOL, likely will affect prognosis. In addition, the expression of tumor suppressor proteins, such as p53, anti-apoptotic proteins like BCL-6, or proteins associated with oncogenesis, including MUM1 (a post-germinal center marker) may also have a role in tumor progression or aggressiveness.[38,39]

The first step in making the diagnosis of PIOL is having a high index of suspicion. Is the patient elderly and complaining of blurry vision and floaters? Does the examination appear like an idiopathic uveitis? Perhaps the patient is immune compromised with declining vision. When we suspect PIOL, it is necessary to obtain an MRI to rule out cerebral involvement as 80% of the patients with ocular involvement will eventuate to cerebral disease.[6,40] A definitive diagnosis of PIOL requires that we identify the atypical, neoplastic lymphocytes.[2,5,15,41,42] Typically, we make our diagnosis from cytologic evaluation of the CSF or vitrectomy. However, if such tissues are non-diagnostic, but the suspicion for PIOL is high, we may consider chorioretinal biopsy if there are obvious sub-RPE lesions.[43–51] When a diagnosis of PIOL is established it is imperative that we involve neuro- and hematooncologists in the patient's care and coordinate follow-up. Care of the patient should never become one-sided. Ophthalmologic examinations and evaluation of treatment is necessary throughout the care of the patient, whether the disease is solely ocular or oculocerebral. The current therapy is centered on chemotherapy with high-dose systemic methotrexate taking center stage.[3] Intravitreal administration of methotrexate may be considered in situations where systemic administration is contraindicated. These situations include cases with bulky ocular disease or recurrent ocular disease.[52-54] When the lymphoma is noted at discovery to involve both the brain and eye(s), systemic high-dose methotrexate is used with consideration of intrathecal administration. In cases of recurrence, chemotherapy may be employed again or radiation therapy may be considered.[3] Newer treatments involving biologics and stem cell transplantation are on the horizon and may prove to be important tools in our repertoire of therapeutic agents.

Finally, the use of animal models plays an integral role in expanding our knowledge of this unique malignancy and offers opportunities to design or test therapeutics.[31,33,55]

References

1. Velez G, Chan CC, Csaky KG. (2002) Fluorescein angiographic findings in primary intraocular lymphoma. *Retina* 22(1): 37–43.
2. Chan CC, Buggage RR, Nussenblatt RB. (2002) Intraocular lymphoma. *Curr Opin Ophthalmol* 13(6): 411–418.
3. Levy-Clarke GA, Chan CC, Nussenblatt RB. (2005) Diagnosis and management of primary intraocular lymphoma. *Hematol Oncol Clin North Am* 19(4): 739–749.
4. Freeman LN, Schachat AP, Knox DL, et al. (1987) Clinical features, laboratory investigations, and survival in ocular reticulum cell sarcoma. *Ophthalmology* 94: 1631–1639.
5. Whitcup SM, de Smet MD, Rubin BI, et al. (1993) Intraocular lymphoma. Clinical and histopathologic diagnosis. *Ophthalmology* 100: 1399–1406.
6. Peterson K, Gordon KB, Heinemann MH, DeAngelis LM. (1993) The clinical spectrum of ocular lymphoma. *Cancer* 72(3): 843–849.
7. Akpek EK, Ahmed I, Hochberg FH, et al. (1999) Intraocular-central nervous system lymphoma: clinical features, diagnosis, and outcomes. *Ophthalmology* 106(9): 1805–1810.
8. Cassoux N, Merle-Beral H, Leblond V, et al. (2000) Ocular and central nervous system lymphoma: clinical features and diagnosis. *Ocul Immunol Inflamm* 8(4): 243–250.

9. Hoffman PM, McKelvie P, Hall AJ, *et al.* (2003) Intraocular lymphoma: a series of 14 patients with clinicopathological features and treatment outcomes. *Eye* **17**(4): 513–521.

10. Hormigo A, Abrey L, Heinemann MH, DeAngelis LM. (2004) Ocular presentation of primary central nervous system lymphoma: diagnosis and treatment. *Br J Haematol* **126**(2): 202–208.

11. Fine HA, Mayer RJ. (1993) Primary central nervous system lymphoma. *Ann Intern Med* **119**(11): 1093–1104.

12. Wolf T, Brodt HR, Fichtlscherer S, *et al.* (2005) Changing incidence and prognostic factors of survival in AIDS-related non-Hodgkin's lymphoma in the era of highly active antiretroviral therapy (HAART). *Leuk Lymphoma* **46**(2): 207–215.

13. MacMahon EM, Glass JD, Hayward SD, *et al.* (1991) Epstein-Barr virus in AIDS-related primary central nervous system lymphoma. *Lancet* **338**(8773): 969–973.

14. Rosenblum ML, Levy RM, Bredesen DE, *et al.* (1988) Primary central nervous system lymphomas in patients with AIDS. *Ann Neurol* **23 Suppl**: S13–16.

15. Char DH, Ljung BM, Deschenes J, Miller TR. (1988) Intraocular lymphoma: immunological and cytological analysis. *Br J Ophthalmol* **72**(12): 905–911.

16. Chan CC. (2003) Molecular pathology of primary intraocular lymphoma. *Trans Am Ophthalmol Soc* **101**: 275–292.

17. Davis JL, Solomon D, Nussenblatt RB, *et al.* (1992) Immunocytochemical staining of vitreous cells. Indications, techniques, and results. *Ophthalmology* **99**(2): 250–256.

18. Vogel MH, Font RL, Zimmerman LE, Levine RA. (1968) Reticulum cell sarcoma of the retina and uvea. Report of six cases and review of the literature. *Am J Ophthalmol* **66**(2): 205–215.

19. Ridley ME, McDonald HR, Sternberg P, Jr., *et al.* (1992) Retinal manifestations of ocular lymphoma (reticulum cell sarcoma). *Ophthalmology* **99**(7): 1153–1160; discussion 1160–1151.

20. Wilson DJ, Braziel R, Rosenbaum JT. (1992) Intraocular lymphoma. Immunopathologic analysis of vitreous biopsy specimens. *Arch Ophthalmol* **110**(10): 1455–1458.

21. Coupland SE, Anastassiou G, Bornfeld N, *et al.* (2005) Primary intraocular lymphoma of T-cell type: report of a case and review of the literature. *Graefes Arch Clin Exp Ophthalmol* **243**(3): 189–197.

22. White VA, Gascoyne RD, Paton KE. (1999) Use of the polymerase chain reaction to detect B- and T-cell gene rearrangements in vitreous specimens from patients with intraocular lymphoma. *Arch Ophthalmol* **117**(6): 761–765.

23. Shen DF, Zhuang Z, LeHoang P, *et al.* (1998) Utility of microdissection and polymerase chain reaction for the detection of immunoglobulin gene rearrangement and translocation in primary intraocular lymphoma. *Ophthalmology* 105(9): 1664–1669.

24. Blay JY, Burdin N, Rousset F, *et al.* (1993) Serum interleukin-10 in non-Hodgkin's lymphoma: a prognostic factor. *Blood* 82(7): 2169–2174.

25. Bost KL, Bieligk SC, Jaffe BM. (1995) Lymphokine mRNA expression by transplantable murine B lymphocytic malignancies. Tumor-derived IL-10 as a possible mechanism for modulating the anti-tumor response. *J Immunol* 154(2): 718–729.

26. Wolf LA, Reed GF, Buggage RR, *et al.* (2002) Levels of IL-10 and IL-6 in the vitreous are helpful for differential diagnosis of primary intraocular lymphoma and ocular inflammation. *ARVO Abstract.* #2221.

27. Wolf LA, Reed GF, Buggage RR, *et al.* (2003) Vitreous cytokine levels. *Ophthalmology* 110(8): 1671–1672.

28. Whitcup SM, Stark-Vancs V, Wittes RE, *et al.* (1997) Association of interleukin-10 in the vitreous and cerebral spinal fluid and primary central nervous system lymphoma. *Arch Ophthalmol* 115: 1157–1160.

29. Cassoux N, Giron A, Bodaghi B, *et al.* (2007) IL-10 measurement in aqueous humor for screening patients with suspicion of primary intraocular lymphoma (PIOL). *Invest Ophthalmol Vis Sci* (in press).

30. Shen D, Zhuang Z, Matteson DM, *et al.* (1998) Detection of interleukin-10 and its gene expression in primary intraocular lymphoma by microdissection and reverse transcription PCR [ARVO Abstract]. *Invest Ophthalmol Vis Sci* 39((4)): S290.

31. Gonzales JA, Shen D, Zhou M, *et al.* (2006) Chemokine and chemokine receptor expression in two models of primary intraocular lymphoma. *ARVO Poster.* #2831.

32. Chan CC, Shen D, Hackett JJ, *et al.* (2003) Expression of chemokine receptors, CXCR4 and CXCR5, and chemokines, BLC and SDF-1, in the eyes of patients with primary intraocular lymphoma. *Ophthalmology* 110(2): 421–426.

33. Chan CC, Fischette M, Shen D, *et al.* (2005) Murine model of primary intraocular lymphoma. *Invest Ophthalmol Vis Sci* 46(2): 415–419.

34. Alizadeh AA, Eisen MB, Davis RE, *et al.* (2000) Distinct types of diffuse large B-cell lymphoma identified by gene expression profiling. *Nature* 403(6769): 503–511.

35. Alizadeh A, Eisen M, Davis RE, *et al.* (1999) The lymphochip: a specialized cDNA microarray for the genomic-scale analysis of gene expression in normal and malignant lymphocytes. *Cold Spring Harb Symp Quant Biol* 64: 71–78.

36. Lossos IS, Alizadeh AA, Eisen MB, *et al.* (2000) Ongoing immunoglobulin somatic mutation in germinal center B cell-like but not in activated B cell-like diffuse large cell lymphomas. *Proc Natl Acad Sci U S A* **97**(18): 10209–10213.
37. Lossos IS. (2005) Molecular pathogenesis of diffuse large B-cell lymphoma. *J Clin Oncol* **23**(26): 6351–6357.
38. Coupland SE, Bechrakis NE, Anastassiou G, *et al.* (2003) Evaluation of vitrectomy specimens and chorioretinal biopsies in the diagnosis of primary intraocular lymphoma in patients with Masquerade syndrome. *Graefes Arch Clin Exp Ophthalmol* **241**(10): 860–870.
39. Chang CC, Kampalath B, Schultz C, *et al.* (2003) Expression of p53, c-Myc, or Bcl-6 suggests a poor prognosis in primary central nervous system diffuse large B-cell lymphoma among immunocompetent individuals. *Arch Pathol Lab Med* **127**(2): 208–212.
40. Coupland SE, Damato B. (2006) Lymphomas involving the eye and the ocular adnexa. *Curr Opin Ophthalmol* **17**(6): 523–537.
41. Hochberg FH, Miller DC. (1988) Primary central nervous system lymphoma. *J Neurosurg* **68**(6): 835–853.
42. Tuaillon N, Chan CC. (2001) Molecular analysis of primary central nervous system and primary intraocular lymphoma. *Curr Mol Med* **1**(2): 259–272.
43. Chan CC, Wallace DJ. (2004) Intraocular lymphoma: update on diagnosis and management. *Cancer Control* **11**(5): 285–295.
44. Whitcup SM, Chan CC, Buggage RR, *et al.* (2000) Improving the diagnostic yield of vitrectomy for intraocular lymphoma [letter; comment]. *Arch Ophthalmol* **118**(3): 446.
45. Chan CC, Palestine AG, Davis JL, *et al.* (1991) Role of chorioretinal biopsy in inflammatory eye disease. *Ophthalmology* **98**(8): 1281–1286.
46. Klingele TG, Hogan MJ. (1975) Ocular reticulum cell sarcoma. *Am J Ophthalmol* **79**(1): 39–47.
47. Michels RG, Knox DL, Erozan YS, Green WR. (1975) Intraocular reticulum cell sarcoma. Diagnosis by pars plana vitrectomy. *Arch Ophthalmol* **93**(12): 1331–1335.
48. Park SS, D'Amico DJ, Foster CS. (1994) The role of invasive diagnostic testing in inflammatory eye diseases. *Int Ophthalmol Clin* **34**(3): 229–238.
49. Siegel MJ, Dalton J, Friedman AH, *et al.* (1989) Ten-year experience with primary ocular 'reticulum cell sarcoma' (large cell non-Hodgkin's lymphoma). *Br J Ophthalmol* **73**(5): 342–346.
50. Martin DF, Chan CC, de Smet MD, *et al.* (1993) The role of chorioretinal biopsy in the management of posterior uveitis. *Ophthalmology* **100**(5): 705–714.
51. Johnston RL, Tufail A, Lightman S, *et al.* (2004) Retinal and choroidal biopsies are helpful in unclear uveitis of suspected infectious or malignant origin. *Ophthalmology* **111**(3): 522–528.

52. Levy-Clarke GA, Byrnes GA, Buggage RR, *et al.* (2001) Primary intraouclar lymphoma diagnosed by fine needle aspiration biopsy of a subretinal lesion. *Retina* 21(3): 281–284.
53. de Smet MD, Vancs VS, Kohler D, *et al.* (1999) Intravitreal chemotherapy for the treatment of recurrent intraocular lymphoma. *Br J Ophthalmol* 83(4): 448–451.
54. Fishburne BC, Wilson DJ, Rosenbaum JT, Neuwelt EA. (1997) Intravitreal methotrexate as an adjunctive treatment of intraocular lymphoma. *Arch Ophthalmol* 115(9): 1152–1156.
55. Smith JR, Rosenbaum JT, Wilson DJ, *et al.* (2002) Role of intravitreal methotrexate in the management of primary central nervous system lymphoma with ocular involvement. *Ophthalmology* 109(9): 1709–1716.
56. Li Z, Mahesh SP, Shen D, *et al.* (2006) Eradication of tumor colonization and invasion by a B cell specific immunotoxin in a murine model for human primary intraocular lymphom. *Cancer Res* 66(21): 10586–10593.

Chapter 15

The Future of PIOL

We are living in an age of rapidly developing technology and information, and this has had an enormous impact on the advancement of science and the practice of medicine. In the arena of cancer, technological advancements and research achievements have enabled us to expand our understanding of factors involved in the development of cancers, oncogenes and tumor suppressor genes that certain cancers express, and how cancers might grow, localize, and metastasize. The progress made in understanding genetics and environmental factors also helps us to prevent and treat cancers with individualized, better-targeting therapies. Recently, we have seen new technologies lending themselves to use in further characterizing PIOL. Much has yet to be learned of this intraocular lymphoproliferation, but it is exciting to think that we are in the midst of truly understanding this disease process. We have made much progress since our first descriptions of the intraocular "reticulum cell sarcoma" of the 1950s.

The immunologic and histologic features of most PIOLs reveal that they belong to the diffuse large B-cell (DLBCL) histologic subtype in the WHO-REAL classification system.[1] As these lymphomas occur outside the setting of lymph nodes and lymphoid structures, they are by definition, extranodal. Yet, with the recent discovery of three pathogenetically and clinically distinct subcategories within the DLBCL histologic subtype of NHLs by DNA microarray technology,[2-5] there is the potential to likewise classify PIOLs as belonging to the activated B-cell (ABC) or germinal center B-cell (GCB) subtypes. We may find that some patients have a PIOL like that of the GCB subtype, while others may have a PIOL resembling the ABC subtype. As our current technology develops and enables us to analyze the gene expression profiles of small samples (as in the case of PIOL), our ability to further characterize PIOLs by their unique genetic signature will increase. This will enable us to stratify our patients into prognostic categories so that we can make better judgments in treating a particular patient with PIOL.

With the sequencing of the human genome, it is now possible to identify single nucleotide polymorphisms (SNPs) that are associated with disease. Genetic variance likely plays an important role in the evolution of some diseases and their response to treatment. For example, SNPs have been associated with age-related macular degeneration (AMD)[6–11] and some have reported methotrexate-toxicity due to SNPs.[12] Analyses of genes important in PIOL (e.g. those associated with IL-10,[13,14] chemokines and their receptors,[15] and drug sensitivity or resistance proteins[16,17]) may reveal that some patients are more susceptible than others to developing PIOL.

Currently, there is no standard of care treatment for PIOL, but high-dose intravenous methotrexate has proven to be the single most important therapy.[18] Intrathecal and intravitreal methotrexate may also become important routes of administration depending upon the bulkiness or refractoriness of disease.[19,20] We may also find intrathecal or intravitreal methotrexate becoming first-line routes of administration like systemic methotrexate. However, we must recall that most cases of PIOL will also lead to cerebral involvement, and this fact requires our consideration when determining the appropriate route of administration for our patients.[21–24] The role of radiation therapy being administered after methotrexate also needs to be further defined.[25,26] May we simply use methotrexate without radiation? Or do we use radiation in the face of refractory or recalcitrant disease? Other therapies, such as biologics[27–29] that include immunologic agents or chemokine receptor antagonists,[30,31] may become important first-line or adjunctive therapies after we have identified the optimal routes of administration and dosing schedules. Issues of toxicity associated with therapeutic agents remain,[20,29,32–37] as to questions with respect to effective treatment of recurrent disease. In addition, the precise genetic nature of the PIOL, which can dictate its sensitivity to a particular therapy, will need to be identified for each patient. Some PIOLs, by virtue of drug resistance proteins, may be less susceptible to mainstay treatments. Therefore, other therapeutic strategies will need to be drawn out. This will constitute a tailored therapy for each patient so that maximal response may be obtained to prolong patients' lives.

Animal models of PIOL that have been developed by our laboratory can help identify important factors involved in the development of PIOL as well as elucidate ways that this disease might be treated.[28,38–40] We can alter various aspects of the animal, such as expression of certain proteins by ocular tissues, to determine the precise relationship between the intraocular tissues, the molecules they express, and the PIOL cells with which they interact.

We should look to the future, then, as an opportunity to not only truly understand PIOL (its unique cytological, histopathological, and immunological features, its genotypic traits, and its epidemiological features), but to also truly make a difference in the way we treat patients with this disease. Diagnosing and caring for PIOL patients requires multiple medical sub-specialists, including ophthalmologist, pathologist, neurooncologist and hematooncologist, all working closely together. Perhaps one day when we are charged with informing a patient that he or she has PIOL, we can not only say that we know why this disease has occurred in our patient, but that we also know how to effectively treat it and our patient can look forward to a bright future. Much work needs to be done to make this future a reality, and it is with this in mind that we continue our relentless pursuit of making the future brighter.

References

1. Tuaillon N, Chan CC. (2001) Molecular analysis of primary central nervous system and primary intraocular lymphoma. *Curr Mol Med* 1(2): 259–272.
2. Alizadeh A, Eisen M, Davis RE, *et al.* (1999) The lymphochip: a specialized cDNA microarray for the genomic-scale analysis of gene expression in normal and malignant lymphocytes. *Cold Spring Harb Symp Quant Biol* 64: 71–78.
3. Alizadeh AA, Eisen MB, Davis RE, *et al.* (2000) Distinct types of diffuse large B-cell lymphoma identified by gene expression profiling. *Nature* 403(6769): 503–511.
4. Lossos IS, Czerwinski DK, Alizadeh AA, *et al.* (2004) Prediction of survival in diffuse large-B-cell lymphoma based on the expression of six genes. *N Engl J Med* 350(18): 1828–1837.
5. Wright G, Tan B, Rosenwald A, *et al.* (2003) A gene expression-based method to diagnose clinically distinct subgroups of diffuse large B cell lymphoma. *Proc Natl Acad Sci USA* 100(17): 9991–9996.
6. Hageman GS, Anderson DH, Johnson LV, *et al.* (2005) A common haplotype in the complement regulatory gene factor H (HF1/CFH) predisposes individuals to age-related macular degeneration. *Proc Natl Acad Sci USA* 102(20): 7227–7232.

7. Tuo J, Smith BC, Bojanowski CM, *et al.* (2004) The involvement of sequence variation and expression of CX3CR1 in the pathogenesis of age-related macular degeneration. *Faseb J* 18(11): 1297–1299.

8. Klein RJ, Zeiss C, Chew EY, *et al.* (2005) Complement factor H polymorphism in age-related macular degeneration. *Science* 308(5720): 385–389.

9. Edwards AO, Ritter R, 3rd, Abel KJ, *et al.* (2005) Complement factor H polymorphism and age-related macular degeneration. *Science* 308(5720): 421–424.

10. Haines JL, Hauser MA, Schmidt S, *et al.* (2005) Complement factor H variant increases the risk of age-related macular degeneration. *Science* 308(5720): 419–421.

11. Zareparsi S, Branham KE, Li M, *et al.* (2005) Strong association of the Y402H variant in complement factor H at 1q32 with susceptibility to age-related macular degeneration. *Am J Hum Genet* 77(1): 149–153.

12. Linnebank M, Pels H, Kleczar N, *et al.* (2005) MTX-induced white matter changes are associated with polymorphisms of methionine metabolism. *Neurology* 64(5): 912–913.

13. Chan CC, Whitcup SM, Solomon D, Nussenblatt RB. (1995) Interleukin-10 in the vitreous of primary intraocular lymphoma. *Am J Ophthalmol* 120(5): 671–673.

14. Merle-Beral H, Davi F, Cassoux N, *et al.* (2004) Biological diagnosis of primary intraocular lymphoma. *Br J Haematol* 124(4): 469–473.

15. Chan CC, Shen D, Hackett JJ, *et al.* (2003) Expression of chemokine receptors, CXCR4 and CXCR5, and chemokines, BLC and SDF-1, in the eyes of patients with primary intraocular lymphoma. *Ophthalmology* 110(2): 421–426.

16. Ferreri AJ, Dell'Oro S, Capello D, *et al.* (2004) Aberrant methylation in the promoter region of the reduced folate carrier gene is a potential mechanism of resistance to methotrexate in primary central nervous system lymphomas. *Br J Haematol* 126(5): 657–664.

17. Hooijberg JH, Broxterman HJ, Kool M, *et al.* (1999) Antifolate resistance mediated by the multidrug resistance proteins MRP1 and MRP2. *Cancer Res* 59(11): 2532–2535.

18. Levy-Clarke GA, Chan CC, Nussenblatt RB. (2005) Diagnosis and management of primary intraocular lymphoma. *Hematol Oncol Clin North Am* 19(4): 739–749.

19. de Smet MD. (2001) Management of non Hodgkin's intraocular lymphoma with intravitreal methotrexate. *Bull Soc Belge Ophtalmol* 279: 91–95.

20. Smith JR, Rosenbaum JT, Wilson DJ, *et al.* (2002) Role of intravitreal methotrexate in the management of primary central nervous system lymphoma with ocular involvement. *Ophthalmology* 109(9): 1709–1716.

21. Char DH, Ljung BM, Miller T, Phillips T. (1988) Primary intraocular lymphoma (ocular reticulum cell sarcoma) diagnosis and management. *Ophthalmology* **95**: 625–630.

22. Char DH, Margolis L, Newman AB. (1981) Ocular reticulum cell sarcoma. *Am J Ophthalmol* **91**(4): 480–483.

23. Rockwood EJ, Zakov ZN, Bay JW. (1984) Combined malignant lymphoma of the eye and CNS (reticulum-cell sarcoma). *J Neurosurg* **61**: 369–374.

24. Chan CC, Buggage RR, Nussenblatt RB. (2002) Intraocular lymphoma. *Curr Opin Ophthalmol* **13**(6): 411–418.

25. Ferreri AJ, Blay JY, Reni M, *et al.* (2002) Relevance of intraocular involvement in the management of primary central nervous system lymphomas. *Ann Oncol* **13**(4): 531–538.

26. Hormigo A, Abrey L, Heinemann MH, DeAngelis LM. (2004) Ocular presentation of primary central nervous system lymphoma: diagnosis and treatment. *Br J Haematol* **126**(2): 202–208.

27. Schaedel O, Reiter Y. (2006) Antibodies and their fragments as anti-cancer agents. *Curr Pharm Des* **12**(3): 363–378.

28. Kim H, Csaky KG, Chan CC, *et al.* (2006) The pharmacokinetics of rituximab following an intravitreal injection. *Exp Eye Res* **82**(5): 760–766.

29. Pels H, Schulz H, Manzke O, *et al.* (2002) Intraventricular and intravenous treatment of a patient with refractory primary CNS lymphoma using rituximab. *J Neurooncol* **59**(3): 213–216.

30. Hendrix CW, Flexner C, MacFarland RT, *et al.* (2000) Pharmacokinetics and safety of AMD-3100, a novel antagonist of the CXCR-4 chemokine receptor, in human volunteers. *Antimicrob Agents Chemother* **44**(6): 1667–1673.

31. Wu L, LaRosa G, Kassam N, *et al.* (1997) Interaction of chemokine receptor CCR5 with its ligands: multiple domains for HIV-1 gp120 binding and a single domain for chemokine binding. *J Exp Med* **186**(8): 1373–1381.

32. Dietlein M, Pels H, Schulz H, *et al.* (2005) Imaging of central nervous system lymphomas with iodine-123 labeled rituximab. *Eur J Haematol* **74**(4): 348–352.

33. Nelson DF, Martz KL, Bonner H, *et al.* (1992) Non-Hodgkin's lymphoma of the brain: can high dose, large volume radiation therapy improve survival? Report on a prospective trial by the Radiation Therapy Oncology Group (RTOG): RTOG 8315. *Int J Radiat Oncol Biol Phys* **23**(1): 9–17.

34. Pels H, Schulz H, Schlegel U, Engert A. (2003) Treatment of CNS lymphoma with the anti-CD20 antibody rituximab: experience with two cases and review of the literature. *Onkologie* **26**(4): 351–354.

35. Flombaum CD, Meyers PA. (1999) High-dose leucovorin as sole therapy for methotrexate toxicity. *J Clin Oncol* **17**(5): 1589–1594.

36. Hoffman PM, McKelvie P, Hall AJ, *et al.* (2003) Intraocular lymphoma: a series of 14 patients with clinicopathological features and treatment outcomes. *Eye* 17(4): 513–521.
37. Abrey LE, DeAngelis LM, Yahalom J. (1998) Long-term survival in primary CNS lymphoma. *J Clin Oncol* 16(3): 859–863.
38. Chan CC, Fischette M, Shen D, *et al.* (2005) Murine model of primary intraocular lymphoma. *Invest Ophthalmol Vis Sci* 46(2): 415–419.
39. Gonzales JA, Shen D, Zhou M, *et al.* (2006) Chemokine and chemokine receptor expression in two models of primary intraocular lymphoma. *ARVO Poster.* #2831.
40. Li Z, Mahesh SP, Shen D, *et al.* (2006) Eradication of tumor colonization and invasion by a B cell specific immunotoxin in a murine model for human primary intraocular lymphom (PIOL)(in preparation).

Chapter 16

Case Illustrations

Case 1

A 75-year-old woman presented with bilateral cataracts, an afferent pupillary defect and questionable disc elevation in the left eye that was worrisome for an anterior ischemic optic neuropathy. A fluorescein angiogram was performed and showed mottling (Fig. 16.1). A borderline elevated erythrocyte sedimentation rate (ESR) was found, and the patient was treated with oral corticosteroids. Visual acuity, however, declined. A temporal artery biopsy was performed and was negative. The patient went on to develop bilateral vitritis, and after cataract extraction in the left eye, ophthalmoscopic exam showed that there was diffuse retinal pigment epithelium (RPE) depigmentation with an edematous optic nerve. Intraocular lymphoma was suspected, and a vitreous biopsy was performed. Microscopic examination of the Giemsa-stained slide showed many large lymphoid cells with large nuclei having irregular borders and scant cytoplasm (Fig. 16.2). These cells were highly suspicious for PIOL, but their lack of preservation precluded a definitive diagnosis by cytology. Assay for IL-10 and IL-6 in the vitreous fluid was 184 pg/ml and 26 pg/ml, respectively, further confirming suspicion for PIOL. Microdissection along with PCR revealed monoclonal rearrangement of the *IgH* gene in the FR3A site (Fig. 16.3). Magnetic resonance imaging (MRI) was subsequently performed, which showed an enhancing mass in the left basal ganglia. The diagnosis of PIOL was confirmed.

Commentary. This case has the classical presentation of PIOL: a bilateral vitritis of unknown etiology with a supposed chorioretinitis appearing in an older patient. Clinical examination can often be non-specific, and even if PIOL is suspected (e.g. as shown by the existence of creamy

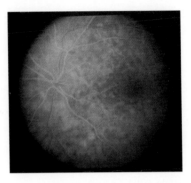

Fig. 16.1 Case 1. Fluorescein angiogram showing multiple hypofluorescent areas in the posterior pole of the left eye. Most of them are small, round lesions with some confluence.

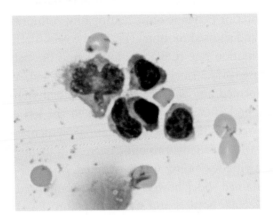

Fig. 16.2 Case 1. Photomicrograph showing cytology of the vitreous sample. Large, atypical lymphocytes with basophilic cytoplasm and large nuclei exhibiting open chromatin are seen (Giemsa, original magnification × 640).

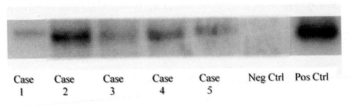

| Case | Case | Case | Case | Case | Neg Ctrl | Pos Ctrl |
| 1 | 2 | 3 | 4 | 5 | | |

Fig. 16.3 Cases 1–5. Polymerase chain reaction (PCR) amplification products demonstrating monoclonal rearrangement of the immunoglobulin heavy chain (*IgH*) gene from the microdissected PIOL cells (lanes 1–5), negative control (lane 6), and positive control (lane 7).

yellow sub-RPE subretinal infiltrates) one needs cytopathologic proof that a malignancy is at play. Often, treatment with corticosteroids is initiated for a presumed idiopathic uveitis. It is not until the "uveitis" is unresponsive to treatment or (in this patient's case) visual acuity shows marked deterioration that a more invasive test, such as a lumbar puncture, diagnostic vitrectomy, or a retinochoroidal biopsy, is pursued. It is also rather common for an MRI to be performed after PIOL has been diagnosed (as in this case). Currently, if PIOL is suspected it is important to perform an MRI and a lumbar puncture with CSF cytology to check for CNS lesions and malignant lymphoma cells.[1] Elevated IL-10 level with a high ratio of IL-10 to IL-6 in the vitreous and the finding of IgH gene rearrangement in the vitreal infiltrating cells support the presence of PIOL cells in the vitreous.[2,3] This patient did go on to develop brain lesions, and the fact that she is over 60 years of age and had involvement of deep brain structures were poor prognostic factors for PCNSL.[4]

Case 2

A 67-year-old woman reported blurred vision in the left eye for three weeks and developed bilateral vitritis and chorioretinitis of unknown etiology (Fig. 16.4).[5] Upon review of systems, it was revealed that she had been worked up for seizures two months prior to presentation. During her work up for the seizures, CSF studies and a computed tomographic (CT)

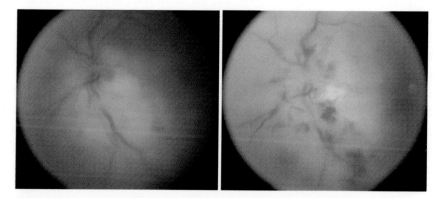

Fig. 16.4 Case 2. Ophthalmoscopic photographs showing subretinal lesion inferior to the optic nerve head (*left*) with progression to a peripapillary 360° infiltrates, edema and multiple hemorrhages (*right*).

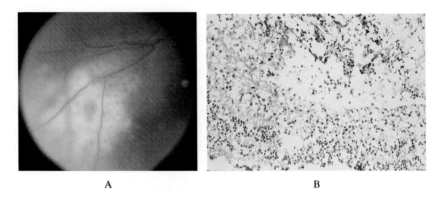

A   B

Fig. 16.5A & B Case 2. (A) Ophthalmoscopic photograph showing a peripheral, creamy yellowish subretinal lesion, which was subsequently biopsied. At the superonasal area of the lesion there is a "leopard spot pattern," a typical feature of PIOL caused by small foci of tumor infiltration. (B) Photomicrograph of frozen section from endoretinal biopsy showing many lymphoid cells in the disorganized retina (hematoxylin and eosin, original magnification × 100).

scan with contrast of the brain were normal. Clinical examination failed to identify any cause for the ocular findings, and as the patient's vision in the left eye significantly worsened and her retinal lesion was progressing without responding to antiviral therapy (Fig. 16.5A), a vitrectomy with internal chorioretinal biopsy was performed in addition to a lumbar puncture. Both the vitrectomy and the CSF specimens failed to reveal any malignant lymphocytes by cytology. Despite this, the IL-10 level in the vitreous and CSF samples were elevated, being 5456 pg/ml and 25 pg/ml, respectively. IL-6 levels in the vitreous and CSF were found to be 193 pg/ml and undetectable, respectively. Thus, for the vitreous sample, the IL-10 to IL-6 ratio was greater than 1.0, suggesting that PIOL could potentially be the culprit involved in this patient's declining visual status. Interestingly, the retinal biopsy showed infiltrating lymphoid cells, although definite malignant cells could not be identified (Fig. 16.5B). However, immunohistochemistry revealed that the overwhelming majority of infiltrating lymphocytes were of B-cell origin (positive for CD19, CD20, and CD22) and that they were monoclonal, staining positive for kappa (κ), but not lambda (λ) light chains (Fig. 16.6). Monoclonality of the B-cell proliferation was further confirmed by the polymerase chain reaction (PCR) showing the same *IgH* gene rearrangement (Fig. 16.3). In light of these findings, a diagnosis of

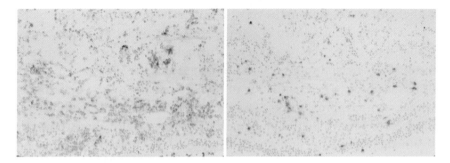

Fig. 16.6 Case 2. Photomicrographs of frozen sections from endoretinal biopsy showing positive kappa (κ) light chain (*left*) and negative lambda (λ) light chain (*right*) (avidin-biotin complex immunoperoxidase, original magnification × 100).

PIOL was attained, and an MRI with gadolinium was performed to check for cerebral involvement. Indeed, a 1 × 1 cm contrast-enhancing mass was discovered in the right frontal lobe. A biopsy of this mass was performed via craniotomy and this confirmed the diagnosis of PCNSL. The patient received radiation, but the left eye developed a retinal detachment. The right eye responded to the radiation therapy, and the visual acuity improved in this eye from hand motion to 20/40 over six weeks. The patient refused systemic chemotherapy, and she died six months later.

Commentary. This case has a presentation like that of a viral retinitis. Therefore, while PIOL can often present as an idiopathic uveitis, findings in the retina produce their own diagnostic challenges. Others have similarly noted that retinal involvement in PIOL can produce a clinical picture comparable to that of a viral retinitis.[6–8] In such instances treatment with anti-viral medication has occurred prior to making the diagnosis of PIOL, much like PIOL mistaken for uveitis is frequently treated first with corticosteroids. The non-diagnostic CSF and vitreous examinations are not unusual in PIOL, and the elevated vitreal IL-10 level with the IL-10 to IL-6 ratio greater than 1 shows how this adjunctive test can be important in prodding us to be persistent in seeking out PIOL in the absence of malignant cells in biopsied tissues. The retinochoroidal biopsy revealed definite monoclonal B-cell infiltration in the retina, and PCR analysis further confirmed this with *IgH* gene rearrangment. It is important, then, that when tissue biopsy is considered there be an experienced pathologist or ocular pathologist involved from the very beginning, before any tissues are biopsied. The rate limiting step is not the surgeon's ability to obtain biopsy tissues, but rather the presence of a pathologist who will perform the histopathologic and molecular examinations that are necessary to establish a diagnosis.[9] The eventuation of PIOL to cerebral disease is an unfortunate reality; approximately 80% of cases presenting initially in the eyes progress to involve the brain as well.[8,10,11] This case also shows how our treatment of PIOL has progressed. This patient was treated with radiation therapy first and later offered systemic chemotherapy. While PIOL and PCNSL are very radiosensitive, severe adverse effects are common. Recently, high-dose systemic methotrexate was identified as the single most important therapeutic agent in treating PIOL and PCNSL and can be followed, depending on the case, by whole brain radiation therapy if the patient is under 60 years of age. Those over the age of 60 years can suffer significant delayed neurotoxicity if radiation therapy is included after methotrexate administration.[12] Complete response in the eye should be assessed by repeat evaluation.[13] While the absence of subretinal infiltrates and vitreous cells is a requirement for noting a complete response, some of the chronic changes that occur to the RPE may not resolve in the setting of a complete response.[13] If recurrence develops after an initial response with methotrexate, we might consider administering higher doses of systemic methotrexate or intravitreal methotrexate injections, again depending on the case.

Case 3

A 46-year-old woman from Brazil noted floaters in her left eye for two months. She was diagnosed with ocular toxoplasmosis (Fig. 16.7) and started on oral corticosteroids and pyrimethamine. Work up revealed that she had a positive toxoplasmosis titer, but she was VDRL- and HIV-negative. Undergoing treatment for toxoplasmosis, the patient showed no improvement from her medication regimen. Therefore, this was discontinued after four weeks. She was then treated for presumed acute retinal necrosis (ARN) with intravenous acyclovir for two weeks followed by oral acyclovir for one week. Despite the antiviral treatment the patient continued to show no improvement. She was put back on toxoplasmosis therapy, including sulfa, pyrimethamine, and corticosteroids, but no improvement was noted. A month later (five months after symptom onset) the patient's chorioretinitis

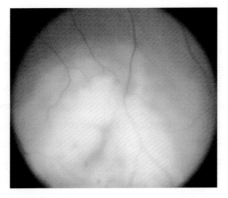

Fig. 16.7 Case 3. Ophthalmoscopic photograph showing huge retinal and subretinal creamy whitish infiltrate in the peripheral retina.

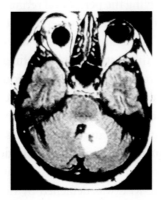

Fig. 16.8 Case 3. Magnetic resonance image (MRI) of the brain showing a lacunar infarct in the cerebellum.

in the left eye progressed, and lesions now appeared in the right eye. An MRI of the brain showed a lacunar infarct (Fig. 16.8), and lumbar puncture with CSF cytopathology revealed no atypical cells. Approximately one month later, the patient developed a retinal detachment in the left eye, and a vitrectomy with silicone oil tamponade was performed. Cytopathology of the vitrectomy specimen failed to show lymphoma cells. The patient was started on intravenous foscarnet, but no improvement was noted. She was then referred to the National Eye Institute (NEI) in the USA where a review of systems revealed a right arm weakness and swaying to the left when she initiated walking. Serological laboratory studies were obtained and were negative for RPR, ANA, c-ANCA, p-ANCA, HIV, lyme titer, and hepatitis. The patient did have a positive toxoplasmosis IgG titer. A fluorescein angiogram was obtained that showed areas of hyperfluorescence at the level of the RPE. A lumbar puncture was performed, and CSF cytology revealed cells suspicious for lymphoma. An infectious disease consult agreed with having the patient on therapy for toxoplasmosis (pyrimethamine and corticosteroids) and acute retinal necrosis (acyclovir). A neurology consultation resulted in a diagnosis of Parkinson's disease. Visual acuity in the right eye was stable, and the left eye was now non-light perception. The chorioretinitis showed progression in the right eye upon ophthalmoscopic examination. To better determine the nature of the patient's ocular processes, whether malignant or infectious, a diagnostic enucleation of the blind left eye was performed. The pathology of the eye disclosed sheets of vitreous condensation, fibrin strands and debris underlying the peripheral retina, pars plana, and pars plicata. Retinal detachment was noted in several places, including the macula, and white-yellowish infiltrates arose between the RPE and neuroretina in several areas, particularly the posterior pole. In the periphery, there were foci of chorioretinal scars with pigmentary demarcation and deposits. The optic disc was flat. Microscopically, the retina was completely detached, except for a few foci in the periphery that had chorioretinal adhesions and scarring. There was also serosanguinous material containing clumps of atypical lymphoid cells and inflammatory cells in the subretinal space. In some areas, fibrovascular inflammatory membrane was formed. Except for the temporal anterior region, the RPE was detached by tightly packed tumor cells characterized by large hyperchromatic and pleomorphic nuclei, and prominent nucleoli (Fig. 16.9). Mitoses were also noted. The RPE cells showed various degrees of atrophy and alternation, and they were infiltrated by tumor cells. In some areas, the tumor cells infiltrated the neuroretina. Bruch's membrane was intact in most places, except at the nasal periphery where there was a small necrotic focus. Some of the ganglion cells were enlarged and had swollen cytoplasm. Moderate-to-intense inflammation was present throughout the choroid. The optic nerve, however, was free of tumor infiltration. Immunohistochemistry was performed, and it revealed that the lymphomatous B-cells were monoclonal κ, rather than λ, light chain positive (Fig. 16.10). Microdissection of the infiltrating B-cells showed that they were monoclonal, having the same *IgH* gene rearrangement as found by PCR (Fig. 16.3).

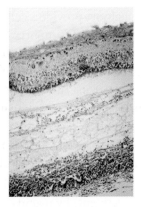

Fig. 16.9 Case 3. Photomicrograph showing PIOL cells located in the subretina between the destroyed retinal pigment epithelium (RPE) and fragmented Bruch's membrane (hematoxylin and eosin, original magnification × 50).

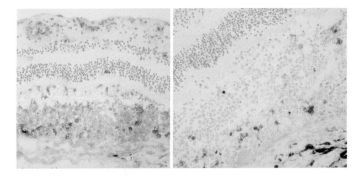

Fig. 16.10 Case 3. Photomicrographs showing PIOL cells staining positive for κ light chain (*left*) and negative for λ light chain (*right*) (avidin-biotin complex immunoperoxidase, original magnification × 200).

Commentary. This patient was younger than we typically would expect for PIOL. However, it is important to consider PIOL even in younger patients.[3,14] Note the typical pathology of PIOL, in which there is subretinal infiltration between Bruch's membrane and the RPE (Fig. 16.9). Lymphomatous infiltration can make its way into the retina as well, as evidenced by this case. Frequently a reactive inflammatory infiltrate is found in the choroid, and these lymphocytes are typically smaller than the PIOL cells. The overwhelming majority of PIOLs are of B-cell origin and that is demonstrated here by immunohistochemistry. It is important to realize that CSF and vitrectomy cytology may not always provide a definitive diagnosis, even if we repeat these tests. Despite this fact, it is important not to become dismayed with initially negative biopsies. Often, a repeat diagnostic vitrectomy is necessary to make the diagnosis of PIOL.[10] However, if vitrectomies prove nondiagnostic and there remains a strong suspicion for PIOL, we may turn to a retinochoroidal biopsy. This is done when there are obvious lesions that can be submitted to sampling and when these lesions fail to respond to therapy and are threatening to advance upon the macula. Alternatively, enucleation may be performed, especially when there is no possibility (as in this case) of restoring vision due to extensive disease progression, and the patient's course can be improved (through treatment) by making a definitive diagnosis. This case also illustrates that while PIOL can frequently be a deadly disease, confinement to the eye without cerebral involvement may prove to be a relatively advantageous situation compared to oculocerebral or solely cerebral disease.

Case 4

A 51-year-old man complained of floaters and decreased vision initially appearing in the right eye and, later, in the left eye.[15] An intermediate uveitis was diagnosed, and was treated with bilateral vitrectomy and scleral buckling over a period of two years. Five years later, the right eye developed episodic increases in intraocular pressure that seemed to correlate with the degree of intraocular inflammation. Importantly, this inflammation would often respond to topical corticosteroids. Eventually the patient developed bilateral multiple white subretinal lesions. An MRI of the brain revealed that there were contrast-enhancing lesions in the left caudate nucleus, and PCNSL with intraocular involvement was suspected. The iris in the right eye had diffuse infiltrative nodules (Fig. 16.11). Ophthalmoscopy revealed a bilateral vitritis, diffuse RPE changes, and macular thickening by dilated ophthalmoscopic examination. A diagnostic vitrectomy showed a B-cell PIOL, and iris biopsy revealed that the stroma was likewise infiltrated with B-cell lymphoma. Microdissection and PCR of the PIOL cells in the iris and vitreous, revealed monoclonal rearrangement of the *IgH* gene (Fig. 16.3). The patient was submitted to both systemic and intrathecal chemotherapy and radiation treatment and showed improvement (Fig. 16.12). Over six years, this patient also had intravitreal injections of methotrexate, allowing for the vitreous to be sampled prior to drug injection for cytokine analysis. When IL-10 levels were

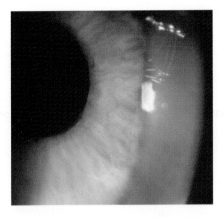

Fig. 16.11 Case 4. Slit lamp photograph showing diffuse infiltrative nodules in the iris.

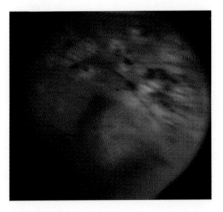

Fig. 16.12 Case 4. Ophthalmoscopic photograph showing small, atrophic chorioretinal scars with some pigmentation representing old PIOL lesions.

high (see Table 16.1), we would treat with intravitreal methotrexate, and the patient would respond. Unfortunately, the patient eventually developed a new cerebral parenchymal lesion after six years and died.

Commentary. This case is an almost classical presentation of PIOL in an immunocompetent patient, but with a twist. While the patient was in his 50s, complaining of decreased vision and floaters, iris stromal involvement eventually occurred, which is extremely rare.[15] This patient had extensive follow up with us at the NEI, and we were able to obtain vitreous

Table 16.1   Vitreous IL-10 and IL-6 Levels in Case 4

Date	IL-10 (pg/ml)	IL-6 (pg/ml)	IL-10/IL-6
12/03/1998	1451	28	51.8
06/09/1999	144	<15.6	>1.0
06/18/1999	1054	124	8.5
07/19/1999	570	<78	>1.0
07/21/1999	1495	596	2.5
07/23/1999	440	566	0.078
07/26/1999	182	290	0.63
08/26/1999	267	130	2.05
09/29/1999	220	38	5.79
11/09/1999	2266	226	10.03
01/10/2000	57	<15.6	>1.0
03/08/2000	14, 412	72	200.17
07/25/2000	<23.4	<15.6	ND[1]
10/04/2000	370	<15.6	>1.0
11/01/2000	350	<15.6	>1.0
11/28/2000	273	<15.6	>1.0
03/22/2002	<31.2	<15.6	ND[1]
04/09/2002	323	<15.6	>1.0
11/08/2002	>3000	48	>1.0
02/05/2003	>3000	84	>1.0
04/21/2003	12, 018	<15.6	>1.0
06/27/2003	19	<62.5	ND[1]
06/09/2004	816.5	186	4.39

[1]ND = not determinable.

or aqueous for assay of IL-10 and IL-6 levels during his visits for intravitreal methotrexate administration. As Table 16.1 shows, we were able to follow this patient's cytokine levels and treated it accordingly over six years. High IL-10 levels, suggesting active disease, prompted intravitreal injection of methotrexate with a subsequent response in the injected eye. Thus, following IL-10 levels can give us an indication as to the adequacy of our treatment regimen. For example, high IL-10 levels that fall in response to methotrexate treatment and stay low (or IL-10/IL-6 ratios less than 1.0) inform us that our treatment regimen is producing some benefit. On the other hand, IL-10 levels that only minimally respond to methotrexate or are refractory to treatment may indicate that the mode of treatment, the amount of drug, or the dosing schedule may not be adequate. Furthermore, while a patient may clinically respond to treatment, high IL-10 levels or IL-10/IL-6 ratios greater than 1.0 may indicate that disease is still present.[16–19]

Case 5

A 29-year-old man with AIDS seen during the pre-highly active anti-retroviral therapy (HAART) era presented with cytomegalovirus (CMV) retinitis (Fig. 16.13) and choroiditis reminiscent of a mycobacterial infection.[5] Later, a subretinal lesion nasal to the fovea was seen in both eyes (Fig. 16.14). Six months later, the patient died from multiple systemic opportunistic infections. A malignancy had not been an issue prior to this patient's death.

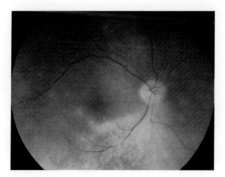

Fig. 16.13 Case 5. Ophthalmoscopic photograph showing classical cytomegalovirus (CMV) retinitis with feathered retinal lesion.

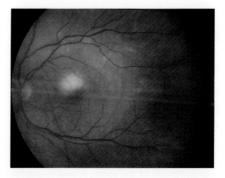

Fig. 16.14 Case 5. Ophthalmoscopic photograph showing a round subretinal lesion confined to the perimacular area.

After the patient died, both eyes were submitted for pathologic autopsy inspection. Findings included old CMV retinitis, chorioretinal scarring, retinal detachments, and an isolated subretinal lesion (Fig. 16.15). In the choroid, *Mycobacterium avium* was found. A cluster of lymphoplasmacytic lymphoproliferation was revealed beneath the retinal detachment (Fig. 16.16). Microdissection of these subretinal clusters of B-cells disclosed *IgH* gene rearrangement and confirmed a diagnosis of PIOL (Fig. 16.3).

Commentary. This case illustrates the difficulties that exist in identifying PIOL in AIDS patients. The presentation of PIOL in the setting of AIDS can be very different from the classical presentation we see in immunocompetent patients (see Case 1). AIDS patients are younger than

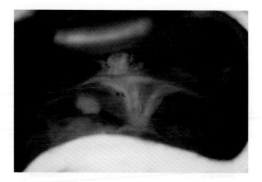

Fig. 16.15 Case 5. Macroscopic photograph of the left eye (see above clinical picture, Fig. 16.14) showing a whitish round lesion under the detached gliotic retina.

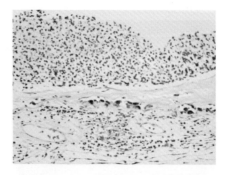

Fig. 16.16 Case 5. Photomicrograph of the above round lesion (see Fig. 16.15) composed of a cluster of small, atypical lymphoid cells in the subretina (hematoxylin and eosin, original magnification × 100).

immunocompetent patients who develop PIOL. In addition, AIDS patients, as this case reveals, often have multiple opportunistic infections that have their own unique presentations in the eye and can mask the presence of concurrent conditions, such as malignant ocular processes. Unfortunately, this patient succumbed to systemic complications arising from multiple opportunistic infections before a malignant ocular disease could be identified. If PIOL had been discovered in this patient prior to death, what treatment might have been initiated? This is not an easy question to answer. Certainly, an idea is developing of how to treat PIOL in immunocompetent patients (see Chapter 10). In AIDS patients, however, it seems that the most important issue regarding treatment is the immunodeficiency itself. The CD4 count must be addressed and typically involves the use of HAART. This patient, however, was being treated before the availability of HAART. Improving the CD4 population in terms of number improves the quality of the immune system and is perhaps the most important factor impacting the development of malignancies in AIDS patients.

Case 6

A 78-year-old pseudophakic man complained of a four-month history of blurry vision in the left eye. His past medical history was ominous, with cutaneous T-cell lymphoma of the leg (three years prior to presentation) and lung cancer being especially prominent. The patient had been treated with radiation for the cutaneous T-cell lymphoma (CTCL) and was status post lobectomy for the lung cancer (the patient had a history of smoking). Visual acuity was measured as 20/25 in the right eye and light perception in the left. Dilated ophthalmoscopy showed that there were trace cells and RPE atrophy superonasal to the fovea in the right eye and 2+ cell 3+ haze with no obvious retinal lesions in the left eye; the view of the fundus in the left, however, was hazy (Fig. 16.17). A fluorescein angiogram was obtained and showed no changes at the level of the RPE. Because of the patient's past history of CTCL and his current ocular presentation with bilateral vitritis, PIOL was suggested. An MRI was obtained and showed no lesions in the brain. A lumbar puncture was performed, and CSF cytology showed that there was a lymphocytosis, but rarely malignant cells were identified (Fig. 16.18). A vitrectomy was then performed and revealed atypical intermediate to

Fig. 16.17 Case 6. Ophthalmoscopic photograph showing hazy vitreous, which made it difficult to visualize the retina.

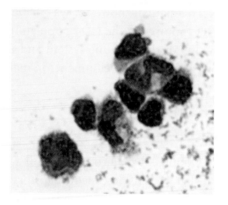

Fig. 16.18 Case 6. Photomicrograph of cerebrospinal fluid (CSF) showing atypical lymphoid cells (Giemsa, original magnification × 640).

large lymphoid cells having large and round or irregular nuclei with prominent nucleoli and scant, basophilic cytoplasm (Fig. 16.19). Immunohistochemistry was performed on these cells and revealed that the overwhelming majority of cells were of T-cell lineage (positive for CD3 with CD4 > CD8) and negative for the B-cell marker CD20. Further adjunctive testing using flow cytometry found that 65% of the T-cells were negative for CD2 and CD5, but positive for CD3 and CD7. Molecular pathology found that there was monoclonal rearrangement of the *TCR-γ* gene (Fig. 16.20), but no rearrangements of the *IgH* gene using FR3A, FR2A, or CDR3 primers. A diagnosis of T-cell lymphoma was made. The patient's previous skin biopsy of CTCL revealed that the infiltrating malignant T-cells were CD3- and CD4-positive

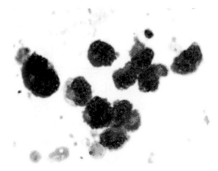

Fig. 16.19 Case 6. Photomicrograph of vitreous showing atypical lymphoid cells with variable size and polymorphic nuclei (Giemsa, original magnification × 640).

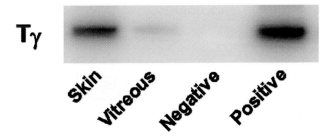

Fig. 16.20 Case 6. PCR amplification products demonstrating monoclonal rearrangement of the T-cell receptor gamma (*TCR-γ*) gene from the microdissected PIOL cells (lane 1, skin; lane 2, vitreous), negative control (lane 3), and positive control (lane 4).

and CD8-, CD30-, and CD20-negative. Interestingly, microdissection and molecular analysis on this skin biopsy showed the same band in the *TCR-γ* gene rearrangement as in the PIOL cells. The patient's visual acuity at this time was 20/80 in the right and 20/320 in the left eye. Treatment for this patient included oncology consultation, oral corticosteroids, sub-Tenon's kenalog injection, and a series of three intravitreal methotrexate injections in the right eye and one injection in the left eye. After treatment, the patient's visual acuity improved in the right to 20/20 and was measured as 20/250 in the left eye. Unfortunately, lesions in the brain developed and the patient rapidly succumbed to his disease.

Commentary. Many of the features of this case are classical of PIOL, although this case is most likely a metastatic CTCL lymphoma into the eye. The patient was older (in his 70s) and presented with a bilateral vitritis.

What is unusual about this case is the T-cell lineage of the PIOL cells. T-cell PIOL is extremely rare and is more often associated with CTCL (e.g., mycosis fungoides) or T-cell acute lymphoblastic leukemia.[20] This patient had a history of treated CTCL of the leg, and it had not recurred during his ocular disease. While B-cell PIOL is typically characterized by large lymphoid cells, the lymphoid cells found in T-cell PIOL can range from small-to-intermediate-to-large in size (Fig. 16.19). This patient's T-cell PIOL had a very unusual immunophenotype. Many features of this case presented dilemmas to treatment. The patient was over the age of 60 years, which is a poor prognostic factor in PCNSL. In addition, the patient had a rare T-cell PIOL where treatment is even less well characterized than for B-cell PIOL. T-cell PIOL and PCNSL seem to be very aggressive as evidenced by this patient's quick demise.

References

1. Levy-Clarke GA, Chan CC, Nussenblatt RB. (2005) Diagnosis and management of primary intraocular lymphoma. *Hematol Oncol Clin North Am* **19**(4): 739–749.
2. Wolf T, Brodt HR, Fichtlscherer S, *et al.* (2005) Changing incidence and prognostic factors of survival in AIDS-related non-Hodgkin's lymphoma in the era of highly active antiretroviral therapy (HAART). *Leuk Lymphoma* **46**(2): 207–215.
3. Chan CC, Wallace DJ. (2004) Intraocular lymphoma: update on diagnosis and management. *Cancer Control* **11**(5): 285–295.
4. Ferreri AJ, Blay JY, Reni M, *et al.* (2003) Prognostic scoring system for primary CNS lymphomas: the International Extranodal Lymphoma Study Group experience. *J Clin Oncol* **21**(2): 266–272.
5. Shen DF, Zhuang Z, LeHoang P, *et al.* (1998) Utility of microdissection and polymerase chain reaction for the detection of immunoglobulin gene rearrangement and translocation in primary intraocular lymphoma [In Process Citation]. *Ophthalmology* **105**(9): 1664–1669.
6. de Smet M, Nussenblatt RB, Davis JL, Palestine AG. (1990) Large cell lymphoma masquerading as a viral retinitis. *Int Ophthalmol* **14**(5–6): 413–417.
7. Ridley ME, McDonald HR, Sternberg P, Jr., *et al.* (1992) Retinal manifestations of ocular lymphoma (reticulum cell sarcoma). *Ophthalmology* **99**(7): 1153–1160; discussion 1160–1151.
8. Char DH, Margolis L, Newman AB. (1981) Ocular reticulum cell sarcoma. *Am J Ophthalmol* **91**(4): 480–483.

9. Martin DF, Chan CC, de Smet MD, *et al.* (1993) The role of chorioretinal biopsy in the management of posterior uveitis. *Ophthalmology* **100**(5): 705–714.
10. Char DH, Ljung BM, Miller T, Phillips T. (1988) Primary intraocular lymphoma (ocular reticulum cell sarcoma) diagnosis and management. *Ophthalmology* **95**: 625–630.
11. Chan CC, Buggage RR, Nussenblatt RB. (2002) Intraocular lymphoma. *Curr Opin Ophthalmol* **13**(6): 411–418.
12. Abrey LE, Yahalom J, DeAngelis LM. (2000) Treatment for primary CNS lymphoma: the next step. *J Clin Oncol* **18**(17): 3144–3150.
13. Abrey LE, Batchelor TT, Ferreri AJ, *et al.* (2005) Report of an international workshop to standardize baseline evaluation and response criteria for primary CNS lymphoma. *J Clin Oncol* **23**(22): 5034–5043.
14. Hormigo A, Abrey L, Heinemann MH, DeAngelis LM. (2004) Ocular presentation of primary central nervous system lymphoma: diagnosis and treatment. *Br J Haematol* **126**(2): 202–208.
15. Velez G, de Smet MD, Whitcup SM, *et al.* (2000) Iris involvement in primary intraocular lymphoma: report of two cases and review of the literature. *Surv Ophthalmol* **44**(6): 518–526.
16. Chan CC, Whitcup SM, Solomon D, Nussenblatt RB. (1995) Interleukin-10 in the vitreous of primary intraocular lymphoma. *Am J Ophthalmol* **120**(5): 671–673.
17. Cassoux N, Merle-Beral H, Lehoang P, *et al.* (2001) Interleukin-10 and intraocular-central nervous system lymphoma. *Ophthalmology* **108**(3): 426–427.
18. Wolf LA, Reed GF, Buggage RR, *et al.* (2003) Vitreous cytokine levels. *Ophthalmology* **110**(8): 1671–1672.
19. Merle-Beral H, Davi F, Cassoux N, *et al.* (2004) Biological diagnosis of primary intraocular lymphoma. *Br J Haematol* **124**(4): 469–473.
20. Coupland SE, Anastassiou G, Bornfeld N, *et al.* (2005) Primary intraocular lymphoma of T-cell type: report of a case and review of the literature. *Graefes Arch Clin Exp Ophthalmol* **243**(3): 189–197.

Author Index

Subject Index